CRASH COURSE

Third Edition

Endocrine and Reproductive Systems

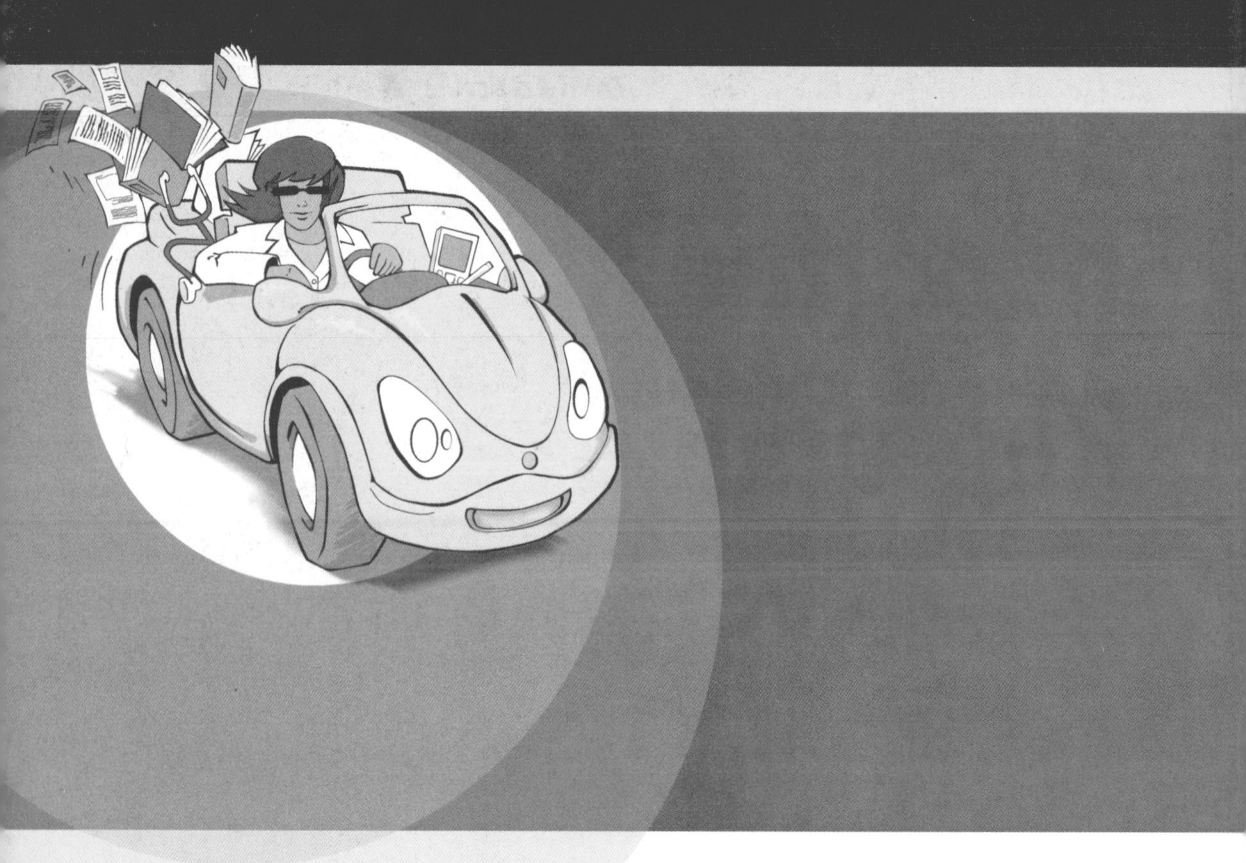

First and second edition authors:

Madeleine Debuse

Stephan Sanders

CRASH COURSE

Third Edition

Endocrine and Reproductive Systems

Series editor

Daniel Horton-Szar

BSc (Hons), MBBS (Hons), MRCGP

Northgate Medical Practice
Canterbury
Kent, UK

Faculty advisor

Roger Searle

Bsc (Hons), PhD

Director of Anatomy & Clinical Skills
Faculty of Medical Sciences
Newcastle University
Newcastle upon Tyne, UK

Alexander Finlayson

BMedSci (Hons)

Newcastle University. Kennedy Scholar, Harvard University

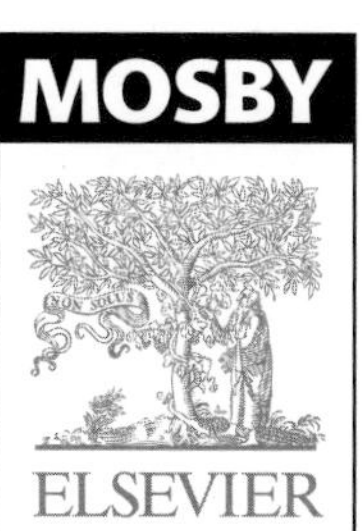

Edinburgh • London • New York • Oxford • Philadelphia • St Louis • Sydney • Toronto 2007

MOSBY
ELSEVIER

Commissioning Editor: Alison Taylor
Development Editor: Lulu Stader
Project Manager: Anne Dickie
Senior Designer: Sarah Russell
Cover: Stewart Larking
Illustrator: Joanna Cameron
Illustration Manager: Merlyn Harvey
Icon Illustrations: Geo Parkin

First edition 1998
Second edition 2003
Third edition 2007

ISBN: 978-0-7234-3427-6

British Library Cataloguing in Publication Data
A catalogue record for this book is available from the British Library

Library of Congress Cataloging in Publication Data
A catalog record for this book is available from the Library of Congress

Note

Knowledge and best practice in this field are constantly changing. As new research and experience broaden our knowledge, changes in practice, treatment and drug therapy may become necessary or appropriate. Readers are advised to check the most current information provided (i) on procedures featured or (ii) by the manufacturer of each product to be administered, to verify the recommended dose or formula, the method and duration of administration, and contraindications. It is the responsibility of the practitioner, relying on their own experience and knowledge of the patient, to make diagnoses, to determine dosages and the best treatment for each individual patient, and to take all appropriate safety precautions. To the fullest extent of the law, neither the Publisher nor the Author assumes any liability for any injury and/or damage to persons or property arising out or related to any use of the material contained in this book.

The Publisher

Printed in China

Preface

When two communities that speak different languages come together, the adults first acquire shared words in order to communicate things which are vital for everyday living. This is known as a pidgeon language. Somehow the children of this first generation in the newly amalgamated community develop a properly mature language, a creole, as good as any other. The same is true of the endocrine system, throughout evolution, various component pathways have been developed and subsequently amalgamated to enable increasingly complicated functions to operate in synchrony. Thus humans integrate their ability to regulate heat balance with water balance, which in turn is dependent on salt and glucose balance. The endocrine system can therefore not be wholly understood by considering the actions of individual hormones in isolation. Rather, in time, the era of 'systems biology' will usher in a new kind of endocrinology where all these interactions are studied using complex mathematical models. Nonetheless, in the mean time, there is much to learn about how each hormone works. A complex understanding of the future is not necessary to significantly alter the lives of patients with endocrine pathologies. Both acute and chronic endocrine problems are well studied and usually have well-developed treatments.

This Crash Course in Endocrinology and Reproduction will provide an overview of key hormones, their regulation, their target sites, the processes which they control and the pathologies which they can be involved in, as well as provide some information about the treatment of endocrine disease. There are frequent clinical sketches throughout to highlight areas of basic science which relate directly to findings in the clinic. *Hic sunt dracones.*

Alexander Finlayson

Whether you are a medical student studying on a traditional, integrated, case-led or problem based learning course the 'core' medical curriculum remains the same. Although what precisely constitutes 'core' knowledge remains to be defined, Medical Schools nowadays adhere to the principle that the factual component of the basic medical sciences underpinning the medical course must be kept to an essential minimum. This revised Crash Course edition has applied the same principle to its contents on the endocrine and reproductive systems; core knowledge must be clinically relevant to health and disease and form a solid foundation for both your present and future understanding of the subject. While excessive and inappropriate detail has no place in the present medical curriculum, the responsibility for learning still lies with you and is lifelong.

The basic science content of the endocrine and reproductive systems has been extensively revised, consolidated and updated, and up and coming treatments and developments flagged. Throughout new topics now considered 'core' have been included, the basic medical sciences have been widely integrated with clinically relevant information and the emerging genetic basis of clinical disorders included. The Self Assessment chapter has a section on extended-matching item questions to reflect the changes in the systems of assessment presently used by Medical Schools.

Regardless of whether you are just starting out on the medical course or are a more senior medical student, how you approach your future clinical practice and professional responsibilities will be critically governed by your grasp of core knowledge. This book aims to present the basic medical sciences underpinning the endocrine and reproductive systems in a concise manageable read but the skills and attitudes that underlie your effective learning of these 'core' facts are equally important.

I wish you every success whilst you are at Medical School and in your future career.

Dr Roger Searle
Faculty Advisor

More than a decade has now passed since work began on the first editions of the Crash Course series, and over four years since the publication of the second editions. Medicine never stands still, and the work of keeping this series relevant for today's students is an ongoing process. These third editions build upon the success of the preceding books and incorporate a great deal of new and revised material, keeping the series up to date with the latest medical research and developments in pharmacology and current best practice.

As always, we listen to feedback from the thousands of students who use Crash Course and have made further improvements to the layout and structure of the books. Each chapter now starts with a set of learning objectives, and the self-assessment sections have been enhanced and brought up to date with modern exam formats. We have also worked to integrate points of clinical relevance into the basic medical science material, which will not only add to the interest of the text but will reinforce the principles being described.

Despite fully revising the books, we hold fast to the principles on which we first developed the series: Crash Course will always bring you all the information you need to revise in compact, manageable volumes that integrate basic medical science and clinical practice. The books still maintain the balance between clarity and conciseness, and providing sufficient depth for those aiming at distinction. The authors are medical students and junior doctors who have recent experience of the exams you are now facing, and the accuracy of the material is checked by senior faculty members from across the UK.

I wish you all the best for your future careers!

Dr Dan Horton-Szar
Series Editor

Acknowledgements

I am very grateful to Dr Roger Searle for his excellent guidance throughout this project. Thank you to Lulu Stader for her patience and gentle encouragement. They have both been great to work with.

Pigmaei gigantum humeris impositi plusquam ipsi gigantes vident, the Latin metaphor for dwarfs standing on the shoulders of giants can definitely be applied to the support I have gained from a few kind teachers. I am forever indebted to Dr Bryan McIver at the Mayo Clinic for being an inspirational endocrine mentor. Thanks also to Dr Phil Leder at Harvard for allowing me the freedom to mix my research with time spent working on the Crash Course. I also appreciate the support of Dr Steve Ball at Newcastle in my study of diabetes insipidus.

On a more personal level, I would like to thank my family, who have supported me steadfastly throughout the last 23 years. Thank you to my mother for taking me to drink bitter lemon at 'The Granary', my dad for taking me on trips in his Morgan and my sisters for putting up with me.

I would like to thank Tessa (superdoc) for continually encouraging me in my work. She is an amazing doctor and an amazing person.

Thank you to the members of 'housegood' (Dan, Josh, Tom, Jamie and Jordan) for providing such an incredibly friendly atmosphere throughout my time at medical school. Thank you to Felix, Katherine, James, and Simon for putting the sparkle into the harsh Bostonian winter.

Figure Acknowledgements

Figure 15.11 Adapted from KL Moore, TVN Persaud, The Developing Human, Clinically Oriented Embryology, 5th edition, by permission of WB Saunders.

Figure 15.12 Adapted from D Llewellyn-Jones, Fundamentals of Obstetrics and Gynaecology, 6th edition, 1994, by permission of Suzanne Abraham and Mosby.

Figure 19.3 Adapted from Lecture Notes on Endocrinology, 5th edition by WJ Jeffcoate. With permission from Blackwell Science, 1993

Figures 19.7, 19.9, 19.12A, 19.15A Reproduced with permission from R Grainger and D Allison, eds, Diagnostic Radiology: A Textbook of Medical Imaging, 4th edition, Churchill Livingstone.

Figures 19.8, 19.10A and B, 19.11A, 19.14 Reproduced with permission from D Sutton, Textbook of Radiology and Imaging, 6th edition, Churchill Livingstone.

Figure 19.13 Reproduced with permission from CRW Edwards et al, eds, Davidson's Principles and Practice of Medicine, 17th edition, Churchill Livingstone.

Figures 19.15B, C and D Reproduced with permission from IPC Murray & PJ Ell, eds, Nuclear Medicine, 2nd edition, Churchill Livingstone.

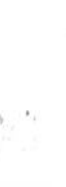

Contents

Glossary

Acromegaly the condition which result from excess growth hormone after fusion of the epiphyses

Adrenarche the initiation of androgen secretion from the adrenal gland

Amenorrhoea the absence of menstruation for 6 months or more

Anorgasmia failure to achieve orgasm

Antidiuretic hormone a hormone which acts on the collecting ducts in the kidneys to increase water retention

Climacteric the time before and after menopause during which symptoms are experienced

Diabetes mellitus a disease caused by insulin deficiency or insulin resistance (reduced sensitivity). The abnormalities result in chronic hyperglycaemia (excess blood glucose) and metabolic disturbance

Diploid cells which contain two copies of each chromosome (one paternal and one maternal) are said to be diploid

Dysmenorrhoea painful menses

Dyspareunia pain during intercourse

Eclampsia the presence of seizure activity in pregnant woman with pre-eclampsia; usually presents in third trimester

Ectoderm outer embryological layer that forms the skin and nervous system

Effector A protein regulated by a hormone that brings about the cellular effects

Endoderm inner embryological layer that forms the intestines and the germ cells

Erectile dysfunction the inability to maintain an erection suitable for vaginal penetration despite normal sexual desire

Fertilization the fusion of the male and female gametes to form a diploid zygote

Galactorrhoea inappropriate secretion of milk from the breasts

Gigantism the condition which results from excess growth hormone prior to fusion of the epiphyses

Gynaecomastia the growth of breasts in men

Haploid gametes contain only one copy of each chromosome and are said to be haploid

Homeostasis the maintenance of a system within tolerable limits

Hormone a chemical substance that is secreted by specialized endocrine cells directly into the blood to exert an effect on distant target cells. This is the traditional definition but many locally secreted chemical messengers are now recognized

Hyperthyroidism an overactive thyroid gland leading to excess thyroid hormones

Hypothalamus a gland located beneath the thalamus. It orchestrates homeostatic processes in the body

Hypothyroidism an underactive thyroid gland leading to a deficiency of thyroid hormone

Labour the onset of painful contractions leading to the progressive effacement and dilatation of the cervix

Menopause the cessation of menstruation and ovulation

Menorrhagia excess menstrual bleeding

Menstrual cycle the process by which the female prepares for possible fertilization of the ovulated secondary oocytes

Mesenchyme support tissue derived from the mesoderm

Mesoderm middle embryological layer that forms many organs and the cardiovascular system

Metabolic syndrome the combination of hyperglycaemia, hyperinsulinaemia, dyslipidaemia, hypertension and central obesity (adipose tissue in an abdominal distribution)

Miscarriage the expulsion of the fetus from the uterus before it is independently viable

Negative feedback the inhibition of hormone by the hormone itself

Oogenesis the production of oocytes

Osteoporosis a common bone disease characterized by inadequate bone mass and fragility. It can be caused by failure to reach peak bone mass, bone resorption or failure to replace lost bone

Ovary oval organ which produces oocytes (female gametes) and sex steroid hormones in response to pituitary gonadotrophins (LH and FSH)

Ovulation the release of oocytes

Pineal gland a gland which coordinates circadian rhythms by secreting the hormone melatonin in response to light signals

Premenstrual syndrome (PMS) describes a negative mood and several physical symptoms that can occur in the luteal phase (days 14–28) of the menstrual cycle

Puberty the process by which a sexually immature child becomes a fully fertile adult

Receptor A protein in target cells that detects hormones

Spermatogenesis is the process by which haploid (23 chromosome) spermatozoa are formed from diploid (46 chromosome) stem cells called spermatogonia

Spermiogenesis the development of the mature structure of a spermatozoan from a spermatid

Steroid hormones small, fat-soluble molecules that can pass through cell membranes. Must circulate bound to plasma proteins because they are insoluble in the blood

Target cell A cell that responds to a specific hormone

Thyrotoxicosis the state of excess thyroid hormone (can occur in the absence of an overactive thyroid gland)

BASIC MEDICAL SCIENCE

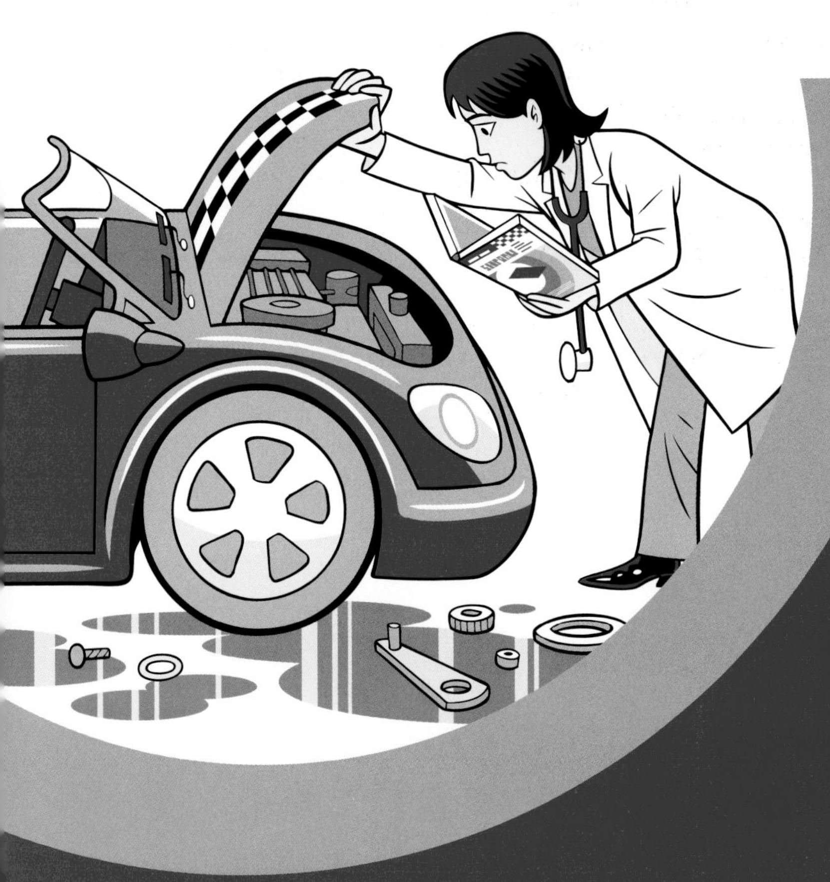

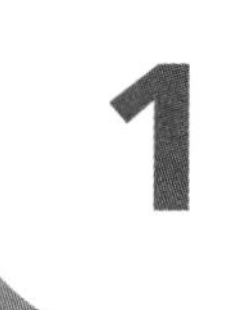

Overview of the endocrine system

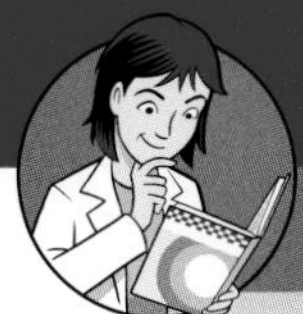

Objectives

By the end of this chapter you should be able to:

- Define the terms hormone, endocrine, target cell, and paracrine.
- Name five hormones, along with the gland that secretes them.
- Outline the role of the hypothalamus in the endocrine system.
- Remember where the hormones of the hypothalamus act.
- Outline the role of the anterior pituitary gland in the endocrine system.
- Remember where the hormones from the anterior pituitary gland act.
- Describe the control of thyroid hormones starting in the hypothalamus.
- Define negative feedback, and give an example of this process.
- Describe the role of amplification in the endocrine system.
- State the three types of hormone, along with an example of each.
- Describe the synthesis and properties of polypeptide hormones.
- Describe the mode of action of a G-protein receptor, along with three examples of hormones that act through these receptors.
- Describe the mode of action of a tyrosine kinase receptor, along with two hormones that act through these receptors.
- Describe the synthesis and properties of steroid hormones.
- Describe the receptors that steroid hormones act on.
- Describe the properties of modified amino-acid hormones.
- Describe the place where neurons can affect the endocrine system.
- List examples of hormones that act on neurons.
- Compare the action of hormones and neurons.

ROLE OF THE ENDOCRINE SYSTEM

The endocrine system allows cells to communicate using chemical messengers called hormones. This communication is essential for the maintenance of homeostasis (Greek for 'staying the same'). Homeostasis is an ongoing process that minimizes change from the ideal physiological conditions, creating a suitable environment for life. As a result, hormones are important components of all major body systems; you cannot escape them.

The endocrine system also regulates long-term changes in the body, including:

- Growth.
- Sexual development.
- Pregnancy.

After reading this chapter, you should be able to:

- Explain what is meant by the term 'hormone'.
- Picture the general organization of the endocrine system.
- Understand how hormone secretion is controlled.
- Describe the synthesis of the main types of hormone.
- Understand how these hormones act through their cellular receptors.
- Discuss the integration and role of the endocrine and nervous systems.

Important words:
Hormone: a chemical signal transported in the blood that is secreted by endocrine cells
Endocrine tissue: a group of cells that secrete hormones
Target cell: a cell that responds to a specific hormone
Receptor: a protein in target cells that detects hormones
Second messenger: a chemical that transmits the hormone message from the receptor to the effector
Effector: a protein regulated by a hormone that brings about the cellular effects

HORMONES AND ENDOCRINE SECRETION

Hormones

Classical definition

Classically, a hormone is described as a chemical substance that is secreted by specialized endocrine cells directly into the blood to exert an effect on distant target cells. This process is endocrine secretion.

Modern definition

Recent research has revealed many locally acting chemical substances that have challenged the classical definition of hormones. Four modes of delivery are recognized (Fig. 1.1). They are:

- Endocrine—chemicals that act on distant cells via the bloodstream, e.g. thyroxine.
- Paracrine—chemicals that act on the surrounding cells without entering the blood, e.g. gut hormones.
- Autocrine—chemicals that act on the cell they are secreted from, e.g. nitric oxide.
- Neurocrine—signals between neurons, e.g. neurotransmitters.

Different textbooks suggest different explanations of the term 'hormone', ranging from the classical definition to a definition that encompasses all chemical signals external to cells. If clinicians talk about hormones, they generally mean chemical signals that pass through the blood (endocrine delivery).

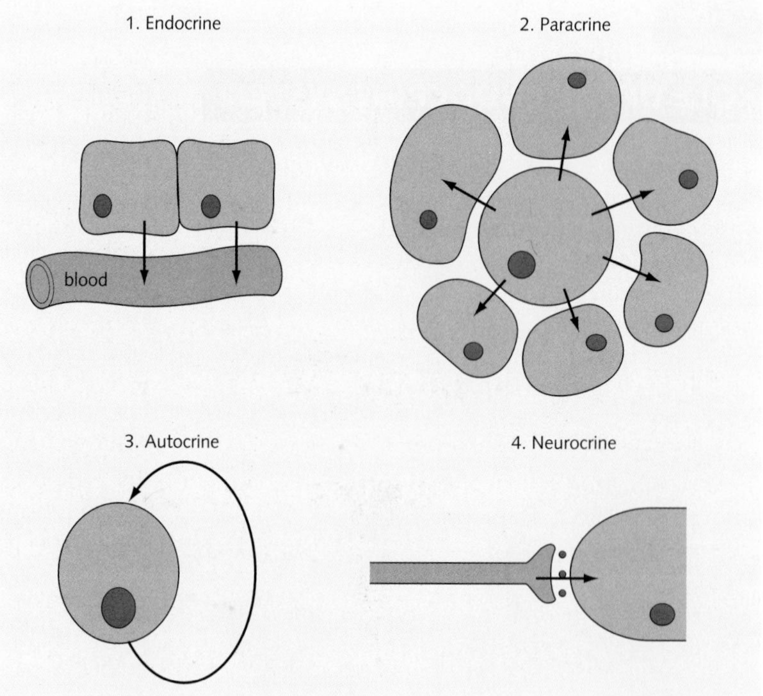

Fig. 1.1 The routes by which chemical signals are delivered to cells.

Types of hormone

Three classes of hormone are secreted into the blood; the characteristics of these are explained later in the chapter:

- Polypeptides (also called proteins).
- Steroids.
- Modified amino acids.

Endocrine tissues

Definition

An endocrine tissue is simply one that secretes a hormone. These tissues respond to signals that either stimulate or inhibit the release of the specific hormone.

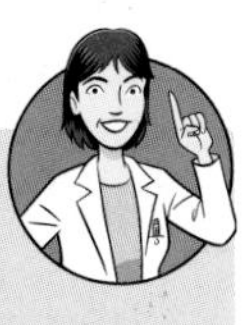

The word 'endocrine' means 'internal secretion', while 'hormone' is derived from the Greek verb '*hormao*' meaning 'I excite'.

Arrangement of endocrine tissues

Endocrine tissues contain cells that secrete hormones; these cells can be arranged in three patterns:

- As an endocrine organ devoted to hormone synthesis, e.g. the thyroid gland.
- As clusters of cells within an organ, e.g. the islets of Langerhans in the pancreas.
- Individual cells scattered diffusely throughout an organ, e.g. the gastrointestinal (GI) tract.

Endocrine organs

The term 'endocrine organ' originally referred to organs in which specialized endocrine cells formed a significant component. These 'traditional' endocrine organs are shown in Fig. 1.2 along with the hormone they secrete. However, we now know that almost all organs contain some endocrine tissue, for example:

- Adipose tissue, secretes leptin.
- Lungs, secrete 5-hydroxytryptamine (5-HT; serotonin).
- Heart, secretes atrial natriuretic factor (ANF).

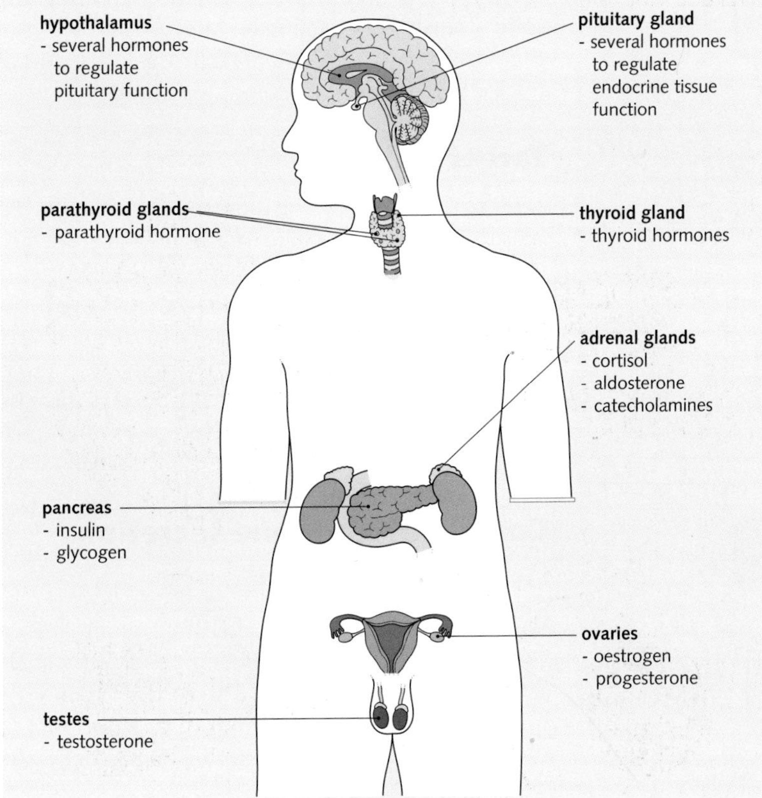

Fig. 1.2 The location of major endocrine organs and the hormones secreted by them.

ORGANIZATION OF THE ENDOCRINE SYSTEM

The regulation and control of many major hormones follows a similar pattern that starts in the brain and ends with a hormone being secreted. Understanding this pattern is the key to understanding how the endocrine system works. There are three steps, each of which involves the secretion of a hormone that stimulates the next step (Fig. 1.3). The control of hormones released by the thyroid gland will be used to illustrate this pathway throughout.

The main components

Hypothalamus

The endocrine system is coordinated by the hypothalamus. This is a part of the brain that acts as a bridge between the nervous system and endocrine system, translating neural messages into chemical (hormonal) signals. It initiates the secretion of hormones by controlling the function of the pituitary gland via 'releasing hormones'. These hormones do not act directly on peripheral endocrine tissues. Hormones secreted from the hypothalamus are released in a pulsatile manner, often with a circadian rhythm (cyclicol through a 24-h cycle). Thyrotrophin-releasing hormone (TRH) is secreted into the blood by the hypothalamus; this initiates the hormone cascade resulting in the release of thyroid hormones.

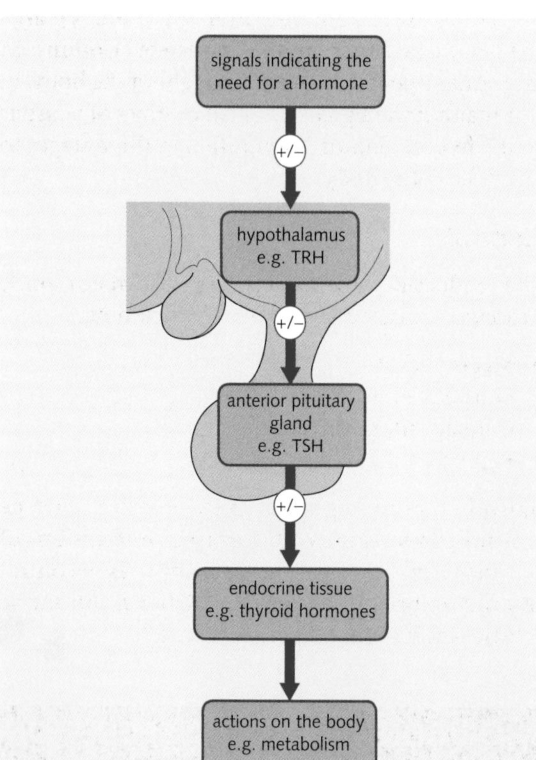

Fig. 1.3 The organization of the endocrine system.(TRH, thyrotrophin-releasing hormone; TSH, thyroid-stimulating hormone.)

Pituitary gland

The pituitary gland is found at the base of the brain beneath the hypothalamus. It releases hormones into the blood in response to signals from the hypothalamus. The hormones from the pituitary gland regulate the function of peripheral endocrine tissues throughout the body. TRH from the hypothalamus acts on the pituitary gland to cause the release of thyroid-stimulating hormone (TSH) into the bloodstream.

Peripheral endocrine tissues

The hormones secreted by the pituitary gland act on peripheral endocrine tissues. These tissues respond by increasing or decreasing secretion of specific hormones into the blood. It is the hormones secreted by these peripheral tissues that affect the state of the body by acting on target cells. TSH from the pituitary gland stimulates the thyroid gland to release thyroid hormones into the blood.

Target cells

Different hormones act on different, specific cells. The cells that respond to a specific hormone are called its target cells; they can be found anywhere in the body. All target cells have receptors to detect the specific hormone, but the effect of the hormone can vary between cells. Thyroid hormones from the thyroid gland act on almost every cell in the body to increase the rate of metabolism through receptors on the cell surface.

Control of hormone secretion

Overall control

Endocrine tissues are regulated by signals from a variety of neural and systemic sources. These signals are processed by cells to determine the rate of hormone secretion. The strength and importance of the signals varies so that hormone secretion fits the needs of the body.

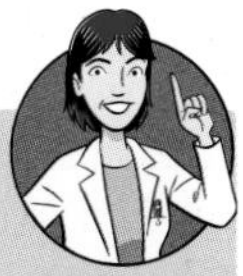

A single hormone may have multiple actions; equally, multiple hormones may have the same action. This is demonstrated by insulin and the regulation of blood glucose, respectively.

Neural control

Higher neural centres can influence the activity of the endocrine system by acting on the hypothalamus. They can increase or decrease the secretion of hypothalamic releasing hormones, which regulate the secretion of pituitary gland hormones. For example, stress or fear will inhibit reproductive hormone secretion, and cold external temperatures will stimulate TRH.

Hormonal feedback

An almost universal feature of endocrine system regulation is feedback from the hormones that are released. The hormones can feed back by two means:

- Directly—e.g. the hormone thyroxine affects the hypothalamus and pituitary.
- Indirectly—e.g. through chemical changes caused by the hormones, such as glucose deficiency.

Feedback is usually inhibitory, thus a hormone can inhibit its own production; this process is called negative feedback. It is an essential mechanism that prevents excess secretion of many hormones. The level at which the feedback acts varies between hormones; however, many hormones act at the level of the hypothalamus and pituitary gland. For example, thyroid hormones feed back to the anterior pituitary where they inhibit the release of TSH (Fig. 1.4).

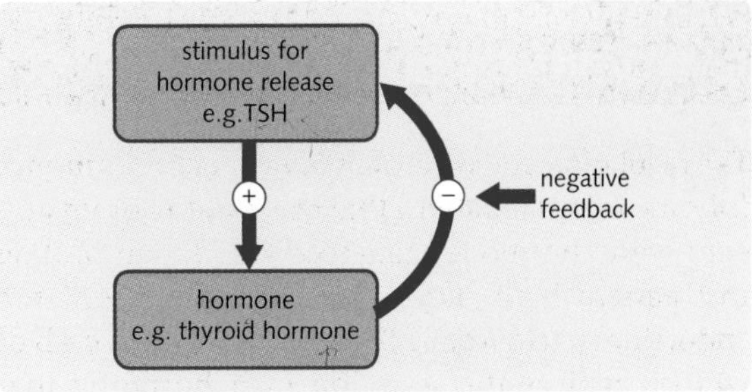

Why is it so complex?

At first glance the endocrine system seems incredibly complex for no obvious reason. Many students wish that the system had fewer hormones and organs, but there are a number of advantages.

Amplification

As described, endocrine signals begin in the hypothalamus and result in a cascade of hormones from different endocrine glands. There is only a small population of cells in the hypothalamus that secrete each hormone; for example, about 2000 neurons secrete gonadotrophin-releasing hormone (GnRH). Because of the small number of cells involved, they are able to respond to important but small neural signals, but they cannot secrete large amounts of hormone.

Fig. 1.4 Negative feedback. (TSH, thyroid-stimulating hormone.)

The very small quantities of hormone secreted directly into the bloodstream by the hypothalamus can be detected by the closely related pituitary gland. This gland is able to secrete a greater quantity of hormone than the hypothalamus, but it is still too small to secrete enough for the whole body.

In response to hormones from the pituitary gland, the peripheral endocrine tissues secrete hormones in large quantities that can act throughout the body. In this manner, the signal of a small number of neurons in the hypothalamus is amplified in three stages to affect the entire body.

Control

The endocrine system regulates all major body processes that are essential for life, including:

- Metabolic rate.
- Nutrient levels.
- Cardiac output and blood pressure.
- Reproduction.

Since they are so important, these processes must be controlled very tightly. The complex interactions of the endocrine system allow for many sites of control in order to prevent excessive or deficient hormone release, and to maintain homeostasis.

HORMONE TYPES AND SECRETION

This section describes the properties and synthesis of the three classes of hormone (Fig. 1.5).

Fig. 1.5 Comparison of different types of hormone

	Polypeptides	Modified amino acids	Steroids
Size	Medium–large	Very small	Small
Ability to cross cell membrane	×	✓	✓
Receptor type	Cell-surface	Cell-surface or intracellular	Intracellular
Soluble in:	Water	Water	Fat
Action	Protein activation	Protein activation or synthesis	Protein synthesis
Transport in the blood	Dissolved in the plasma	Dissolved in the plasma or bound to plasma proteins	Bound to plasma proteins

Polypeptide hormones

As their name suggests, polypeptide hormones are proteins that act as hormones. The size of the polypeptide varies widely, from 3 to 200 amino-acid residues; they cannot pass through cell membranes due to their size and water-soluble nature. Protein hormones are the most numerous type (often a safe bet in an exam). Accordingly they are secreted by many glands, including:

- Hypothalamus—TRH, GnRH, growth-hormone releasing hormone (GHRH), etc.
- Pituitary—TSH, follicle-stimulating hormone (FSH), luteinizing hormone (LH), oxytocin, etc.
- Pancreas and GI tract—insulin, glucagon, cholecystokinin (CCK), etc.

Synthesis

Polypeptide hormones are synthesized in the same manner as any other protein. DNA in the nucleus is transcribed to mRNA and translated into the protein by ribosomes. The protein is then processed by the Golgi apparatus and stored in secretory granules. Many hormones undergo changes in the Golgi apparatus or secretory granules, including:

- Cleavage reactions to free a smaller polypeptide hormone from the larger prohormone.
- Addition of carbohydrate groups to form glycoproteins.

Secretion

The secretory granules are released by exocytosis, in which the membrane of the granule fuses with the membrane of the cell causing the contents to be ejected. This process is triggered by calcium entering the cell. Polypeptide hormone release is controlled mainly by regulating secretion rather than synthesis.

Polypeptide-secreting cells

Polypeptide-secreting cells all have a similar histological appearance (Fig. 1.6):

- Large, prominent nuclei.
- Small amount of cytoplasm.
- Prominent Golgi apparatus.
- Abundant rough endoplasmic reticulum (RER).
- Large numbers of secretory granules.
- Surrounded by fenestrated blood sinusoids.

Steroid hormones

Steroids are small, fat-soluble molecules that can pass through cell membranes but must circulate bound to plasma proteins, since they are insoluble in the blood. They are secreted by:

- Adrenal cortex—cortisol and aldosterone.
- Ovaries—oestrogen and progesterone.
- Placenta—oestrogen and progesterone.
- Testes—testosterone.

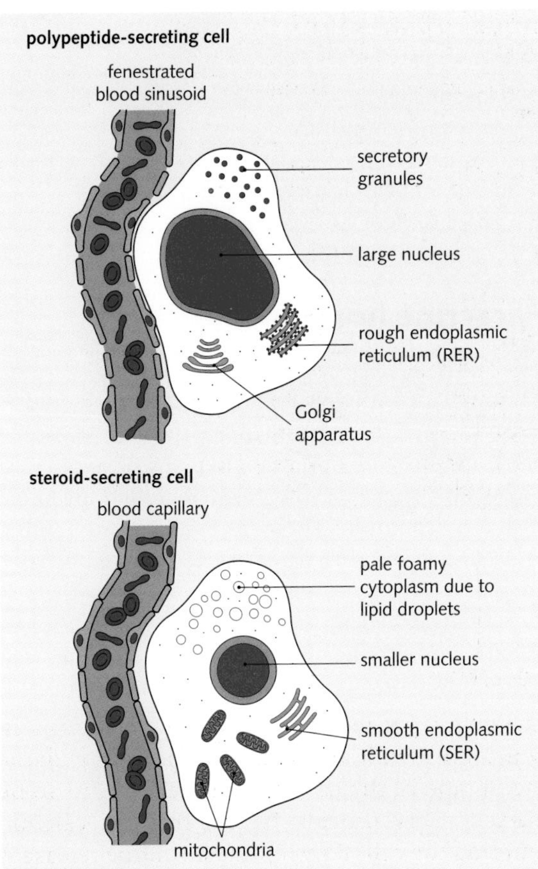

Fig. 1.6 Appearance of a polypeptide-secreting cell and steroid secreting cell.

Synthesis

Steroids are derived from cholesterol by a series of reactions in the mitochondria and smooth endoplasmic reticulum (SER). Cholesterol is acquired from the diet or synthesized within the cells; it is stored within lipid droplets seen in the cytoplasm of steroid cells. All steroids have the same basic structure formed by four rings of carbon (Fig. 1.7), but individual hormones differ in the following ways:

- Side chains attached to these rings.
- Bonds within the rings (double or single).

The exact sequence of reactions to synthesize each hormone varies, since there are many different enzyme pathways. However, the vast majority of steroid hormones share two common steps.

Step 1

Cholesterol is converted into pregnenolone by the desmolase enzyme found within the mitochondria of steroid-producing cells. Desmolase removes six carbon atoms from the cholesterol side chain of ring D. This reaction is the rate-limiting step in steroid synthesis.

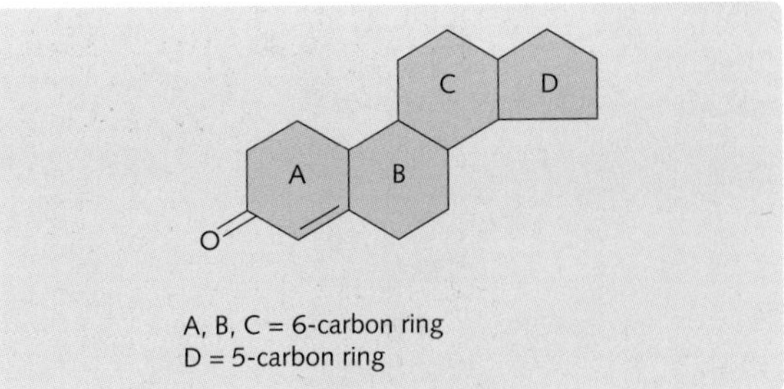

Fig. 1.7 Basic structure of a steroid hormone.

Step 2

Pregnenolone is converted to progesterone by enzymes found in the mitochondria and cytoplasm. This reaction involves:

- Isomerization—the double bond moves from ring B to ring A.
- Oxidation—the hydroxyl group (OH) of ring A becomes a keto group (O).

Further steps are very variable, but the general pattern is shown in Fig. 1.8.

Secretion

The steroid hormone is released immediately, so the rate of release is determined by the rate of synthesis, especially the synthesis of pregnenolone.

Steroid-secreting cells

Steroid-secreting cells also have a similar histological appearance to each other (see Fig. 1.6):

- Small, rounded nuclei.
- Large amount of cytoplasm.
- Large numbers of lipid droplets (foamy appearance).
- Abundant SER.
- Many mitochondria.
- Surrounded by blood capillaries.

Modified amino acids

Several hormones are formed by altering the structure of amino acids, producing small, water-soluble hormones that can cross cell membranes. They are secreted by the:

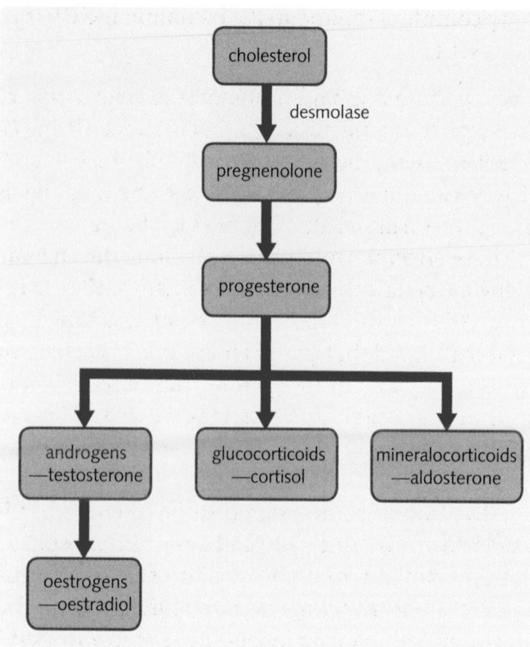

Fig. 1.8 Steroid synthesis. The initial stages are the same for all steroid hormones.

- Thyroid gland—thyroid hormones.
- Adrenal medulla—catecholamines (noradrenaline and adrenaline).
- Hypothalamus—dopamine.
- Pineal gland—melatonin.

Synthesis

These hormones are synthesized from two amino acids:

- Tyrosine—precursor of thyroid hormones, dopamine, and catecholamines.
- Tryptophan—precursor of melatonin and 5-HT.

The reactions to modify these amino acids vary significantly between hormones, so the synthesis is described in the individual chapters. The hormones are stored in secretory granules except thyroid hormones, which uniquely are stored in follicles.

Secretion

The granules are released by exocytosis in the same way as polypeptide hormones. The rate of release is regulated mainly by secretion.

Modified amino-acid-secreting cells

The cells that secrete modified amino-acid hormones vary more than the cells secreting polypeptide or steroid hormones, however the following features are often found:

- Large nuclei.
- Many mitochondria.
- Abundant RER.
- Prominent Golgi apparatus.
- Large numbers of secretory granules.
- Surrounded by blood capillaries.

Paracrine hormones

Eicosanoids

Although eicosanoids are not always considered as hormones and do not form one of the main classes of hormone, they are important in many physiological processes. They are therefore included in most endocrine courses. They are small, lipid-soluble molecules that act in a paracrine (local) manner. They are derived from a phospholipid found in the cell membrane called arachidonic acid, which is broken down by the enzyme phospholipase A_2. There are two pathways, which synthesize different groups of eicosanoids:

- Cyclooxygenase pathway—forms prostaglandins and thromboxanes.
- Lipoxygenase pathway—forms leukotrienes.

Eicosanoids are released immediately and readily cross cell membranes. Their action varies between cells and the specific eicosanoid molecule that is formed.

> Endocrine disruptors are synthetic chemical compounds which act in the body to mimic or antagonize the function of a hormone. They can do this by altering endogenous hormone production, delivery or direct action. A well characterized example of a disruptor is DDT but studies suggest that other pesticides and chemicals may also play a role.

HORMONE RECEPTORS

Target cells possess unique receptors that bind specific hormones; without these receptors the hormones can have no effect. The number of receptors per cell can be increased or decreased to alter the strength of the hormone's effect. Receptors are found in two locations:

- Cell-surface receptors—for polypeptides and catecholamines; they activate or inhibit enzymes, which may affect protein synthesis.
- Intracellular receptors—for steroids and thyroid hormones; they stimulate or inhibit protein synthesis directly.

The response to a hormone varies between target cells, so that the same hormone can have different actions on different tissues. This variation is partly due to different receptor types but also the response to receptor stimulation.

Hormones that act via cell-surface receptors can respond faster than those stimulating intracellular receptors because the activation of pre-existing enzymes takes less time than synthesizing new proteins. This explains why catecholamines released for the 'fight-or-flight' response use cell-surface receptors even though they can cross cell membranes.

Cell-surface receptors

Cell-surface receptors are necessary for polypeptide hormones, which cannot cross the cell membrane, and catecholamines. The receptor must transmit the external signal into the cell where it can have an effect, therefore cell-surface receptors are glycoproteins that cross the cell membrane to create extracellular and intracellular domains. When the hormone binds to the receptor, it triggers a cascade of changes within the cell that alter protein activity. There are two types of cell-surface receptor involved in the endocrine system:

- G-protein coupled receptors.
- Tyrosine kinase receptors.

G-protein coupled receptors

G-protein coupled receptors are extremely common throughout the endocrine system. They consist of two main elements:

- Receptor.
- G-protein.

The receptor is a glycoprotein with a hormone binding site on the extracellular surface and a G-protein binding site on the intracellular surface. When the hormone binds, the receptor changes shape affecting the attached G-protein.

The G-protein is an enzyme that can break down guanosine triphosphate (GTP), hence the name. It is made of two functional subunits:

- α-subunit—bound to guanosine diphosphate (GDP) in the resting state.
- $\beta\gamma$-complex—bound to the α-subunit if GDP is present.

When the hormone binds, causing the receptor to change shape, the α-subunit exchanges the GDP for GTP. The G-protein splits into the two subunits described above, both of which leave the receptor and bind to effector proteins also found on the inside of the cell membrane.

These effector proteins often include the enzyme adenylate cyclase that synthesizes cyclic AMP (cAMP) from ATP. cAMP acts as a second messenger: a chemical signal that can enter the cell to activate or inhibit enzymes to bring about the effects of the hormone. The activated enzymes are often kinases, which add phosphate to other proteins, thereby activating them.

When the hormone signal stops, the α-subunit breaks down GTP into GDP and inorganic phosphate. The $\beta\gamma$-complex rejoins the α-subunit to form the G-protein, and this once again binds to the receptor. The effector proteins are no longer stimulated and cAMP is no longer produced. Fig. 1.9 shows the action of a G-protein receptor.

Other G-protein coupled receptors can use different effectors or second messengers including:

- Inhibition of adenylate cyclase.
- Stimulation of inositol triphosphate.
- Activation of ion channels.

Tyrosine kinase receptors

Insulin and insulin-like growth factors act through tyrosine kinase receptors. These receptors are glycoproteins with kinase activity (ability to add phosphate groups) that is triggered by the binding of the hormone. The receptors mediate their activity by the addition of phosphate groups to particular tyrosines on 'substrate' proteins within the cell. The activated 'substrate' protein acts as a secondary messenger within the cell to induce cell signalling cascades. This mechanism is shown in Fig. 1.10.

Intracellular receptors

Hormones that readily cross the cell membrane, especially steroids, use intracellular receptors. The receptors stimulate protein synthesis directly, so they are also called transcription factors.

The hormone binds to the receptor in the cytoplasm causing a change in shape that activates the receptor. The hormone and receptor enter the nucleus together, where they bind to specific sections of DNA called hormone response elements. This

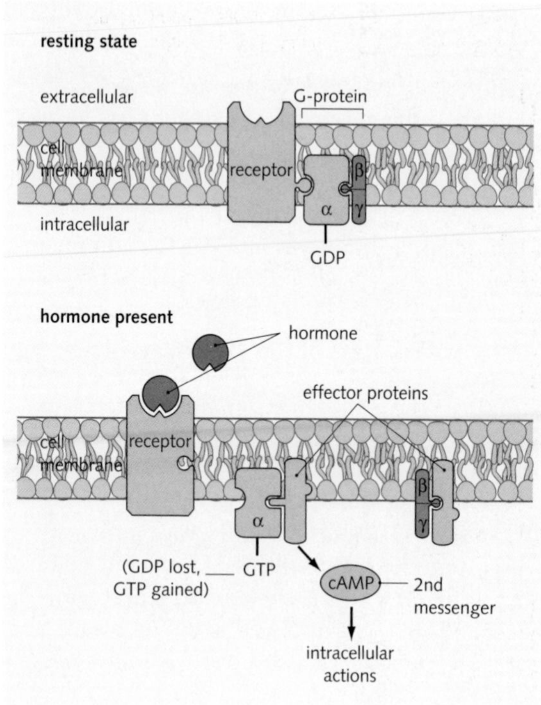

Fig. 1.9 Mechanism of action of a G-protein receptor. (cAMP, cyclic adenosine monophosphate; GDP, guanosine diphosphate; GTP, guanosine triphosphate.)

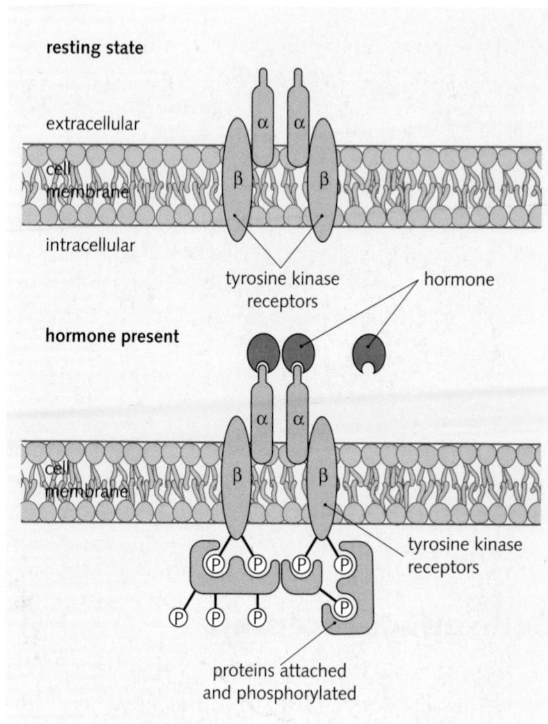

Fig. 1.10 Mechanism of action of a tyrosine kinase receptor.

binding stimulates or inhibits the transcription of specific genes causing changes in protein synthesis. It is this change that brings about the effects of the hormone. This action is shown in Fig. 1.11.

Receptor-mediated control

Hormone receptors are an important site of endocrine regulation. The number of active receptors can be increased or decreased to alter the strength of an endocrine signal. This allows the cell to respond to the deficiency or excess of a hormone. This control can be very subtle, for example, GnRH receptors in the pituitary gland are downregulated if GnRH secretion is not pulsatile. This effect is used clinically to suppress the reproductive hormones.

RELATIONSHIP OF THE NERVOUS AND ENDOCRINE SYSTEMS

Integration

The nervous and endocrine systems have a very close relationship, since they both use chemical signals to communicate between cells, and they may share a common evolutionary origin. The overlap between some hormones and neurotransmitters also supports this idea (e.g. somatostatin is found in both systems). The close relationship allows the two systems to coordinate responses to maintain homeostasis.

Neural control of hormones

The nervous system can control the endocrine system through two routes:

- Hypothalamus.
- Autonomic nervous system (sympathetic and parasympathetic).

The endocrine system often acts as a long-term output from the brain to complement the action of short-term neural responses. This is demonstrated by the three responses to stress listed in the order they take effect:

- Noradrenaline is released from sympathetic nerves.
- Preformed adrenaline is released from the adrenal medulla.
- Cortisol is synthesized by the adrenal cortex.

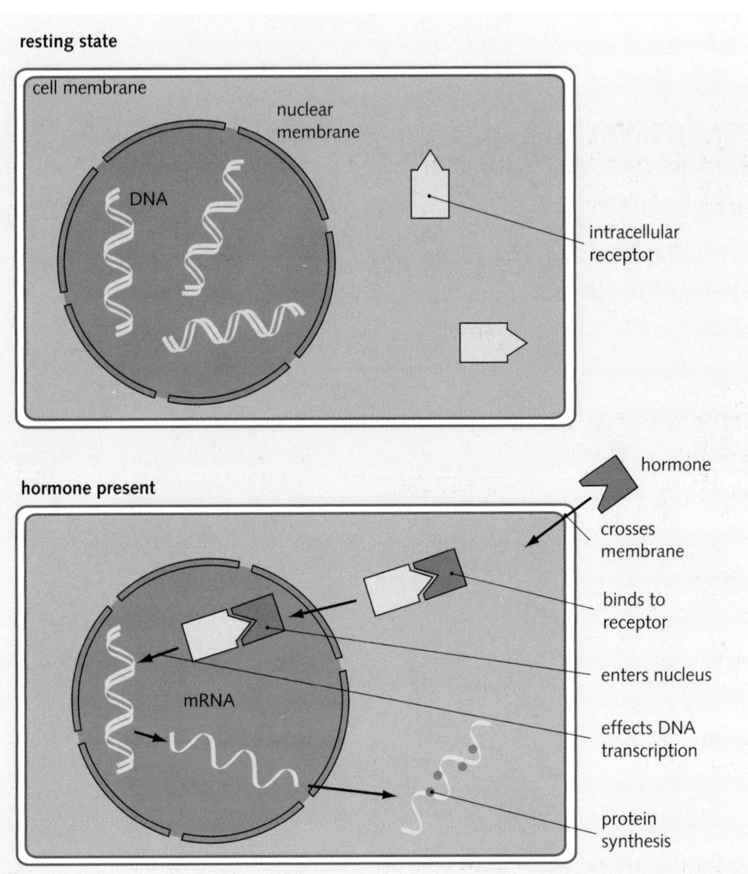

Fig. 1.11 Mechanism of action of an intracellular receptor.

Hormonal control of neurons

To complete this circuit, the hormones of the endocrine system also affect the nervous system. Negative feedback to the hypothalamus has already been described. However, many hormones affect other areas of the brain, for example:

- Thyroid hormone deficiency causes depression.
- Leptin and insulin regulate feelings of hunger.
- Adrenaline increases mental activity.
- Melatonin regulates the feeling of tiredness.

Comparison between the nervous and endocrine systems

While the two systems function closely they have different modes of action. The hypothalamus combines these actions since it is an endocrine tissue composed of nerve cells called neurosecretory cells.

As endocrine hormones are very widespread in their distribution, the manifestations of endocrine disease vary greatly. Endocrine disease can be seen in patients of all ages, from congenital abnormalities in newborns through a plethora of adult and old-age endocrine problems. Patients with cancer can have endocrine dysfunction as part of the primary cancer (i.e. the cancer releases a hormone) or as a side effect of therapy. Endocrine disease can also occur in patients with infections, including HIV. Increasingly, associations are being demonstrated between endocrine disease and atherosclerotic cardiovascular disease. Therefore, the endocrine system is important to understand as it plays a key role in many other branches of medicine.

Nervous system

The nervous system uses very localized chemical signals at synapses to transmit membrane depolarization between neurons. The effects of the nervous system are very rapid but of short duration and expensive metabolically (i.e. the neurotransmitters and depolarization require a lot of energy). The specific target cell is determined mostly by the location of chemical release rather than the receptors.

Endocrine system

The endocrine system uses very generalized chemical signals, though a few endocrine tissues can depolarize. These signals require less energy than neural signals. The signals travel throughout the body in the bloodstream, and the target cell is determined mainly by the presence and specificity of receptors. The signals of the endocrine system tend to be slower but with a longer duration.

The hypothalamus and the pituitary gland

2

Objectives

By the end of this chapter, you should be able to:

- Describe the function of the hypothalamic–pituitary axis.
- Appreciate that the hypothalamus acts as an interface between the endocrine system and the environment.
- Explain how the hypothalamus regulates the anterior pituitary gland, including relevant vasculature.
- List the hormones secreted by the hypothalamus, along with their effects.
- Explain the structure–function relationship of the hypothalamus to the posterior pituitary.
- Describe the anatomical relationships of the pituitary gland and recognize their clinical significance.
- Explain the embryological development of the pituitary gland and how this affects hypothalamic control.
- List the hormones of the anterior pituitary gland, along with their effects.
- List the hormones of the posterior pituitary gland, along with their effects.
- Name the most common types of pituitary adenoma.
- List the effects of compression by a pituitary tumour and state the order in which they occur.
- List the symptoms of hyperprolactinaemia in males and females.
- List three treatment options for adenomas.
- Describe the investigations of pituitary hormone excess and deficiency.
- Describe the difference between a suppression and stimulation test, along with an example of each.
- Recognize which pituitary hormone deficiency is life threatening.
- Describe the treatment of panhypopituitarism.
- Name and describe the disorders of excess and deficient ADH secretion.
- Draw a diagram to illustrate the reflex that initiates lactation.

Endocrine hormones must both maintain homeo-stasis and adapt to changing demands. To achieve this, they are regulated by a system of complex feedback loops that can be modulated by changing environments. The hypothalamic–pituitary axis is the hub of these feedback loops and also the interface between the neural impulses generated by environmental stimuli and the chemical milieu of the endocrine system.

The hypothalamus receives neural stimuli and integrates this information to generate chemical signals that signal to the pituitary. The hypothalamus also has non-hypothalamo-hypophyseal outputs (i.e. not involving the pituitary), which affect hunger, thirst and sexual behavior.

Hypothalamic releasing and inhibitory hormones are carried, in the hypophyseal portal vessels, to the anterior pituitary, where they regulate the release of anterior pituitary hormones. Most of these anterior pituitary hormones regulate other endocrine organs (e.g. thyroid-stimulating hormone); however, some affect parts of the body directly (e.g. prolactin).

The posterior part of the pituitary gland functions in a slightly different way because it is a direct extension of the hypothalamus. Neurosecretory cells in the hypothalamus synthesize hormones that are transported along their axons. These hormones are released into capillaries within the posterior pituitary gland to affect body parts directly.

The secretory activity of the hypothalamus and pituitary gland can also be affected by hormones released from other endocrine organs (e.g. thyroxine from the thyroid gland). This feedback helps to control hormone levels, and it is a key component of endocrine function.

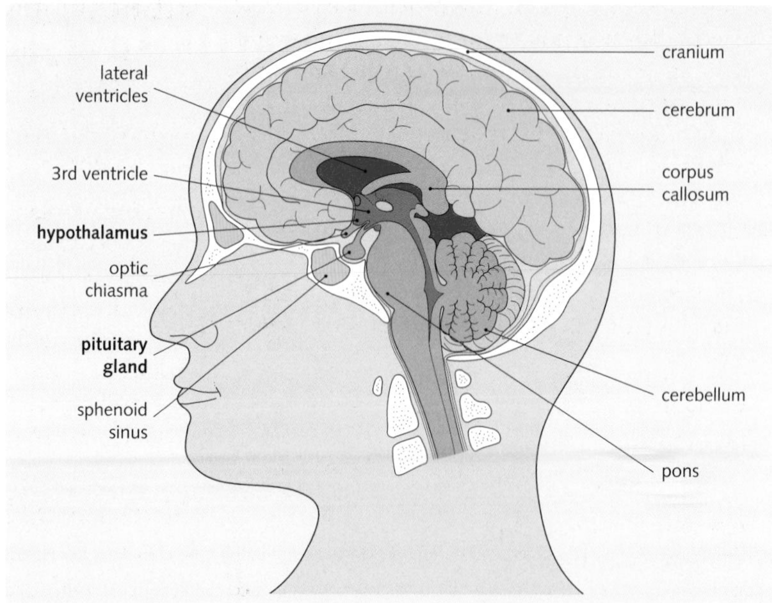

Fig. 2.1 Medial sagittal section of head showing the location of the hypothalamus and pituitary gland.

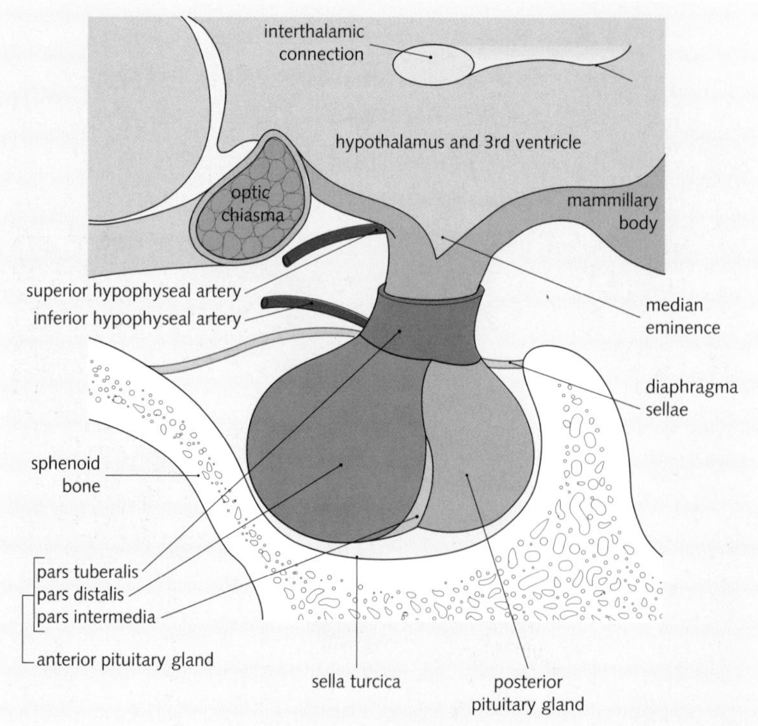

Fig. 2.2 Anatomical relationship of the pituitary gland and the hypothalamus to surrounding structures.

At first glance, the hypothalamus and pituitary gland seem needlessly complicated to perform a simple task. There are two main reasons for this arrangement:

- It allows intricate regulation of hormone levels.
- It amplifies the initial signal so that a few neurons can affect cells throughout the body.

ANATOMY

Hypothalamus

The hypothalamus is located at the base of the forebrain beneath the thalamus, and together they form the lateral walls of the third ventricle (see Fig. 2.1). The optic chiasma is anterior to the hypothalamus and the mammillary bodies are found posteriorly. The inferior part of the hypothalamus—called the median eminence—gives rise to the pituitary stalk, which is continuous with the posterior pituitary gland. This arrangement is shown in Fig. 2.2. The inputs and outputs of the hypothalamic–pituitary axis are shown in Figs 2.3 and 2.4.

The hypothalamus receives multiple inputs about the homeostatic state of the body. These arrive by two means:

- Circulatory, e.g. temperature, blood glucose, hormone levels.
- Neuronal, e.g. autonomic function, emotional.

It responds to these inputs by the secretion of hormones that either regulate the release of hormones from the anterior pituitary or are released directly from the posterior pituitary (e.g. antidiuretic hormone—ADH).

Pituitary gland

The pituitary gland is divided into two lobes with distinct embryological origins, structure, and function:

- Anterior pituitary or adenohypophysis.
- Posterior pituitary or neurohypophysis.

The pituitary gland lies in a bony hollow of the sphenoid bone (the sella turcica), and it is covered by the fibrous diaphragma sellae. The optic chiasma lies above this diaphragm directly superior to the anterior lobe. The posterior lobe is connected to the median eminence of the hypothalamus by the pituitary stalk (infundibulum). The cavernous sinuses, including the cranial nerves III–VI, lie laterally (see Figs 2.1 and 2.2).

Blood supply

Neurohormones from the hypothalamus are secreted into the extracellular fluid (ECF) at the median eminence. The median eminence is supplied by the superior hypophyseal artery, which forms a plexus

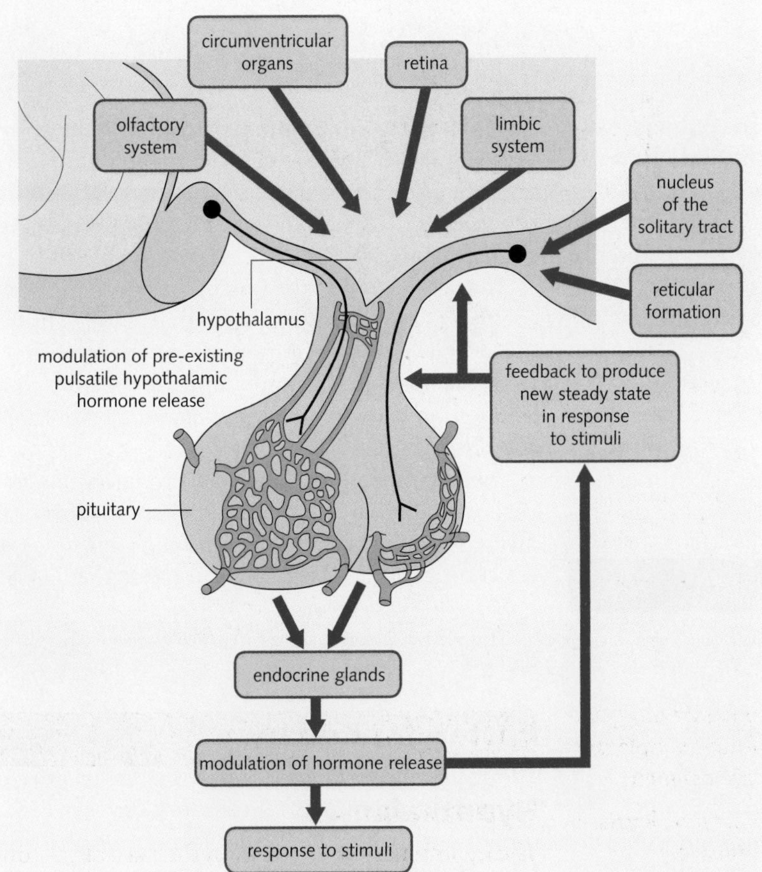

Fig. 2.3 The hypothalamic–pituitary system.

Fig. 2.4 Inputs to the hypothalamus

Circumventricular organs	Limbic system	Nucleus of the solitary tract	Reticular formation	Olfactory system
Monitor circulatory chemicals that normally have no access to the central nervous system. Include the organum vasculosum of the lamina terminalis (OVLT), which detects changes in osmolarity. Information from the OVLT is relayed, after processing in the hypothalamus, to the posterior pituitary, where ADH, the hormone that regulates blood osmolarity, is released.	The limbic system is responsible for emotion. It includes the amygdala (fear centre) and the hippocampus. Integration of these signals via the hypothalamus leads to endocrine responses to emotional changes, for instance sexual behaviour.	Conveys visceral sensory information, such as blood pressure (BP) and gut distension, which is important in the feedback control of BP/hunger/satiety.	Relays information from the spinal cord to the hypothalamus.	Conveys information about smell to the hypothalamus, which can initiate the endocrine and neural changes that lead to feeding responses such as salivation.

capable of picking up these neurohormones. From here, the hypophyseal portal veins carry the hormones to the adenohypophysis where they are released from a secondary capillary plexus. Hormones secreted from the median eminence pass directly to the anterior pituitary in the bloodstream, as shown in Fig. 2.5.

The posterior pituitary gland is supplied by the inferior hypophyseal arteries. These vessels do not communicate with the median eminence.

The veins draining the pituitary gland drain to the cavernous sinuses and from here carry the hormones to the systemic circulation.

DEVELOPMENT

Hypothalamus

The hypothalamus develops from the embryological forebrain; it can be identified at week 6 of gestation.

Anterior pituitary

The anterior pituitary develops as an outgrowth of the ectoderm of the primitive oral cavity called Rathke's pouch. It grows upwards until it fuses with the down-growing infundibulum of the hypothalamus. The anterior pituitary is composed of non-neural secretory epithelial tissue, and it is not directly connected to the hypothalamus.

The connection to the roof of the developing oral cavity is gradually lost, along with its blood supply. The portal veins from the hypothalamus grow down to replace this blood supply, and are the only communication between the hypothalamus and the anterior pituitary.

As the connection to the primitive mouth is lost, nests of epithelial cells may be left behind. These can give rise to cysts or tumours, which may secrete ectopic hormones (e.g. craniopharyngiomas—see p. 27).

The embryology of the pituitary gland is shown in Fig. 2.6.

Posterior pituitary

The posterior pituitary is derived from the neuroectoderm of the primitive brain tissue. It develops as an outgrowth from the hypothalamus called the infundibulum. Axons from neurosecretory cells in the

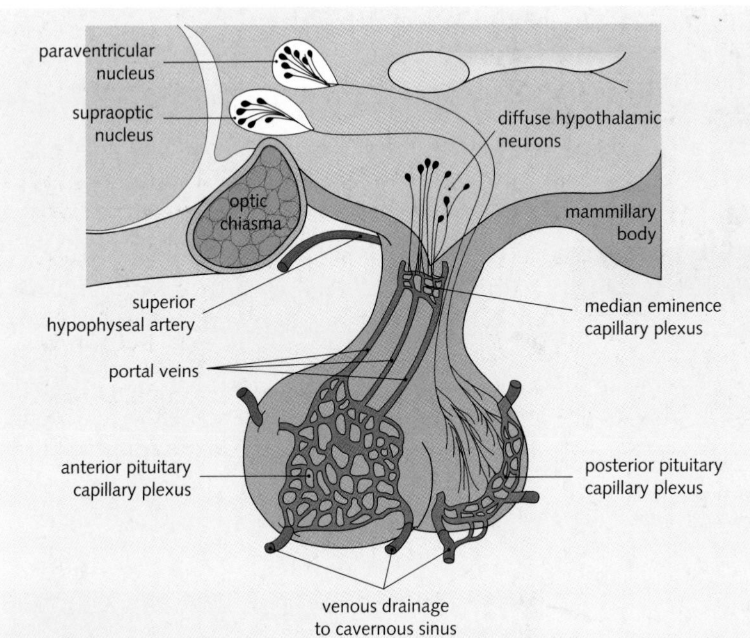

Fig. 2.5 Communication between the hypothalamus and pituitary gland; note the difference between the anterior and posterior pituitary gland.

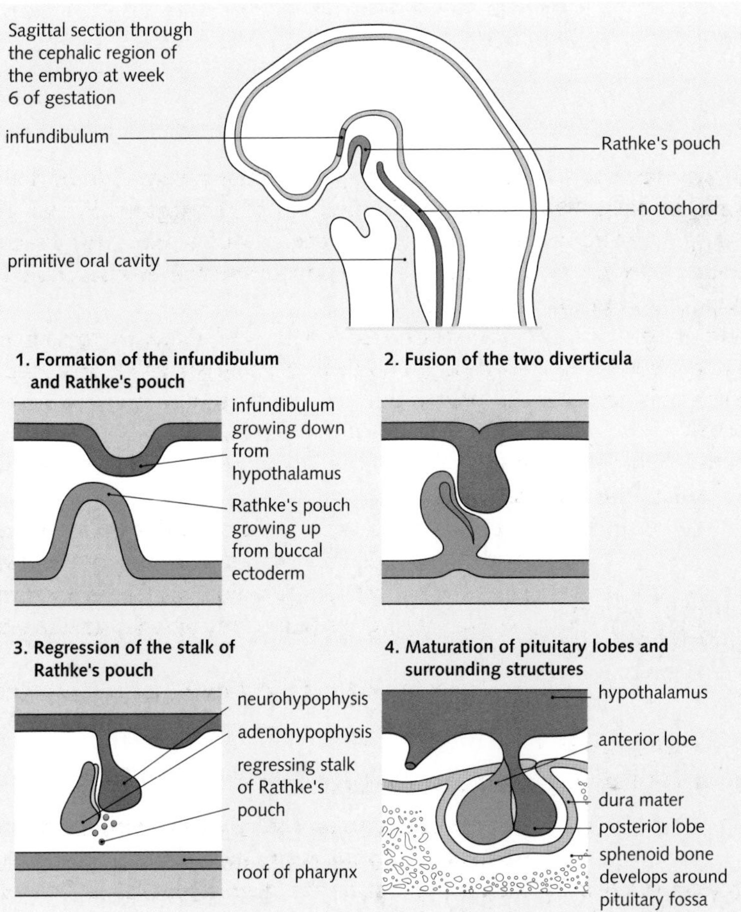

Fig. 2.6 Embryological development of the anterior and posterior lobes of the pituitary gland.

hypothalamus pass downwards in the stalk of the pituitary gland and terminate in the posterior pituitary. A direct neuronal connection between the hypothalamus and posterior pituitary is formed, and this is the only means of communication between these structures.

MICROSTRUCTURE

Hypothalamus

There are a number of different secretory neurons in the hypothalamus, each specialized to secrete specific hormones. Neurons that secrete the same chemical may be arranged in clusters called nuclei, or they may be scattered diffusely. Some neurons can secrete more than one hormone.

Anterior pituitary

The anterior pituitary is composed of cords of secretory cells in a rich network of capillaries. Six types of secretory cell can be distinguished using immuno-histochemistry. These are listed with the hormones that they synthesize:

- Somatotrophs—growth hormone (GH).
- Gonadotrophs—luteinizing hormone (LH) and follicle-stimulating hormone (FSH).
- Corticotrophs—adrenocorticotrophic hormone (ACTH).
- Thyrotrophs—thyroid-stimulating hormone (TSH).
- Lactotrophs—prolactin.
- Chromophobes—inactive secretory cells.

In the past, cells were differentiated by their pH; the terms acidophil and basophil in older textbooks refer to this.

The anterior pituitary is divided into three distinct areas (see Fig. 2.2):

- Pars distalis—the majority of the gland.
- Pars tuberalis—a layer of mostly functionally inactive gonadotroph cells around the pituitary stalk in humans.
- Pars intermedia—a thin layer of corticotroph cells between the anterior and posterior pituitary. It is poorly developed in adult humans. During pregnancy, peptide hormones γ-melanocyte-stimulating hormone (MSH) and α-MSH are processed from the larger precursor protein proopiomelanocortin (POMC)

Posterior pituitary

The posterior pituitary is composed of two cell types, but it contains no secretory cells:

- Non-myelinated axons, originating from the hypothalamus.
- Pituicytes, which are stellate (star-shaped) glial support cells.

Within the axons, there are microtubules and mitochondria that are involved in the transport of neurosecretory granules. These granules travel from the hypothalamus to the axon terminals in the posterior pituitary, where they are stored before release. The axon terminals lie close to blood sinusoids, where the neurosecretory granules are released into the systemic circulation (Fig. 2.7).

HORMONES

Hormones of the hypothalamus

The hypothalamus secretes very small quantities of hormones into the portal veins to exert control over the anterior pituitary. The quantity is so small that the hormones can rarely be detected in systemic blood, but by travelling in the portal veins directly to the anterior pituitary, their concentration is high enough to produce an effect. This system allows for a rapid response and amplification of the signal. The hypothalamic hormones are often released in a pulsatile manner. The pulses vary in amplitude and rate, often with a circadian rhythm (see Chapter 6). Hormones that influence the anterior pituitary are secreted by short parvocellular neurons. The hypothalamic neurons, which travel directly to the posterior pituitary, are the magnocellular neurons.

Hormones that regulate anterior pituitary function

The hormones secreted by the hypothalamus are small peptides (between 3 and 44 amino-acid residues), except for dopamine, which is derived from the amino acid tyrosine. These hormones are shown in Fig. 2.8, along with their effects.

The factors that regulate the secretion of these hormones are discussed independently in the individual chapters. They act on the secretory cells in an excitatory (e.g. thyrotrophin-releasing hormone—TRH) or inhibitory (e.g. growth-hormone inhibitng hormone—GHIH) manner. There is some overlap in function between these peptides; for example,

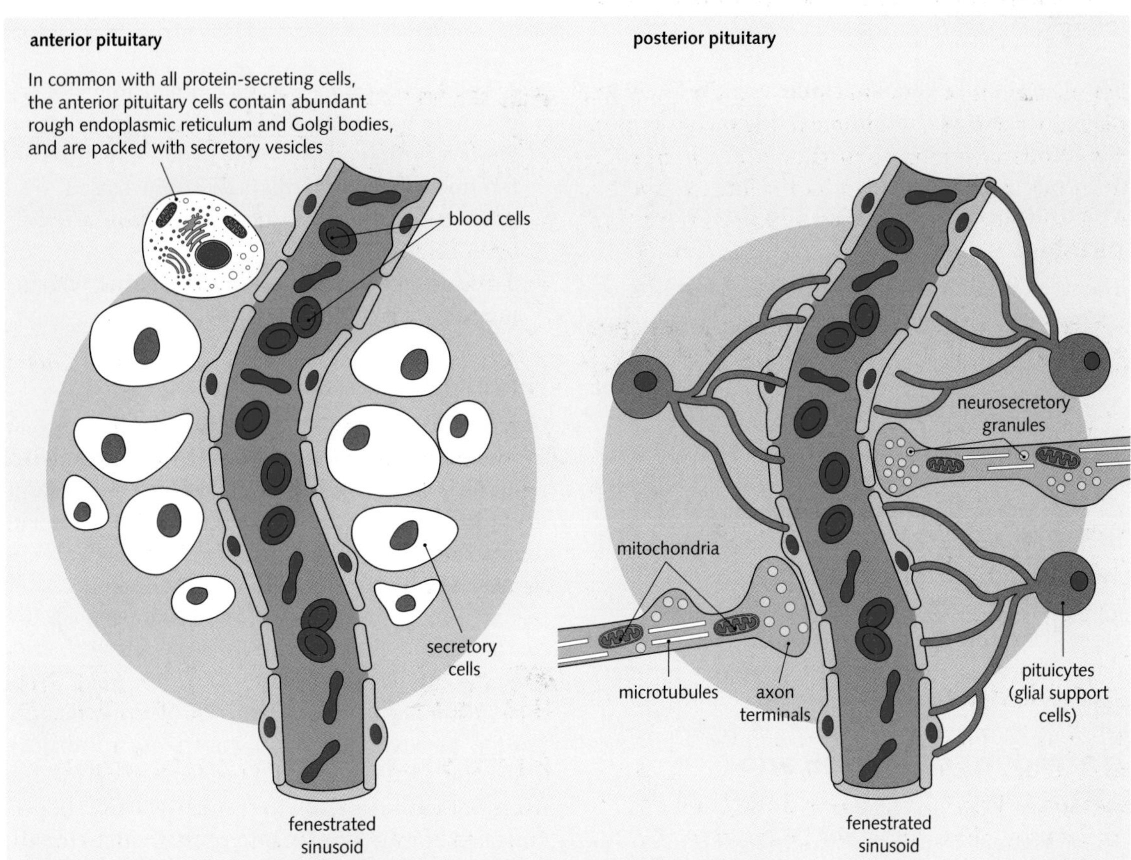

Fig. 2.7 Histology of the anterior and posterior pituitary gland.

Fig. 2.8 Hormones secreted by the hypothalamus and their effects on the secretion of the anterior pituitary hormones

Hormone	Target cells in the anterior pituitary gland	Effect on the anterior pituitary gland
Growth-hormone releasing hormone (GHRH)	Somatotrophs	↑ GH release
Growth-hormone inhibiting hormone (GHIH also called somatostatin)	Somatotrophs and thyrotrophs	↓ GH and TSH release
Corticotrophin-releasing hormone (CRH)	Corticotrophs	↑ ACTH release
Gonadotrophin-releasing hormone (GnRH)	Gonadotrophs	↑ LH and FSH release
Thyrotrophin-releasing hormone (TRH)	Thyrotrophs and lactotrophs	↑ TSH and prolactin release
Prolactin-releasing factors (PRF)	Lactotrophs	↑ Prolactin release
Dopamine (prolactin-inhibiting hormone)	Lactotrophs	↑ Prolactin release

ACTH, adrenocorticotrophic hormone; FSH, follicle-stimulating hormone; GH, growth hormone; LH, luteinizing hormone; TSH, thyroid-stimulating hormone.

TRH can stimulate prolactin release. It is likely that other hypothalamic hormones will be discovered in the future.

Hormones released from the posterior pituitary

The small peptides ADH and oxytocin are synthesized in the cell bodies of magnocellular neurons arranged into two nuclei in the hypothalamus:

- Supraoptic nucleus.
- Paraventricular nucleus.

Both nuclei secrete both hormones, but the supraoptic tends to secrete more ADH whereas the paraventricular favours oxytocin. The hormones pass along the axons bound to glycoproteins. They pass through the median eminence to the posterior pituitary where they are stored before release. Their actions are described in the section 'Hormones of the posterior pituitary', below.

Hormones of the anterior pituitary

The hormones secreted by the anterior pituitary are large peptides (about 200 amino acid residues) or glycopeptides.

The six main hormones are:

- Growth hormone (GH).
- Thyroid-stimulating hormone (TSH also called thyrotrophin).
- Adrenocorticotrophic hormone (ACTH).
- Luteinizing hormone (LH).
- Follicle-stimulating hormone (FSH).
- Prolactin (PRL).

The hormones synthesized by the anterior pituitary are released into the systemic circulation. They act in two ways:

- Regulation of other endocrine organs—TSH, ACTH, GH, LH and FSH.
- Direct effects on distant organs—prolactin.

GH and prolactin are large peptides whereas the others are glycopeptides. The individual hormones are discussed in more detail in later chapters (see also Figs 2.9 and 2.10). The secretion and release of these hormones often follows the pulsatile pattern of the releasing hormones from the hypothalamus.

The pars intermedia of the anterior pituitary gland also secretes a number of less important hormones including:

- α-MSH and γ-MSH, which stimulate melanocytes in skin in human fetal life and during pregnancy. Patients with high ACTH are hyperpigmented but it is unclear whether this is due to increased production of MSH or the melanotropic activity of ACTH.
- β-Endorphin, an endogenous morphine, which may have a role in the control of pain.

Hormonal feedback

In response to the small quantities of releasing hormones secreted by the hypothalamus, the anterior pituitary is stimulated to secrete hormones in quantities large enough to act on endocrine organs throughout the body. The release of pituitary hormones is also regulated by hormones from other endocrine glands, mainly through negative feedback echanisms, e.g. thyroxine from the thyroid inhibits the release of TSH from the anterior pituitary.

Hypothalamic regulation of prolactin release is unique because the main control is inhibitory: dopamine secreted from the hypothalamus inhibits release of prolactin from the pituitary. This is important if a tumour stops the hypothalamic releasing hormones from reaching the anterior pituitary. The levels of most pituitary hormones will fall, while the levels of prolactin will increase.

Hormones of the posterior pituitary

Two major hormones are synthesized in the hypothalamus and released into the systemic circulation from the posterior pituitary:

- Antidiuretic hormone (ADH) also called arginine vasopressin (AVP).
- Oxytocin.

Both hormones are peptides consisting of nine amino-acid residues that vary by a single residue. The main actions of these hormones are shown in Figs 2.11 and 2.12.

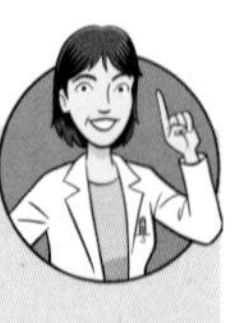

The hormones of the anterior pituitary can be remembered using the mnemonic 'Fresh Pituitary Tastes Almost Like Guinness'.

Fig. 2.9 Hormones synthesized and secreted by the anterior pituitary and their effects

Hormone	Synthesized by	Stimulated by	Inhibited by	Target organ	Effect	Chapter
GH	Somatotrophs	GHRH	GHIH and IGF-1	Liver	Stimulates IGF-1 production and opposes insulin	9
TSH	Thyrotrophs	TRH	T_3	Thyroid gland	Stimulates thyroxine release	3
ACTH	Corticotrophs	CRH	Glucocorticoids	Adrenal cortex	Stimulates glucocorticoid and androgen release	4
LH+FSH	Gonadotrophs	GnRH, sex steroids	Prolactin, sex steroids	Reproductive organs	Release of sex steroids	11
Prolactin	Lactotrophs	PRF and TRH	Dopamine	Mammary glands and reproductive organs	Promotes growth of these organs and initiates lactation	11
MSH	Corticotrophs	–	–	Melanocytes in skin	Stimulates melanin synthesis	–
Beta-endorphin	Corticotrophs	–	–	Unknown	May be involved in pain control	–

ACTH, adrenocorticotrophic hormone; CRH, corticotrophin-releasing hormone; FSH, follice-stimulating hormone; GH, growth hormone; GHRH, growth-hormone releasing hormone; GnRH, gonadotrophin-releasing hormone; GHIH, growth-hormone inhibiting hormone; LH, luteinizing hormone; MSH, melanocyte-stimulating hormone; TRH, thyrotrophin-releasing hormone; TSH, thyroid-stimulating hormone.

Antidiuretic hormone

ADH acts mainly on the collecting ducts of the kidney to prevent water excretion. It also has a vasoconstricting action at high doses, hence the name vasopressin. Low blood volume detected by peripheral baroreceptors stimulates very high ADH release to increase blood pressure.

A small proportion of ADH is released into the portal veins, where it stimulates corticotrophs in the anterior pituitary gland to secrete ACTH.

Oxytocin

When a baby suckles the mother's breast, stretch receptors in the nipple send signals to the brain via sensory nerves. These signals reach the paraventricular neurons causing depolarization and oxytocin release from the posterior pituitary. The oxytocin reaches the myoepithelial cells of the breast, which contract pushing milk out of the breast. This reflex is illustrated in Fig. 16.7).

DISORDERS OF THE HYPOTHALAMUS

Primary diseases of the hypothalamus are very rare, but they tend to cause deficiency of hypothalamic hormones and the corresponding pituitary hormones. Dopamine deficiency has the opposite effect, resulting in excessive prolactin secretion from the anterior pituitary. The main causes of hypothalamic hormone deficiency are:

- Trauma/surgery.
- Radiotherapy.
- Congenital gonadotrophin-releasing hormone (GnRH) deficiency (Kallmann's syndrome) causing infertility.
- Congenital GHRH deficiency causing dwarfism.
- Primary glial cell tumours of the hypothalamus.

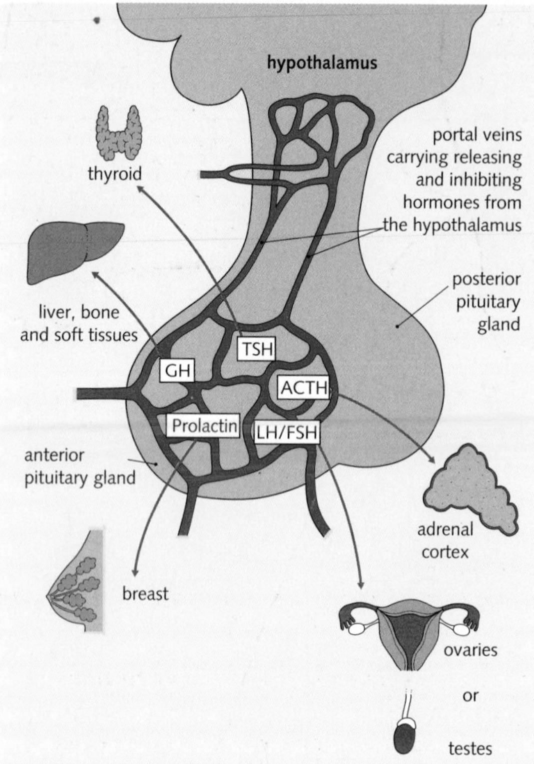

Fig. 2.10 Hormones of the anterior pituitary gland and their respective target organs. (ACTH, adrenocorticotrophic hormone; FSH, follicle-stimulating hormone; GH, growth hormone; LH, luteinizing hormone; TSH, thyroid-stimulating hormone.)

Lesions in the hypothalamus can cause many other abnormalities, including disorders of consciousness, behaviour, thirst, satiety and temperature regulation. These disorders usually occur together with hypopituitarism and diabetes insipidus.

In addition to endocrine abnormalities, pituitary tumours can present with the effects of a space-occupying lesion. These include headaches from stretching of the dura mater. Paradoxically, pituitary tumours can cause panhypopituitarism due to compression of functioning cells. Tumours of the pituitary gland are surrounded by the bone of the sella turcica, so they can only expand upwards into the optic chiasma, causing visual field defects. Further expansion compresses cranial nerves III, IV, V and VI in the wall of the cavernous sinus.

DISORDERS OF THE ANTERIOR PITUITARY

Aetiology

The nine I's of pituitary pathology are:

- Iatrogenic, e.g. surgery or radiotherapy.
- Invasion, i.e. tumours.
- Infarction, e.g. Sheehan's syndrome.
- Idiopathic, i.e. no underlying cause known.
- Injury, e.g. severe head trauma.
- Infection, e.g. tuberculosis (very rare).
- Infiltration, e.g. sarcoidosis (very rare).
- Immunological, e.g. lymphocytic hypophysitis (very rare).
- Inherited, e.g. congenital hormone deficiency (very rare).

Tumours

The majority of pituitary gland disorders are caused by benign tumours of the secretory cells called adenomas. Disease occurs as a result of three processes:

- Hyperpituitarism—excess pituitary hormone secretion.
- Hypopituitarism—insufficient pituitary hormone secretion.
- Compression of surrounding structures—caused by space-occupying lesions.

These tumours are classified into two groups: functioning and non-functioning adenomas. Functioning adenomas present early whilst still very small. These microadenomas cause disease by excess hormone release, which can be fatal if untreated. They also cause compression, so other pituitary hormones may be deficient (Fig. 2.13).

Non-functioning adenomas usually present at a later stage as larger macroadenomas. These cause disease indirectly by compressing surrounding structures, often causing insufficient pituitary hormone release when they compress the portal vessels or secretory cells.

Hyperpituitarism

Prolactinomas

All the anterior pituitary secretory cells can form tumours; however, the vast majority are prolactinomas i.e. tumours of the prolactin-secreting cells (Fig. 2.14). They are more common in women in whom they tend to present earlier, before visual

Fig. 2.11 Hormones secreted by the posterior pituitary and their effects

Hormone	Synthesized by	Stimulated by	Inhibited by	Target organ	Effect	Chapter
Antidiuretic hormone (ADH)	Supraoptic vasopressinergic neurons	Raised osmolarity; low blood volume	Lowered osmolarity	Kidney	Increases the permeability of the collecting duct to reabsorb water	7
Oxytocin	Paraventricular oxytocinergic neurons	Stretch receptors in the nipple and cervix; oestrogen	Stress	Uterus and mammary glands	Smooth muscle contraction leading to birth or milk ejection	13

disturbance occurs, with amenorrhoea and infertility. Excess prolactin secretion—hyperprolactinaemia—causes galactorrhoea and infertility. Infertility is the result of prolactin interfering with the release of GnRH, which inhibits LH and FSH release and causes hypogonadism (Fig. 2.15).

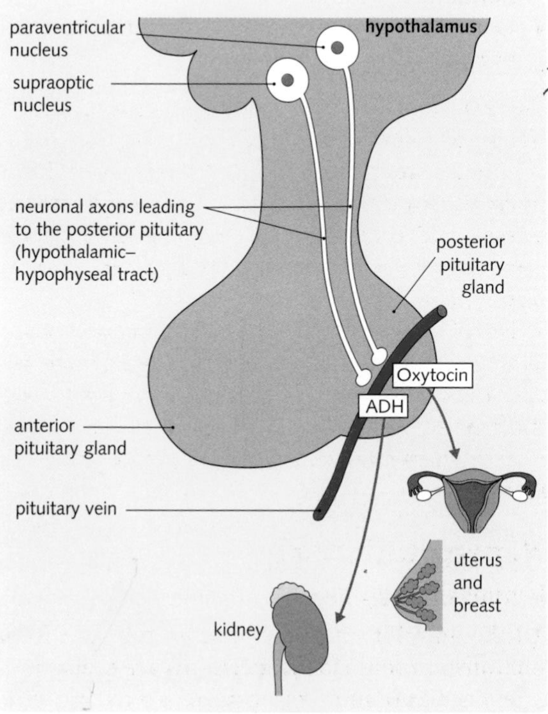

Fig. 2.12 Hormones of the posterior pituitary gland and their respective target organs. (ADH, antidiuretic hormone.)

Investigations

A number of symptoms and investigations are assessed to achieve a diagnosis:

- Are there symptoms of a specific endocrine abnormality?
- Visual field assessment is carried out to detect compression of the optic chiasma.
- Are there abnormal hormone levels in the blood? If an excess is suspected, all pituitary hormones should be tested as an adenoma can cause related deficiencies.
- Suppression tests are carried out—these assess pituitary response to hormone analogues or inhibiting factors to locate the lesion on the endocrine axis. Generally adenomas display reduced negative feedback.
- Magnetic resonance imaging (MRI) or computed tomography (CT) scans are used to detect abnormal anatomy.

Prolactin-secreting adenomas are the most common type of functioning adenoma and secrete excess prolactin by definition. Hyperprolactinaemia and galactorrhoea can also be caused by dopamine antagonists used to treat patients with movement disorders. Furthermore, renal failure can be associated with hyperprolactinaemia due to impaired prolactin secretion. Non-functioning adenomas can also produce hyperprolactinaemia by removing dopaminergic inhibition of prolactin release.

Fig. 2.13 Anterior pituitary hormones and the disorders caused by their deficiency and excess

Hormone	Deficiency	Excess
GH	Dwarfism in children or adult GH deficiency syndrome	Gigantism in children, acromegaly in adults
LH and FSH	Gonadal insufficiency (decreased sex steroids)	Extremely rare but causes infertility
ACTH	Adrenocortical insufficiency (decreased cortisol and adrenal androgens)	Cushing's disease (increased cortisol and adrenal androgens)
TSH	Hypothyroidism (decreased thyroid hormones)	Extremely rare but causes hyperthyroidism (increased thyroid hormones)
Prolactin	Hypoprolactinaemia (failure in postpartum lactation)	Hyperprolactinaemia (impotence in males, amenorrhoea in females and decreased libido)

ACTH, adrenocorticotrophic hormone; FSH, follicle-stimulating hormone; GH, growth hormone; LH, luteinizing hormone; TSH, thyroid-stimulating hormone.

Fig. 2.14 Adenomas of the anterior pituitary gland and their effects

Tumour	Hormone excess	Percentage of all pituitary tumours	Disease	Chapter
Prolactinoma	Prolactin	50%	Hyperprolactinaemia	2
Non-secretory prolactinoma	None	20%	Hypopituitarism	2
Somatotrophic cell adenoma	GH	20%	In children: gigantism In adults: acromegaly	9
Corticotrophic cell adenoma	ACTH	5%	Cushing's disease	4
Gonadotrophic cell adenoma	LH and FSH	Very rare	Infertility	–
Thyrotrophic cell adenoma	TSH	Very rare	Hyperthyroidism	3

ACTH, adrenocorticotrophic hormone; FSH, follicle-stimulating hormone; GH, growth hormone; LH, luteinizing hormone; TSH, thyroid-stimulating hormone.

The main suppression tests for anterior pituitary levels are to measure:

- GH in response to an oral glucose tolerance test, which normally suppresses GH levels.
- ACTH in response to dexamethasone, a steroid that normally suppresses CRH and ACTH release.

Treatment

There are four methods of treating excess hormone production, but they all carry the risk of causing hypopituitarism:

- Bromocriptine (dopamine agonist) to reduce prolactin secretion.
- Octreotide (synthetic somatostatin) to reduce GH secretion.

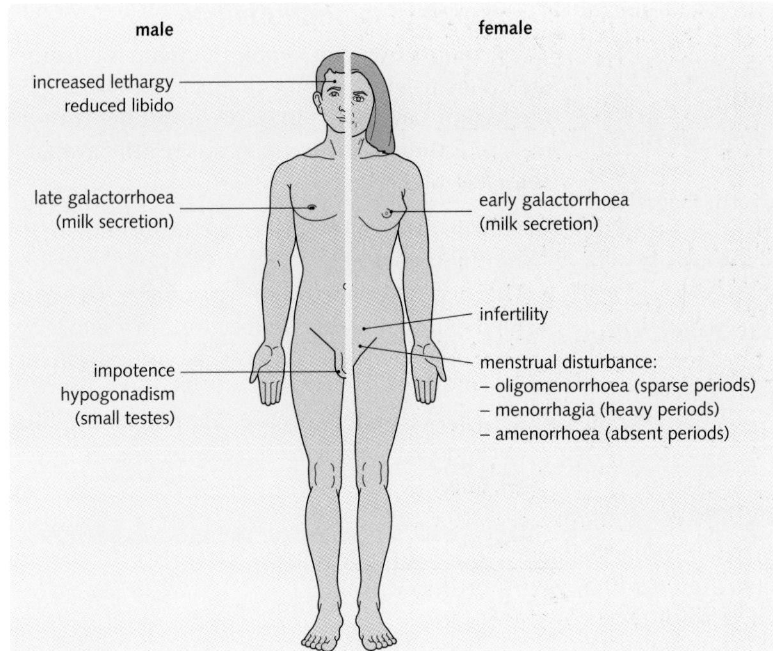

Fig. 2.15 Symptoms and signs of hyperprolactinaemia. Women tend to present earlier with endocrine symptoms.

- Surgical removal of pituitary adenoma.
- Irradiation to prevent adenoma recurrence.

Hypopituitarism

Pituitary insufficiency (hypopituitarism) often presents with insidious-onset depression, tiredness, and hypogonadism as most hormone levels fall and prolactin levels rise. When there is a deficiency of more than one pituitary hormone it is called panhypopituitarism. The causes of pituitary insufficiency are more varied than those of hyperpituitarism. However, the most common cause is the treatment of hyperpituitarism.

Non-functioning adenomas

About 20% of pituitary tumours do not produce hormones and so are called non-functioning adenomas (sometimes called chromophobe adenomas). They are almost always non-active prolactinomas. Since there is no excess hormone production they present late with symptoms caused by compression of surrounding structures, which become progressively severe:

- Headaches.
- Pituitary hormone deficiencies.
- Hypogonadism due to hyperprolactinaemia.
- Loss of peripheral vision due to compression of the optic nerve (bitemporal hemianopia).
- Cranial nerve palsies (starting with nerve IV).
- Raised intracranial pressure.

The tumour can cause hormone deficiencies by direct compression of the secretory cells or by compressing the portal veins that bring the hypothalamic releasing factors. Secretion of anterior pituitary hormones is inhibited in a characteristic order: GH, LH and FSH, ACTH, TSH (see Fig. 2.13 for symptoms). Unless the compression is very severe, prolactin secretion often increases initially since dopamine inhibition is lost. This excess prolactin secretion is not from the cells of the adenoma but it causes the symptoms shown in Fig. 2.15.

Other tumours

Tumours in surrounding tissues can also compress the pituitary gland causing panhypopituitarism, the most common being:

- Craniopharyngiomas.
- Gliomas (especially in the optic chiasma).

Craniopharyngiomas are rare tumours formed in the remnants of Rathke's pouch left behind when the connection with the developing oral cavity regressed. They can form above, below or within the sella turcica.

Gliomas are primary tumours of the glial support cells found throughout the brain.

Infarction of the pituitary gland

Infarction of the pituitary gland causes necrosis of all secretory cells with resultant panhypopituitarism, including loss of prolactin secretion. Sheehan's syndrome is a rare cause of pituitary infarction . Sheehan's is caused by a severe drop in blood pressure during obstetric haemorrhage. The pituitary gland is enlarged during pregnancy, which makes it particularly susceptible to hypotension and hypoxia. The ensuing panhypopituitarism causes a failure to lactate, amenorrhoea and eventually death if untreated.

Compression of the pituitary gland

Empty sella syndrome is a condition where the sella turcica partially fills with cerebrospinal fluid, causing the pituitary gland to be compressed. It is not always pathological (some cerebrospinal fluid is found within the sella in at least 50% of normal individuals). Causes include congenital incompetence of the diaphragma sellae, pituitary surgery or irradiation, postpartum pituitary infarction (Sheehan's syndrome) and coexisting pituitary tumour.

Other causes of pituitary failure

Pituitary failure can also result from infiltrative processes such as sarcoidosis and haemochromatosis, and infective processes such as TB and syphilis.

Diagnosis of hypopituitarism

Diagnosis of hypopituitarism involves the same steps as for hyperpituitarism; however, stimulation is used instead of suppression:

- Symptoms.
- Visual field assessment.
- Basal hormone levels in the blood.
- Stimulation tests.
- MRI or CT scan.

The main stimulation tests for anterior pituitary levels are to measure:

- GH in response to an insulin tolerance test, which normally increases GH levels.
- Cortisol in response to hypoglycaemia or the ACTH analogue Synacthen®.
- LH and FSH in response to GnRH or the anti-oestrogen clomiphene.

Treatment of hypopituitarism

The main treatment of hypopituitarism is hormone replacement, which requires frequent monitoring. All the major anterior pituitary hormones can be replaced, though prolactin is not readily available since it is rarely needed:

- Subcutaneous GH replacement using human recombinant GH.
- Oral thyroxine once cortisol replacement has begun.
- Oral or intramuscular testosterone in males.
- Oral oestrogen and progesterone cyclically in females.
- Intramuscular human chorionic gonadotrophin, LH and FSH are given if male or female fertility is required.

Surgery may be required to remove adenomas, gliomas or craniopharyngiomas.

Pituitary apoplexy is the result of sudden infarction or haemorrhage of the pituitary. It is usually the result of a pre-existing adenoma compressing the blood supply at the median eminence. Apoplexy refers to a sudden neurological event. When panhypopituitarism results from apoplexy, ACTH and TSH levels can be life threatening due to adrenal crisis and myxoedema, respectively. Apoplexy usually presents with acute onset headache, optic paresis, visual field defects, altered mental status and vomiting. This is one of only a few endocrine emergencies and requires neurosurgical intervention.

DISORDERS OF THE POSTERIOR PITUITARY

Diabetes insipidus

A deficiency of ADH (vasopressin) secretion prevents osmotic control of the kidney, so that very dilute polyuria occurs. Up to 20 litres of urine can be passed in a day, causing a potentially fatal dehydration and constant thirst. It is rare and usually idiopathic, but it can be caused by trauma, surgery or tumours (Fig. 2.16).

An ADH stimulation test is used to distinguish between deficient ADH and unresponsive kidneys. The condition is treated with desmopressin, a long-acting vasopressin analogue, to control fluid loss.

Fig. 2.16 Posterior pituitary hormones and the disorders caused by their deficiency and excess

Hormone	Deficiency	Excess
ADH	Diabetes insipidus (polyuria, hypotension)	Syndrome of inappropriate ADH secretion (SIADH)
Oxytocin	Failure to progress in labour and difficulty with breastfeeding	No effect

ADH, antidiuretic hormone.

Excess antidiuretic hormone secretion

The syndrome of inappropriate secretion of ADH (SIADH) can be caused by neurological, endocrine, malignant or infective diseases, but it can also be idiopathic, postoperative or caused by medications. Excess ADH causes water retention resulting in hypo-osmotic hyponatraemia (low sodium). The symptoms progress from malaise and weakness to confusion and coma. If untreated, it can be fatal. Oedema does not occur (see Fig. 2.16).

The thyroid gland

3

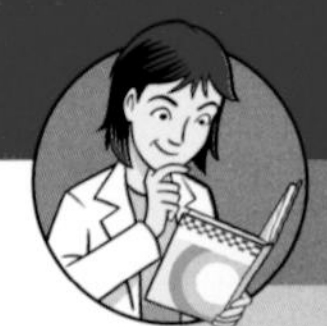

Objectives

By the end of this chapter you should be able to:

- Describe the anatomical shape and location of the thyroid and parathyroid glands, and explain why the thyroid gland moves during swallowing.
- Describe the blood supply to the thyroid gland, and describe the nerves that are related to these vessels.
- Describe how the cells of the thyroid gland are arranged, and how this relates to hormone synthesis.
- Envisage how the thyroid and parathyroid glands develop in the embryo.
- List the hormones secreted by the thyroid gland, and describe their actions.
- Describe thyroid hormone synthesis.
- Explain the endocrine control of the thyroid gland.
- State the main causes, symptoms and signs of thyrotoxicosis.
- State the main causes, symptoms and signs of hypothyroidism.
- Describe the treatment of hyperthyroidism and hypothyroidism.

Hormones convey information that maintains homeostasis. Levels of thyroid hormone do not fluctuate greatly under normal physiological conditions, and the hormone therefore acts more like a substrate that maintains cellular processes than a hormone that regulates cellular processes. Nonetheless, pathological fluctuations in thyroid hormone levels cause significant problems, which makes this system an important area of study.

The thyroid, from the Greek '*thyreoeides*', meaning shield shaped, is made up of two lobes and a bridging 'isthmus'. The gland consists of spherical 'follicles', which are composed of an outer basement membrane, a peripheral layer of follicular cells and a core of proteinaceous colloid. The thyroid hormones are synthesized and stored in these follicles and are dependent on an adequate iodine supply. The thyroid gland acts as a store of iodine and, in evolutionary terms, has allowed animals to migrate away from the ocean, the primary source of iodine. Thyroid hormone levels are regulated by a multiplex negative feedback loop with control from the hypothalamic–pituitary axis and autoregulation within the thyroid itself. The end product of this process is the production of the two thyroid hormones (Fig. 3.1):

- T_4—a prohormone that acts as a plasma reservoir.
- T_3—the active hormone.

Disease of the thyroid gland is the second most common endocrine disorder, after diabetes. Thyroid disease ranges from the production of too much or too little of the thyroid hormones, to the development of neoplasia. Excessive release of thyroid hormones in the presence of normally functioning downstream pathways is referred to as hyperthyroidism. These patients tend to be hyperactive, heat sensitive and to lose weight. Insufficient thyroid hormone is called hypothyroidism, and is associated with a slow metabolism, making patients feel lethargic and gain weight.

ANATOMY

Overview

The thyroid gland is palpable in about 50% of women and 25% of men. It is located in the neck, inferior to the larynx and cricoid cartilage. It has two lobes, each about 5 cm long and joined by a narrow isthmus. The lobes lie either side of the trachea and oesophagus, and the isthmus crosses the trachea anteriorly, usually over the second and third tracheal cartilages (Fig. 3.2).

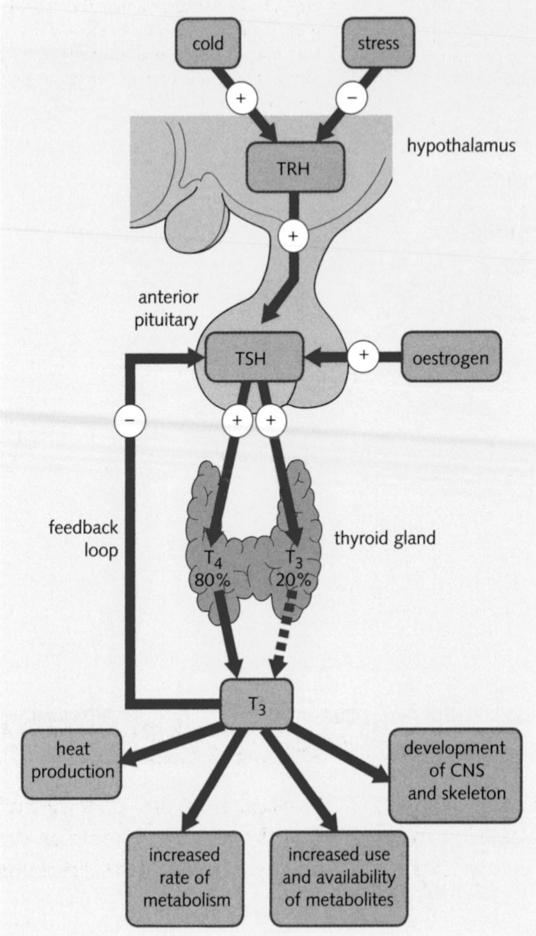

Fig. 3.1 Hormonal regulation of the thyroid hormones. (T_3, tri-iodothyronine; T_4, thyroxine; TRH, thyrotrophin-releasing hormone; TSH, thyroid-stimulating hormone.)

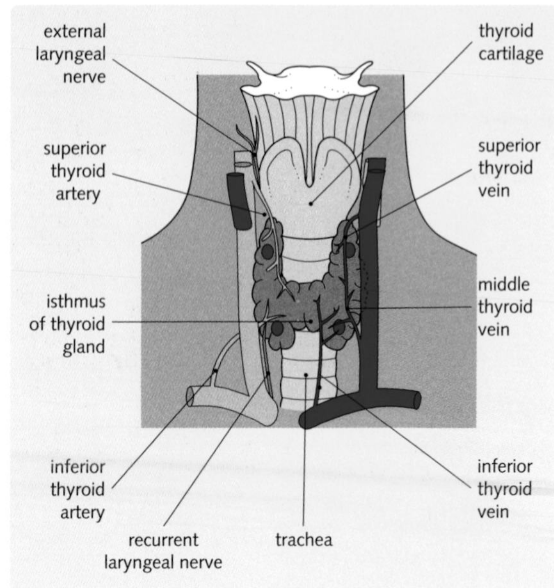

Fig. 3.2 Anterior view of the neck, showing the location and blood supply of the thyroid gland.

The thyroid gland is surrounded by a fibrous capsule derived from the pretracheal layer of the deep cervical fascia (Fig. 3.3). Extensions of this capsule into the body of the thyroid create septae, which divide the gland into lobules. This connective tissue firmly connects the thyroid to the larynx and explains why the thyroid moves on swallowing.

Blood supply, nerves, and lymphatics

The thyroid is highly vascular, and a bruit (the sound of turbulent blood flow) is sometimes heard in overactive glands. It is supplied by two arteries that anastomose (join) within the gland: the inferior and superior thyroid arteries.

The inferior thyroid artery is a branch of the thyrocervical trunk that arises from the subclavian arteries. It ascends behind the carotid sheath to enter the thyroid posteriorly. The right recurrent laryngeal nerve is intimately related to this artery near the inferior pole of the thyroid gland. Surgery to the thyroid gland can damage this nerve, causing temporary difficulty with speaking. To minimize the risk to this nerve, the artery is ligated far away from the thyroid gland during thyroidectomy.

The superior thyroid artery is usually the first branch of the external carotid artery. The external laryngeal nerve is related to this artery, but it is at less risk than the recurrent laryngeal during thyroid surgery. The superior thyroid artery is ligated close to the thyroid gland to reduce this risk (Fig. 3.2).

A third artery, called the thyroid ima artery, is present in 10% of people. It supplies the isthmus and it arises near the aortic arch, although the exact origin varies.

The thyroid gland is drained by three veins:

- Superior thyroid vein.
- Middle thyroid vein.
- Inferior thyroid vein.

The first two veins drain into the internal jugular, whereas the inferior vein drains into the brachiocephalic veins.

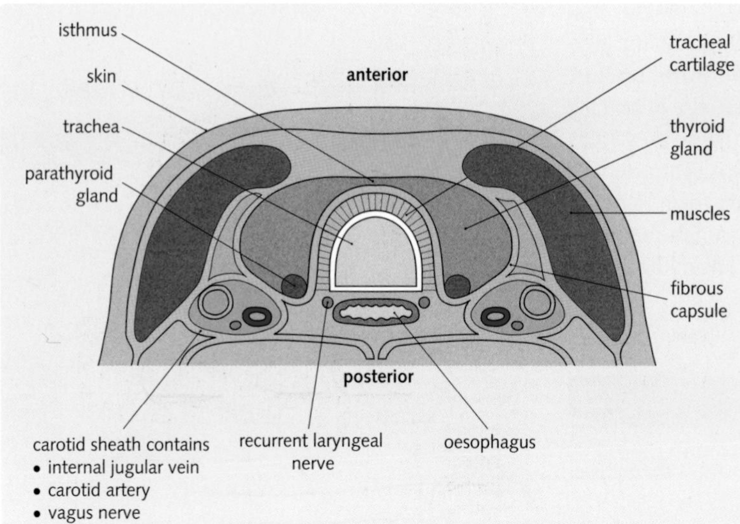

Fig. 3.3 Horizontal section of the anterior neck at the level of the sixth cervical vertebra, showing the location of the thyroid and parathyroid glands and their surrounding structures.

Thyroid lymphatics drain into four groups of nodes:

- Prelaryngeal lymph nodes.
- Pretracheal lymph nodes.
- Paratracheal lymph nodes.
- Deep cervical lymph nodes.

MICROSTRUCTURE

The thyroid is composed of about one million spherical follicles or acini. Each follicle is lined by a single layer of secretory epithelial cells (follicular cells) around a colloid-filled space. These cells secrete thyroglobulin into the lumen of the follicle, and thyroid hormones are synthesized from thyroglobulin at the cell–colloid boundary. When the thyroid gland is not actively secreting hormones, the size of the colloid store and the follicle itself increase in diameter.

When the follicular cells enter an active secretory phase, microvilli form on their inner surface and thyroglobulin is absorbed. The colloid store shrinks as a result. The absorbed thyroglobulin is broken down to release thyroid hormone. The histology of the thyroid gland is shown in Fig. 3.4.

Another type of secretory cell is found between the follicles. These parafollicular cells (C cells) synthesize and secrete calcitonin.

DEVELOPMENT

The thyroid gland develops from an endodermal extension in the floor of the pharynx known as the thyroglossal duct. The thyroglossal duct descends

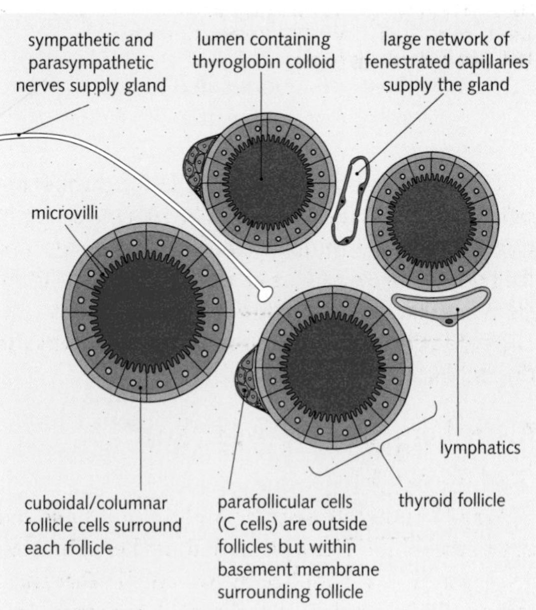

Fig. 3.4 Histology of the thyroid gland.

through the tongue and usually degenerates when the thyroid develops. The vestigial marking of the thyroglossal duct is the foramen cecum of the tongue. Remnants of thyroglossal duct anywhere else in its track can develop into a thyroglossal cyst. These present as neck lumps that rise when the tongue is protruded. In 50% of people a remnant of this duct forms a small pyramidal lobe extending superiorly from the isthmus. The parafollicular (C) cells are derived from the neural crest.

HORMONES

The thyroid gland synthesizes and secretes three hormones:

- Thyroxine (T_4).
- Tri-iodothyronine (T_3).
- Calcitonin.

Calcitonin is involved with calcium homeostasis (discussed in Chapter 8).

Synthesis

T_4 and the less abundant but more potent T_3 are synthesized in a step-by-step process that takes place in both the colloid and the follicular cells. Thyroid hormones are lipophilic, and therefore must be bound up as residues of the thyroglobulin molecule during synthesis in order to restrict their movements. Thyroglobulin in the colloid acts as a precursor and storage form of thyroid hormones. T_3 and T_4 are synthesized by three or four iodination reactions, respectively, of tyrosyl residues in thyroglobulin. Their structures are shown in Fig. 3.5.

Thyroid hormones are formed in the lumen of follicles, not in the cells. The process of T_3 and T_4 synthesis involves the processing of tyrosine and iodine followed by a reaction to bind them together. These steps are also shown in Fig. 3.6.

Tyrosine processing is relatively simple, since tyrosine molecules are already within the cell:

Thyroglobulin synthesis Tyrosine is converted into the glycoprotein thyroglobulin, which contains approximately 110 tyrosine residues.

The processing of iodine involves two stages as plasma iodine concentrations are very low:

Iodine trapping Plasma iodide ions (I^-) are actively transported from the plasma into the follicular cells

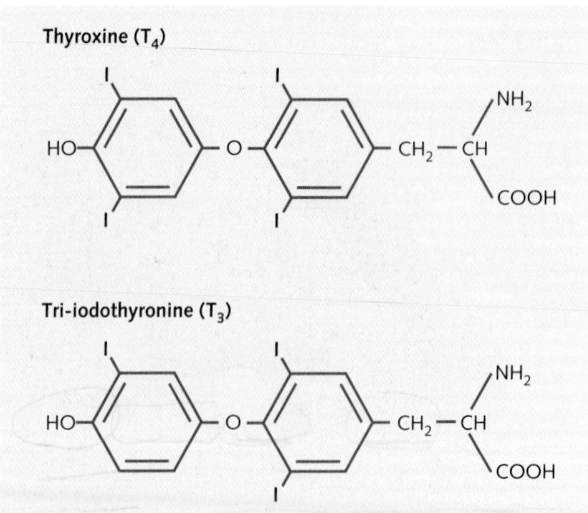

Fig. 3.5 Structures of T_3 and T_4.

against a steep concentration gradient by the Na/I symporter (NIS). This is a rate-limiting step.

Iodide oxidation I^- is rapidly oxidized into iodine (I_2) by thyroid peroxidase (TPO) anchored on the luminal surface of the follicular cell membrane.

The two components are then combined in the colloidal lumen:

Iodination of thyroglobulin Reactive iodine rapidly attaches to the tyrosine molecules within the extracellular thyroglobulin in a process that is catalysed by TPO. Monoiodotyrosine (MIT or T_1) and diiodotyrosine (DIT or T_2) are formed.

Coupling Tyrosine molecules within thyroglobulin are then coupled together. Combinations of T_1 and T_2 can form thyroid hormones:

- T_3 is made from $T_1 + T_2$.
- T_4 is made from $T_2 + T_2$.

Only a small proportion of coupling reactions form T_3 and T_4.

The thyroid hormones can now be released on demand:

Secretion Under the direction of thyroid-stimulating hormone (TSH or thyrotrophin), iodinated thyroglobulin is taken into the follicular cells by pinocytosis and degraded by lysosomal enzymes. Coupled tyrosine molecules are released, including some T_3 and T_4. Some T_4 is converted to T_3 in the follicular cell cytoplasm by the enzyme type 1,5′deiodinase. Whilst the secreted ratio of T_4:T_3 is usually 20:1 conversion to T_3 is promoted by TSH stimulation and can result in the so-called T_3

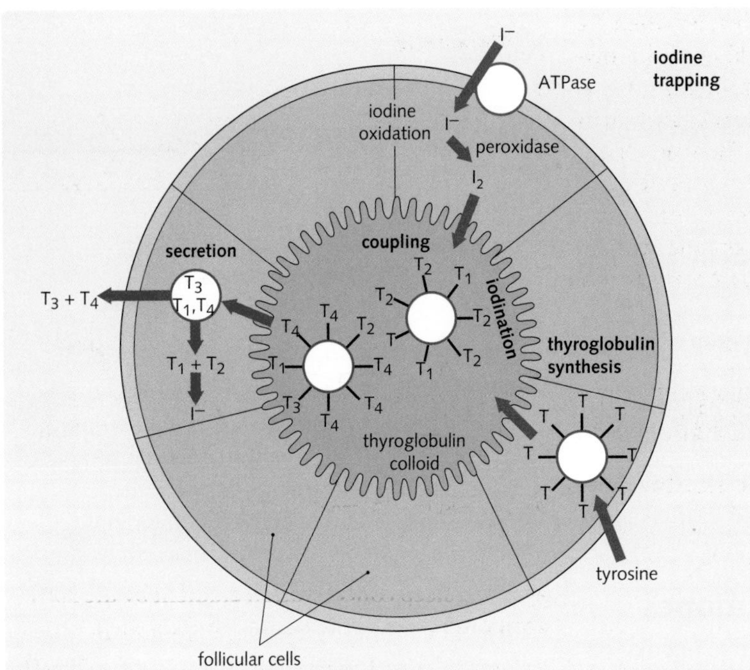

Fig. 3.6 Steps in the synthesis and secretion of T_3 and T_4. (T_3, tri-iodothyronine; T_4, thyroxine.)

thyrotoxicosis. MIT and DIT are also released, but they are deiodinated by iodotyrosine deholgenase to recycle iodine.

The majority of plasma T_3 is formed by the deiodination of T_4, and *not* from the thyroid gland. This is important in the treatment of hypothyroidism, since only T_4 is given

Iodine metabolism

Iodine is acquired from the diet mainly from iodized salt, meat and vegetables. About 150 mg of iodine is needed per day, though only a fraction of this is absorbed. The thyroid gland cells are the only cells that can actively absorb and utilize plasma iodine; a considerable quantity of iodine is stored in the thyroid as preformed thyroid hormones. Iodine is returned to the plasma by the breakdown of these thyroid hormones. Iodine is excreted mainly via the kidneys.

Thiacarbimide drugs, such as carbimazole, used in the treatment of hyperthyroidism, inhibit thyroid peroxidase. This inhibition results in decreased oxidation of iodide, decreased iodination of iodides and ultimately reduced thyroid hormone production.

Regulation

Hypothalamic thyrotrophin-releasing hormone (TRH) stimulates the release of thyroid-stimulating hormone (TSH) from thyrotrophs in the anterior pituitary gland and also causes upregulation of TSH gene transcription. TSH acts on extracellular receptors (TSH-R) on the surface of thyroid follicle cells, activating the G-protein–adenyl-cyclase–cAMP and phophatidylinositol (PIP_2) pathways. Ultimately, TSH stimulates the following processes in the thyroid gland:

- Iodine uptake.
- Transcription of thyroglobulin and thyroid peroxidase.
- Iodination.

- Coupling.
- Type 1 5′deiodinase conversion of T_4 to T_3.
- Pinocytosis and secretion of thyroid hormones.

As a result, T_3 and T_4 are synthesized and secreted more rapidly (see Fig. 3.1). TSH also has long-term actions on the thyroid gland by increasing its size and vascularity to improve hormone synthesis.

A number of factors affect thyroid hormone release. Three main factors stimulate secretion:

- Long-term exposure to cold temperatures acting on the anterior pituitary.
- Oestrogens acting on the anterior pituitary.
- Adrenaline acting directly on the thyroid gland.

TSH forms part of a negative feedback loop, as its release is inhibited by increased serum T_3 and T_4 and also by somatostatin, glucocorticoids and chronic illness.

Transport of thyroid hormones

The thyroid hormones circulate bound to plasma proteins produced in the liver, which protect the hormones from enzymic attack:

- 70% are bound to thyroid-binding globulin (TBG).
- 30% are bound to albumin.

Only 0.1% of T_4 and 1% of T_3 are carried unbound—it is this free (unbound) fraction that is responsible for their hormonal activities.

Both T_3 and T_4 can cross cell membranes, though a carrier transport may be involved.

The concentration of circulating T_4 is much higher than that of T_3 (50:1). There are two reasons for this:

- The thyroid secretes more T_4 than T_3.
- T_4 has a longer half-life (7 days vs 1 day).

Actions

Fig. 3.7 describes some of the differences between T_4 and T_3. T_4 is a relatively inactive, stable molecule that can be thought of as a prohormone. T_3 is the active hormone, since it is readily available and it has more effect on receptors. The benefit of producing both hormones is that T_4 can maintain a background level of activity, whilst T_3 levels can adapt rapidly to changing environments.

Peripheral tissues can regulate local T_3 levels by increasing or decreasing T_3 synthesis. T_4 is converted to T_3 by deiodination, i.e. removal of one iodine atom catalysed by deiodinase enzymes. Two main forms of this enzyme have been found:

Fig. 3.7 Comparison of T_3 and T_4

	T_3	T_4
Proportion of secreted thyroid hormone	10%	90%
Percentage free in plasma	1%	0.1%
Relative activity	10	1
Half-life (days)	1	7

- Type 1—mostly in liver and kidney but also in other tissues. It supplies plasma with T_3 and is inhibited by the propylthiouracil that is used to treat hyperthyroidism.
- Type 2—intracellular enzymes that maintain constant T_3 in the central nervous system (CNS) and pituitary gland in the face of rising plasma T_4.

A further deiodinase enzyme can remove a different iodine molecule from T_4 to form reverse T_3 (rT_3). This is an inactive molecule that is rapidly cleared from the circulation by the kidney and liver. Production of rT_3 is favoured by low energy stores and illness when energy stores need to be conserved.

Free plasma T_3 enters cells and binds to intracellular T_3 receptors, which are capable of binding specific sequences (or thyroid response elements) of DNA. Accordingly, after a lag of several hours, the expression of various thyroid response genes is up- or downregulated. The intracellular actions are described in Fig. 3.8 and related to physiological effects.

In general, T_3 promotes energy production in every cell in the body. This causes heat production and maintains metabolism.

The thyroid gland is the only endocrine gland to store its hormone in an extracellular compartment. 2–3 months' supply of thyroid hormone are stored within the follicles, and this delays the onset of symptoms in deficiency diseases.

Feedback

T_3 receptors are also found in the pituitary gland and the hypothalamus, where they inhibit transcription of the gene for TRH prohormone and the release of

Fig. 3.8 Intracellular and physiological actions of T_3

Site of action	Intracellular effects	Physiological results
Cell membrane	Stimulates the Na^+/K^+ATPase pump	Increased demand for metabolites, e.g. glucose
Mitochondria	Stimulates growth, replication and activity; basal metabolic rate is raised	Increased heat production, oxygen demand, heart rate and stroke volume
Nucleus	Increases expression of enzymes necessary for energy production	Lipolysis, glycolysis and gluconeogenesis increased to raise blood metabolite levels and cellular metabolite use
Neonatal cells	Essential for cell division and maturation	Essential for normal development of CNS and skeleton

TSH, respectively. Excess T_3 inhibits TSH release while a deficiency of T_3 stimulates TSH release. This feedback mechanism helps to maintain T_3 levels, and therefore stabilizes metabolic rate.

DISORDERS OF THE THYROID GLAND

The thyroid gland is prone to a number of diseases that can alter its function and structure. These diseases frequently have wide-ranging systemic effects because thyroid hormones regulate the metabolism of almost every cell in the body. The main categories of disease are:

- Hyperthyroidism—excess of thyroid hormone production.
- Hypothyroidism—deficiency of thyroid hormone production.
- Goitre formation.
- Adenoma (benign growths) of the thyroid.
- Carcinoma of the thyroid.

Hyperthyroidism

Hyperthyroidism is defined as an overactive thyroid gland, leading to excess thyroid hormones (T_4 and T_3). When this becomes symptomatic it is called thyrotoxicosis. Thyrotoxicosis can occur in the absence of true hyperthyroidism. This phenomenon is seen during inflammation of the thyroid (thyroiditis), which stimulates the release of stored hormone or can be the result of excess exogenous thyroid hormone (thyrotoxicosis factitia) or ectopic hormone production (ovarian struma or metastatic thyroid cancer). It is a common disorder affecting 1/50 females and 1/250 males. The symptoms and signs of thyrotoxicosis are illustrated in Fig. 3.9.

Presentation is usually slow with a history lasting over 6 months.

An acute exacerbation of symptoms is called a thyrotoxic crisis; it is usually brought on by infection in previously undiagnosed patients. Surgery or radioactive ablation of the thyroid gland can also be responsible as the damaged thyroid follicles release their contents. The main causes of hyperthyroidism are:

- Diffuse toxic goitre: Graves' disease—an autoimmune disease involving autoantibody stimulation of TSH receptors.
- Toxic multinodular goitre—nodular enlargement of the thyroid in the elderly.
- Toxic nodule—autonomously functioning thyroid nodule; most are adenomas (benign thyroid hormone producing tumours).
- Lymphocytic thyroiditis—inflammation causes release of stored hormones (followed by hypothyroid phase).
- Subacute thyroiditis—thyroiditis associated with a painful goitre.

Diagnosis

Thyroid function tests are the main component of diagnosis. Serum TSH, free T_3, and free T_4 are measured by radioimmunoassay (RIA). Raised T_3 and T_4 indicate that hyperthyroidism is present. Raised TSH

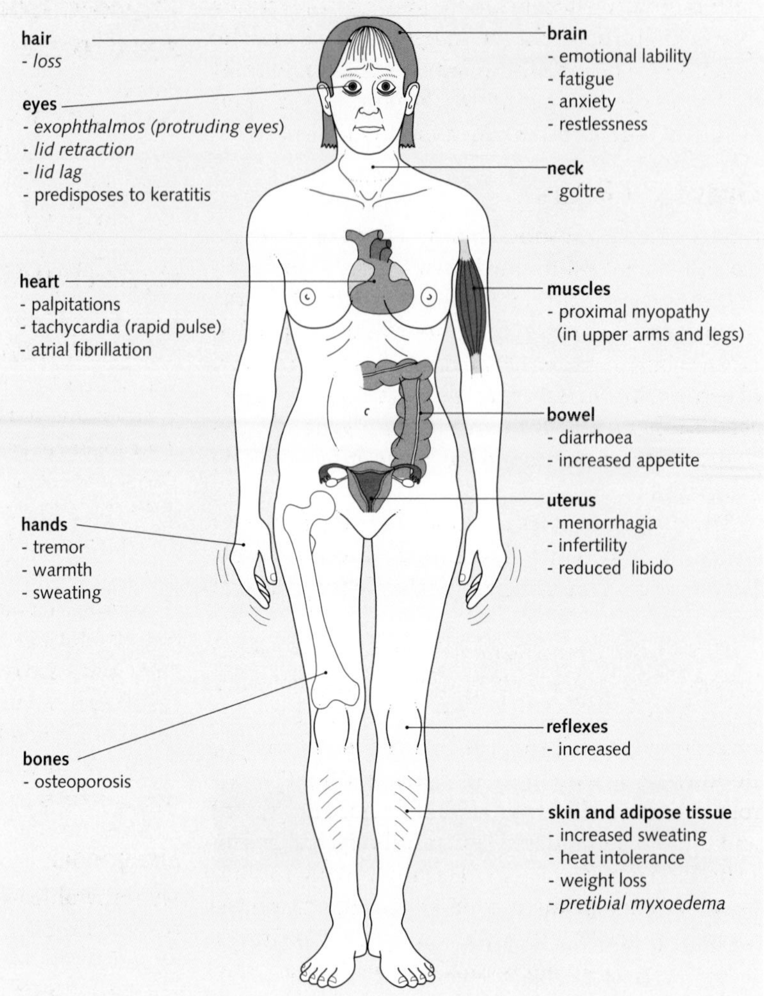

Fig. 3.9 Symptoms and signs of thyrotoxicosis (hyperthyroidism). The features in italic are only found in Graves' disease.

suggests the fault lies in or above the pituitary gland, whereas low TSH points to a thyroid organ lesion.

Other tests include:

- Autoantibody detection, e.g. Graves' disease.
- Radioisotope scanning to show the size of the thyroid gland and any abnormal 'hot' areas such as a toxic adenoma.
- ECG for sinus tachycardia or atrial fibrillation.

Treatment

There are three methods of treatment:

- Carbimazole—this drug inhibits the peroxidase reactions of T_3 and T_4 synthesis. It takes 3–4 weeks to have an effect. Two principal regimes exist for antithyroid therapy. The titration regime involves giving increasing doses of anti-thyroid drug until the patient becomes euthyroid. The alternative is the 'block and replace', which involves full-dose carbimazole and thyroxine replacement.
- Radioactive iodine therapy—^{131}I is only taken up by thyroid tissue; it kills the cells leading to reduced T_3 and T_4 synthesis. The response is slow and carbimazole may be required. The benefits include a reduced chance of relapse and taking away the need to take carbimazole, which carries risk of agranulocytosis, in the long term.
- Partial thyroidectomy—the thyroid gland is surgically removed leaving some tissue and the parathyroid glands. Used in patients with relapsing disease or allergy to medical treatment. Carries risk of recurrent laryngeal nerve palsy and hypocalcaemia due to the removal of parathyroid glands.

Both radioactive iodine and partial thyroidectomy carry a high risk of long-term hypothyroidism. The remaining thyroid tissue may be insufficient to meet the body's needs, especially as the patient ages. Their treatment is described under hypothyroidism.

Graves' disease

Graves' disease, the most common form of thyrotoxicosis, is an autoimmune disease in which autoantibodies against the TSH receptors stimulate the receptors so that thyroid hormones are produced in excess. Graves' disease is the most common cause of hyperthyroidism; it is especially common in middle-aged women (♀:♂, 8:1) and it has a genetic component with some human leucocyte antigen (HLA) association.

The disease follows either a relapsing-remitting course or one with fluctuating severity. Rarely Graves' disease can progress to hypothyroidism with time.

Graves' disease can cause the classical picture of hyperthyroidism with bulging eyes (exophthalmos), goitre (with bruit) and swollen legs (pretibial myxedema). It is diagnosed by detection of autoantibodies along with low TSH and raised T_3. The thyroid autoantibodies, thyroglobulin antibody (Tg Ab) and thyroid peroxidase (TPO) antibody, are present in both Graves' disease and Hashimoto's thyroiditis. However, stimulating thyroid-stimulating hormone receptor (TSH-R) antibodies are specific to Graves' disease. The treatment is consistent with other causes of hyperthyroidism, but radioactive iodine and surgery are especially likely to cause hypothyroidism.

Eye disease is an important symptom of Graves' disease as it can lead to compromised vision due to optic nerve compression and corneal ulcers. Inflammation of the orbit causes the eye to protrude, which can lead to discomfort and double vision. This symptom may occur before thyroid hormone levels rise.

> The major symptoms of hyperthyroidism can be remembered as: '**D**on't **E**vade **F**eeling **H**ot **A**nd **S**weaty **P**atients' i.e. **D**iarrhoea, **E**motional lability, **F**atigued, **H**eat intolerance, increased **A**ppetite, **S**weating, and **P**alpitations.

Thyroid hormone resistance syndrome

This is a rare condition that occurs due to a mutation in one of the thyroid receptor genes. In most cases the raised levels of T_3 and T_4 compensate for the resistance, but 'generalized resistance' can present with congenital hypothyroidism.

Hypothyroidism

Hypothyroidism is defined as an underactive thyroid gland leading to deficient thyroid hormones (T_4 and T_3). When this becomes symptomatic, it is called myxoedema. It is slightly less common than hyperthyroidism, affecting 1/100 females and 1/500 males. The symptoms and signs of myxoedema are illustrated in Fig. 3.10. Presentation is even more gradual than in hyperthyroidism, with many symptoms frequently being ignored.

Thyroid hormones are essential between birth and puberty for the normal development of the CNS. Deficiency can cause irreversible mental retardation called cretinism. TSH levels are checked in all newborns for this relatively common abnormality; the levels will be raised if the thyroid gland is not functioning correctly.

Diagnosis

Hypothyroidism is not investigated as thoroughly as hyperthyroidism, since treatment does not vary. Free T_3 and T_4 levels are low, whereas TSH levels are usually raised. If TSH is low then a lesion of the hypothalamus or pituitary is likely. Autoantibodies can be detected in Hashimoto's thyroiditis.

Treatment

All hypothyroidism is treated with thyroxine (T_4) administered as an oral tablet in varying doses. The dose is increased over several months, with regular monitoring of TSH levels until they are within the normal boundaries. This process is slow, since it takes 4 weeks for TSH levels to reflect an increased dose due to the long half-life of thyroxine. Thyroxine therapy is usually maintained for life.

Overtreatment of hyperthyroidism

Radioactive ablation and surgical removal of the thyroid gland initially cure hyperthyroidism, but with time, the remaining thyroid tissue is often insufficient. Hypothyroidism can develop and life-long thyroxine treatment is required.

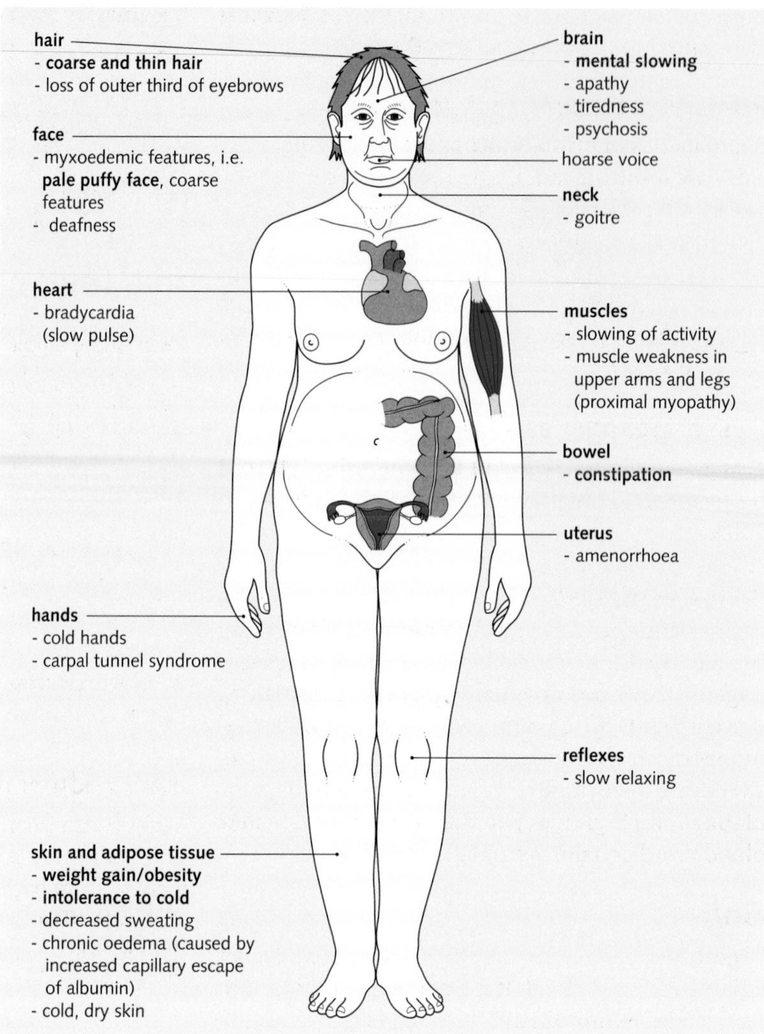

Fig. 3.10 Symptoms and signs of myxoedema (hypothyroidism). The main features are shown in bold.

Many drugs can also cause reversible hypothyroidism including lithium amiodarone and excess iodine.

Hashimoto's thyroiditis

When the thyroid gland is inflamed, the disease is called thyroiditis. This can be caused by autoimmune or viral processes. Hashimoto's thyroiditis is a destructive autoimmune disease that is especially common in middle-aged women. It is mediated by autoantibodies against rough endoplasmic reticulum (microsomal antibodies) or thyroglobulin. The presence of these antibodies can be tested to confirm the diagnosis. The thyroid gland is infiltrated by lymphocytes that cause the gland to enlarge, forming a goitre.

The initial destruction of the thyroid gland can release the thyroglobulin colloid causing temporary hyperthyroidism. The patients usually progress to a euthyroid (normal) state and finally develop progressive hypothyroidism.

Subacute (de Quervain's) thyroiditis

De Quervain's thyroiditis is inflammation of the thyroid gland caused by a virus. It is common in young or middle-aged women, in whom it causes a tender swollen gland along with a febrile illness. The inflammation causes an initial increase in thyroid hormone release followed by destroying the follicles, which causes hypothyroidism and leakage of the thyroglobulin colloid. An immune reaction against this colloid causes the formation of granulomas, so this disease is also called granulomatous thyroiditis.

Primary atrophic hypothyroidism

Spontaneous or primary atrophic hypothyroidism is a disease resulting in hypothyroidism in the elderly. The biochemical profile may include the presence of TSH-R blocking autoantibodies, but in this condition the thyroid fibroses and shrinks so that there is no goitre. It is suspected that this disease is the end-stage of many thyroid diseases, including Hashimoto's and de Quervain's thyroiditis.

Dyshormonogenesis

This is an inherited defect in the synthesis of thyroid hormones, and can present with hypothyroidism and goitre.

Iodine deficiency

Iodine deficiency was once a common cause of goitre in regions where the soil lacked iodine (e.g. Derby, England), but nowadays iodine is added to salt to prevent this. Deficient iodine means that thyroid hormones cannot be synthesized with a resultant rise in TSH levels. TSH causes thyroid enlargement by stimulating follicle growth and the development of new blood vessels, so the thyroid gland enlarges.

Goitres

A goitre is a swelling in the neck caused by an enlarged thyroid gland. It is a common finding, and it is usually asymptomatic; however, large goitres can compress the oesophagus and trachea. If a goitre is associated with hyperthyroidism it is described as 'toxic'. Non-toxic goitres secrete normal or reduced levels of thyroid hormones. Non-toxic goitres are usually the result of excessive TSH stimulation in the presence of hypothyroidism. Goitres are treated by correcting the underlying pathology or by surgical removal for cosmetic reasons or to prevent compression of surrounding structures.

Iodine deficiency

The goitre formed by this process is diffusely enlarged and smooth. It is sometimes called an endemic goitre because it occurred in certain regions.

Graves' disease

The constant stimulation of TSH receptors in Graves' disease causes a goitre in a similar manner to iodine deficiency with similar characteristics. The gland becomes very vascular, to the extent that a bruit can be heard using a stethoscope.

Graves' ophthalmopathy is caused by lymphocytic infiltration of the periorbital tissues and activation of fibroblasts to secrete osmotically active hyaluronic acid. This increases the pressure and pushes the eye forward, resulting in proptosis. This pressure change also causes muscle fibrosis and diplopia due to weakening of the extraocular muscles. The eye disease may precede the onset of thyroid dysfunction, and does not respond to correction of thyroid status. Treatment involves radiotherapy and surgery.

Puberty and pregnancy

Higher levels of thyroid hormones are required in puberty and pregnancy so the thyroid gland often enlarges to meet the increased demand. This enlargement is a physiological response, not a pathological process. The goitre regresses once the demand lessens.

Multinodular goitre

Many elderly people have an enlarged thyroid that contains many nodules of varying sizes. These nodules are formed from hyperplasia (increased number) of thyroid cells. The excess cells sometimes cause excess thyroid hormone production, i.e. hyperthyroidism. The disease is then called toxic multinodular goitre.

Thyroiditis

Inflammation of the thyroid gland can cause swelling, and infiltration by lymphocytes can also cause enlargement. The goitre formed is usually slightly nodular, but it may be tender if the inflammation is acute.

Thyroid gland neoplasia

Thyroid lumps are common and usually benign; however, they must be investigated. Solitary thyroid lumps are found in 5% of women and it is very difficult to distinguish between benign (80%) and malignant (20%) on clinical grounds. A fine-needle aspiration should be performed along with thyroid function tests. Aspiration alone will not distinguish a follicular adenoma from a follicular carcinoma but low TSH suggests the former as malignant nodules are not usually hyperfunctioning.

Causes of solitary thyroid lumps include:

- Thyroid cysts.
- Nodule of multinodular goitre.
- Follicular adenoma.
- Malignancy.

Five separate forms of cancer can arise in the thyroid gland, but three of these are derived from the follicle cells. These tumours are summarized in Fig. 3.11.

Medullary carcinomas of the parafollicular cells often secrete ectopic hormones, including:

- Calcitonin—usually asymptomatic.
- Adrenocorticotrophic hormone (ACTH)—Cushing's syndrome.
- 5-hydroxytryptamine (5-HT; serotonin)—carcinoid syndrome.

The molecular biology of thyroid cancer

A great deal has been learnt about the molecular biology of thyroid cancer. 50% of papillary thyroid cancers have a translocation that causes constitutive activation of the *RET* proto-oncogene. *RET* is a transmembrane receptor with tyrosine kinase activity, which when active can drive oncogenesis (the development of neoplasia). In follicular thyroid cancer (FTC), 40% of cases have an activating point mutation of the *RAS* proto-oncogene. 60% of FTCs were shown to produce an abnormal 'fusion protein' (PAX-8/PPARγ), which is the result of two gene fragments coming together by translocation and producing a single gene product. Medullary thyroid cancer often occurs as part of the multiple endocrine neoplasia syndrome and as such is often associated with *RET* mutations. The more aggressive form, anaplastic thyroid cancer, is often associated with a *p53* mutation. This new knowledge of the events driving thyroid neoplastic transformation has opened up novel avenues for therapy.

Occasionally thyroid disorders can present as emergencies. A thyrotoxic crisis (thyroid storm) is an acute episode of hyperthyroidism with pyrexia, and can cause life-threatening arrhythmias. Thyroid storms can be precipitated by radioactive iodine treatment, thyroid surgery or by severe illness. Treatment is aimed at preventing cardiovascular complications, and the mainstays are antithyroid therapy and beta-blockers. Undertreated hypothyroidism can progress to a life-threatening myxoedema coma. This rare condition is characterized by bradycardia and hypotension. Plasma levels of glucose and sodium can also drop, and type II respiratory failure may develop.

Fig. 3.11 Characteristics of the five primary thyroid gland malignancies

Type	Cell type	Age group	Route of metastasis	Prognosis
Papillary	Follicle cells	All	Cervical lymphatics	Excellent
Follicular	Follicle cells	Middle-aged	Blood to bone, lung and brain	Good
Medullary	Parafollicular cells	Middle-aged and elderly	Cervical lymphatics	Variable but usually good
Malignant lymphoma	Lymphatics	Elderly	Local invasion	Poor
Anaplastic	Follicle cells	Elderly	Local invasion	Very poor

The adrenal glands

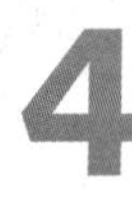

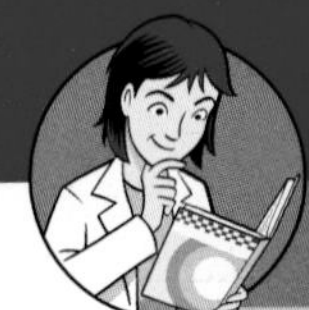

Objectives

By the end of this chapter you should be able to:

- List the five major hormones secreted by the adrenal gland.
- Describe the shape and location of each adrenal gland.
- Describe the innervation of the adrenal medulla and the developmental origins of this relationship.
- State the functions of the adrenal cortex.
- Name the blood vessels that supply and drain the adrenal gland.
- List the three layers of the adrenal cortex and state which group of hormones each layer secretes.
- Explain the role of mineralocorticoids.
- Describe the regulation and actions of mineralocorticoids.
- State the main target tissues and intracellular actions of mineralocorticoids.
- Explain the roles of glucocorticoids.
- Describe the regulation of glucocorticoid release including variation through the day.
- List the physiological actions of glucocorticoids.
- Explain the role of androgens.
- Describe the actions of adrenal androgens in males and females.
- List the symptoms of Conn's syndrome.
- List the main causes of hyperaldosteronism; which are most common?
- Describe the diagnosis of excess glucocorticoids. What makes this more complicated?
- State the difference between Cushing's disease and Cushing's syndrome.
- State the most common cause of Cushing's syndrome.
- Describe congenital adrenal hyperplasia including the symptoms in males and females.
- List the symptoms of Addison's disease.
- Describe the regulation and action of catecholamine hormones from the adrenal medulla.
- Recognize a patient presenting with a phaeochromocytoma.

The adrenal glands are divided functionally and anatomically into two parts, the adrenal medulla and the adrenal cortex. The medulla contains phaeochromocytes, which secrete catecholamines, and the cortex produces steroid hormones, namely mineralocorticoids, glucocorticoids and androgens. The catecholamines play an important part in functions associated with the autonomic nervous system. Mineralocorticoids, glucocorticoids and androgens are important in electrolyte balance, metabolism and sexual development, respectively. These functions are also determined by other endocrine hormones [e.g. vasopressin (posterior pituitary), insulin (pancreas) and testosterone (testis)]. The adrenal glands are therefore essential organs which act in concert with the endocrine system at large.

The adrenal cortex is derived from embryonic mesoderm. Its function is regulated by adrenocorticotrophic hormone (ACTH) from the pituitary gland, and it responds by secreting three types of steroid hormone:

- Glucocorticoids to deal with stress.
- Mineralocorticoids to regulate blood volume.
- Androgens for sexual development.

The adrenal medulla is derived from ectodermal neural crest tissue, and it consists of sympathetic nerve cells; it is under the direct control of the sympathetic nervous system, and it responds by secreting two modified amino acid hormones:

- Adrenaline (epinephrine).
- Noradrenaline (norepinephrine).

The most important hormones produced by the adrenal glands are glucocorticoids, such as cortisol. They are regulated by hypothalamic and anterior pituitary hormones to form the hypothalamic–pituitary–adrenal (HPA) axis (Fig. 4.1). Synthetic versions of these hormones are commonly used to treat inflammatory illness and they are referred to as 'steroids' or 'corticosteroids'.

An excess of glucocorticoids causes Cushing's syndrome, and a deficiency causes Addison's disease.

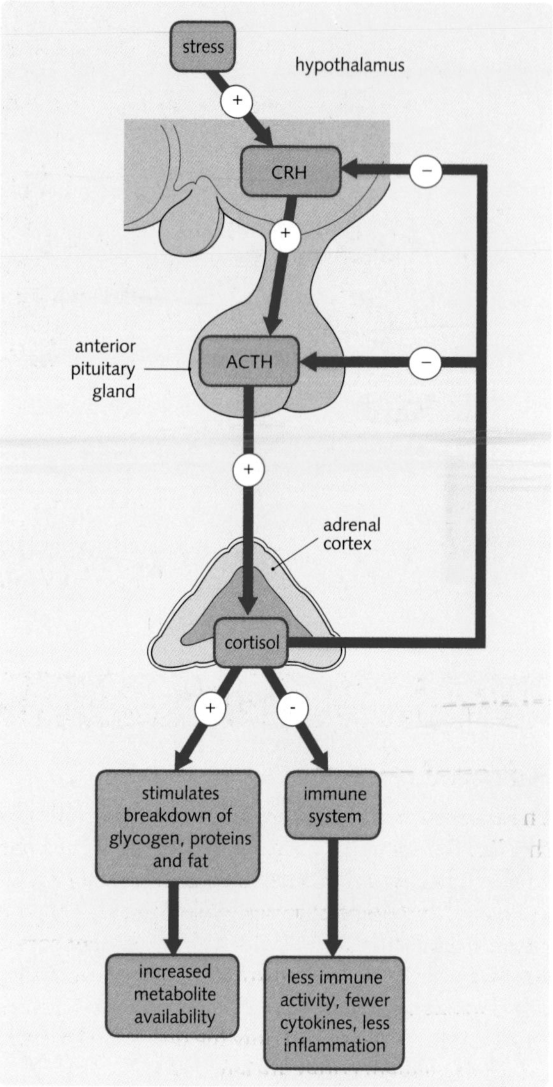

Fig. 4.1 Hormonal regulation of cortisol. (ACTH, adrenocorticotrophic hormone; CRH, corticotrophin-releasing hormone.)

ANATOMY

The two adrenal (or suprarenal) glands, are located above the kidneys. Both glands are retroperitoneal and are embedded in adipose tissue.

Right adrenal gland

The right adrenal gland is pyramidal in shape, lying between the inferior vena cava and the right crus (a large tendon) of the diaphragm. The liver is located superiorly.

Left adrenal gland

The left adrenal gland is crescent shaped; it lies medially to the left crus of the diaphragm. Anteriorly, the body of the pancreas and the splenic artery are adjacent. The stomach is situated superiorly, separated by the peritoneum. The location of both glands is shown in Fig. 4.2.

Blood supply, nerves and lymphatics

The outer cortex receives no significant innervation; instead it is regulated by ACTH from the pituitary gland and other blood-borne factors. The left adrenal vein drains into the left renal vein and is longer than the right adrenal vein, which drain into the inferior vena cava.

The medulla is innervated directly by the splanchnic nerves, which arise from the thoracic spinal cord and do not synapse before reaching the adrenal medulla. The nerves are therefore preganglionic sympathetic nerves that release acetylcholine, while all other tissues receive only postganglionic sympathetic innervation. The cause of this relationship is apparent from their development (see below).

The glands receive a rich blood supply from the superior, middle and inferior adrenal arteries, which are branches of the inferior phrenic artery, the aorta and renal artery, respectively. They left and right adrenal glands are drained by the left and right adrenal veins which, in turn, drain into the left renal vein and inferior vena cava, respectively. Lymphatic drainage passes to the para-aortic nodes.

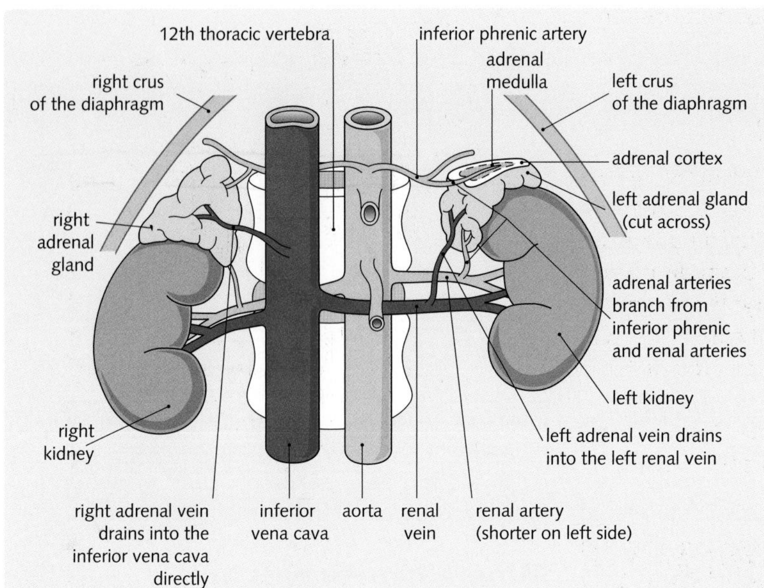

Fig. 4.2 Location and blood supply of the adrenal glands.

DEVELOPMENT

Adrenal cortex

The adrenal cortex develops from mesodermal cells that lie adjacent to the urogenital ridge. The fetal zone of the cortex develops first. Later, more mesodermal cells surround the fetal cortex to form the permanent cortex found in adults. At birth, the permanent cortex has two layers while a third (the zona reticularis) develops by the third year. At around this time the fetal cortex regresses until only the developed medulla and permanent cortex are left.

Adrenal medulla

The adrenal medulla is derived from ectodermal neural crest cells of the embryo. They form part of the amine precursor uptake and decarboxylation (APUD) system. These cells contribute to many diverse structures, including all the noradrenaline-secreting postganglionic neurons in the sympathetic nervous system. The secretory cells in the adrenal medulla secrete either adrenaline or noradrenaline, and they are essentially highly specialized neurons (Fig. 4.3). The medullary precursor cells also form paraganglia in the Organ of Zuckerkandl located around the origin of the inferior mesenteric artery and the aortic bifurcation, which act as accessory medullary tissue and are a common site of extra-adrenal catecholamine-secreting tumours.

MICROSTRUCTURE

Adrenal cortex

The adult adrenal cortex makes up about 90% of the adrenal gland by weight. It is functionally and anatomically divided into three layers, which secrete the following groups of steroid hormone (Figs 4.4 and 4.5):

- Outer zona glomerulosa secretes mineralocorticoids.
- Middle zona fasciculata secretes glucocorticoids.
- Inner zona reticularis secretes androgens and glucocorticoids.

These hormone groups will be explained later in the chapter.

The cells of the zona fasciculata and zona reticularis are arranged in columns around blood sinusoids. The blood in these sinusoids passes directly into the adrenal medulla.

Adrenal medulla

The adrenal medulla comprises two types of neuroendocrine cell:

- Noradrenaline-secreting cells (20%).
- Adrenaline-secreting cells (80%).

Both types contain neuroendocrine granules that store the hormone. In older textbooks, these cells are called chromaffin cells because they turn a dark brown colour

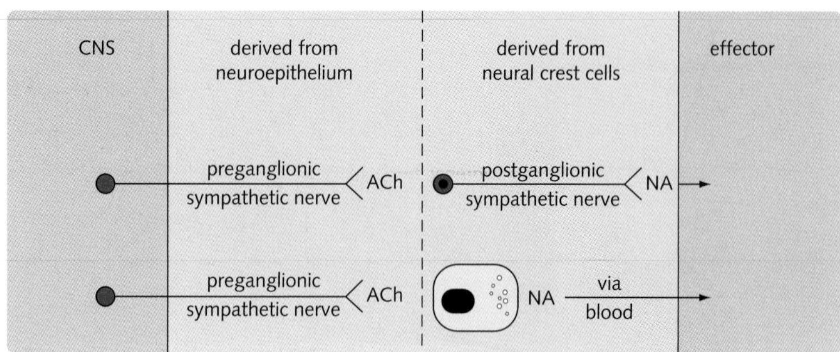

Fig. 4.3 Comparison between the adrenal medulla and the sympathetic nervous system (ACh, acetylcholine; CNS, central nervous system; NA, noradrenaline).

if exposed to oxygen after fixation in chrome salts. The cells are arranged around blood sinusoids.

Medullary cells require the steroid cortisol to convert noradrenaline to adrenaline. Cortisol is produced in the cortex, and it travels in the cortical capillaries to the medulla. Separate medullary arteries supply oxygenated blood directly.

HORMONES OF THE ADRENAL CORTEX

The adrenal cortex secretes three groups of steroid hormones:

- Mineralocorticoids, e.g. aldosterone, deoxycortisone.
- Glucocorticoids, e.g. cortisol.
- Androgens, e.g. dehydroepiandrosterone (DHEA).

Steroid hormones are synthesized from cholesterol. Steroid hormones are small lipid-soluble molecules that cross membranes readily. Inside cells, they act on intracellular receptors to regulate gene expression. The synthesis and mechanism of action of steroid hormones are discussed in more detail in Chapter 1.

Mineralocorticoids and aldosterone

Regulation of aldosterone

Mineralocorticoids help to regulate the electrolyte balance of plasma; their name is derived from this action on the body's minerals. Aldosterone is the main mineralocorticoid secreted by the zona glomerulosa. Aldosterone release is stimulated by:

- Angiotensin II.
- High plasma potassium.
- ACTH.

Angiotensin II is released in response to low blood volume as part of the renin–angiotensin system (see Chapter 7 and Fig. 4.6). ACTH from the anterior pituitary gland is less important as a regulator, so pituitary

Fig. 4.4 Microstructure of the adrenal gland and the major hormones secreted in each region

Region	Name	Cell structure	Hormones synthesized
Outer cortex	Zona glomerulosa	Cells arranged in clumps (Latin, glomerulus: little ball)	Mineralocorticoids (mainly aldosterone)
Middle cortex	Zona fasciculata	Cells arranged in cords alongside blood sinusoids; (Latin, fasciculus: bundle)	Glucocorticoids (mainly cortisol)
Inner cortex	Zona reticularis	Network of smaller cells (Latin, reticularis: network)	Glucocorticoids and androgens (DHEA)
Centre of gland	Adrenal medulla	Loose network of neurosecretory cells surrounded by blood sinusoids	Catecholamines (adrenaline and noradrenaline)

DHEA, dehydroepiandrosterone.

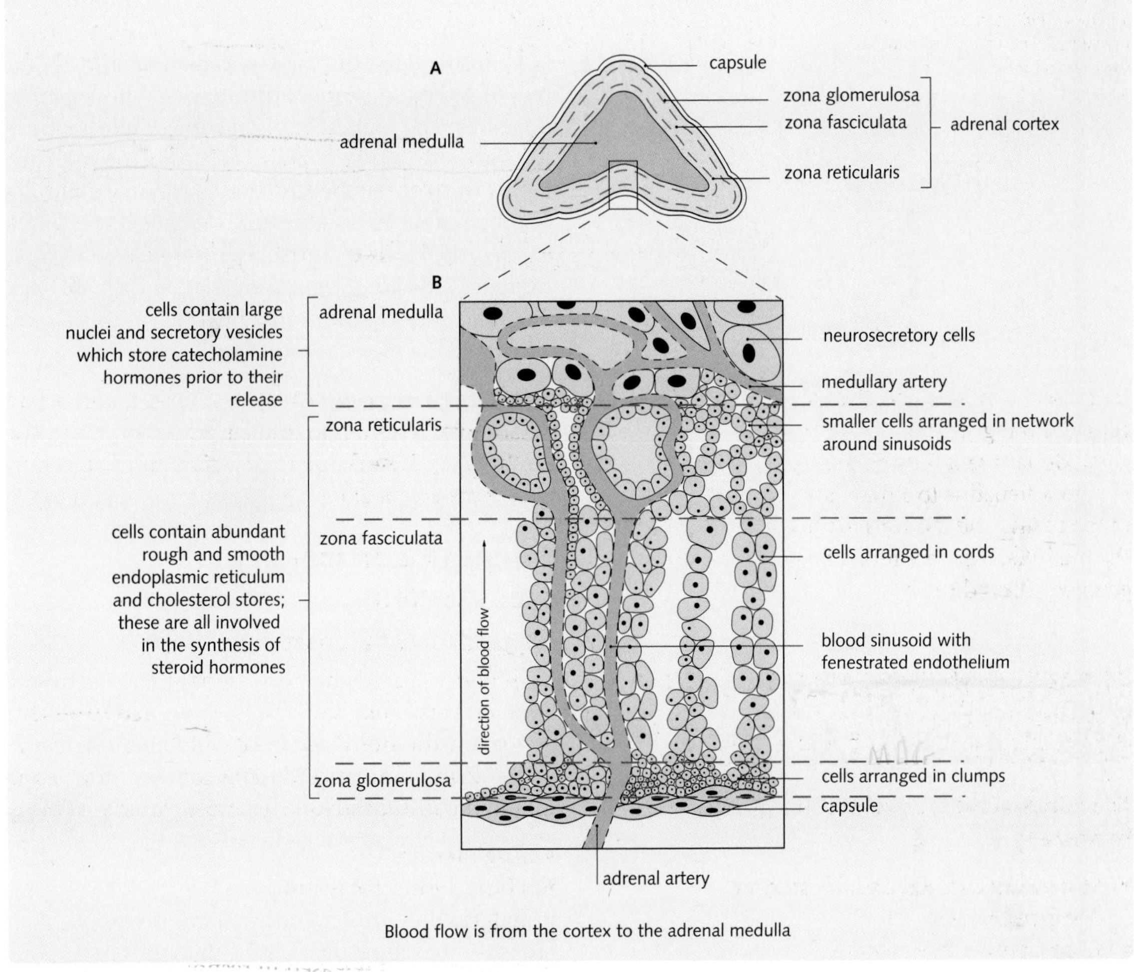

Fig. 4.5 Microstructure of a cross-section through the adrenal glands showing the cell types and regions.

failure does not severely impair aldosterone secretion. An excess of aldosterone due to an adrenal adenoma is called Conn's disease.

Actions of aldosterone

Aldosterone acts mainly on the distal convoluted tubule (DCT) and the collecting duct of the kidney. It causes reabsorption of sodium ions in exchange for potassium and hydrogen ions. Water is also reabsorbed and blood volume is increased. Other hormones are involved in this mechanism and they are discussed in more detail in Chapter 7 on fluid balance.

Intracellular actions of aldosterone

To cause these physiological effects, aldosterone acts on the nucleus via an intracellular receptor. Only cells that express this receptor can respond to aldosterone. Aldosterone upregulates the expression of four genes in the cells of the DCT and collecting duct. The actions of the gene products (proteins) are described in Fig. 4.7.

Aldosterone circulates in the plasma with 60% bound to albumin and 40% free, and therefore active. The high proportion of free hormone causes aldosterone to be rapidly degraded by the liver, giving a short half-life of about 15 minutes.

Glucocorticoids and cortisol

Glucocorticoids regulate the metabolism of carbohydrate, protein and, to a lesser extent, fat. Glucocorticoids also have potent anti-inflammatory and immunosuppressive effects. The major glucocortcoid in humans is cortisol. Cortisol also plays an important part in metabolic adaptation in response to stressful stimuli.

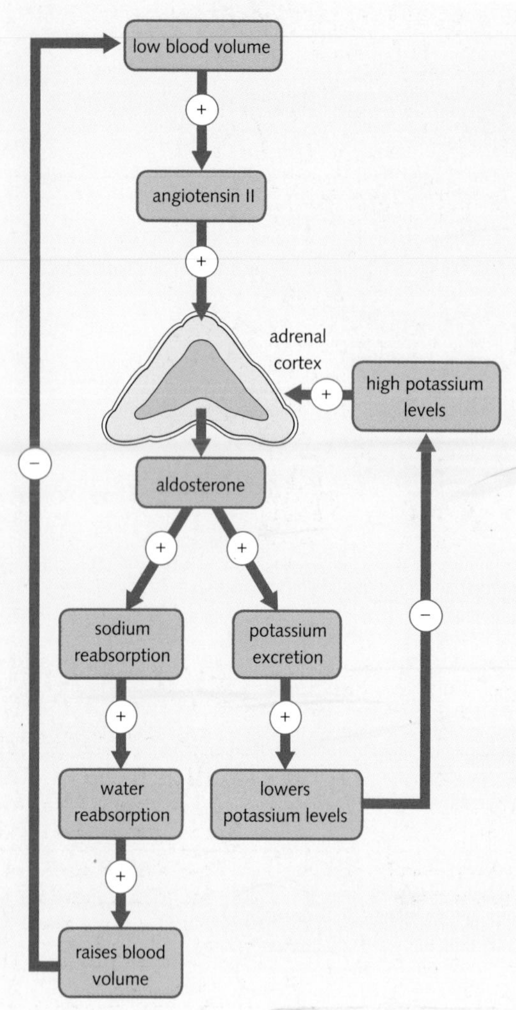

Fig. 4.6 Control of aldosterone secretion.

During fasting, glucorticoids act to maintain plasma glucose levels.

Regulation of cortisol

Corticotrophin-releasing hormone (CRH) is secreted by the hypothalamus and stimulates the anterior pituitary to produce proopiomelanocortin (POMC), which is converted to ACTH and leads to increased ACTH release. ACTH, in turn, acts on G-protein coupled receptors on the wall of the adrenal cells to stimulate steroidogenesis. Vasopressin can increase the ability of CRH to cause ACTH release. Cortisol has a negative feedback effect on the hypothalamus (inhibits CRH transcription) and anterior pituitary gland (inhibits POMC transcription) to inhibit CRH and ACTH release.

Cortisol release displays a circadian rhythm, i.e. the rate of secretion changes through a 24-hour period (Fig. 4.8). The highest levels of cortisol release are in the early morning, peaking at about 6 a.m., then falling throughout the day. This circadian variation is initiated in the hypothalamus by changing sensitivity to cortisol levels. Cortisol exerts a weaker negative feedback effect in the morning, so CRH release rises. The circadian rhythm must be taken into account when making plasma cortisol measurements.

Actions of cortisol

Physical and psychological stressors (e.g. trauma, haemorrhage, fever) increase ACTH and cortisol secretion, which, in turn, regulate metabolic adaptations to these stimuli. This effect is very important, and cortisol deficiency can rapidly become life threatening under stressful conditions. The response to stress is called the general adaptation syndrome (GAS), and it is divided into three phases:

Alarm reaction A stressful stimulus causes:

- Noradrenaline release from sympathetic nerves.
- Adrenaline and noradrenaline release from adrenal medulla.
- Cortisol release from adrenal cortex.

Resistance The effects of cortisol are slower to initiate, as they are dependent on transcription. However they are longer lasting than those of adrenaline and noradrenaline; this allows the resistance to stress to be maintained. It also counteracts the effects of other hormones (e.g. insulin) to maintain substrates required to combat stress.

Exhaustion Prolonged stress causes continued cortisol secretion, and it results in muscle wastage, immune system suppression and hyperglycaemia.

Cortisol affects almost every cell in the body. The physiological effects are described in Fig. 4.9. The main actions of cortisol are:

- Increase of energy metabolite levels in the blood.
- Suppression of the immune system and inhibition of allergic and inflammatory processes.

There is some overlap between the actions of mineralocorticoids and glucocorticoids. Cortisol can have mineralocorticoid actions and aldosterone can act as a glucocorticoid.

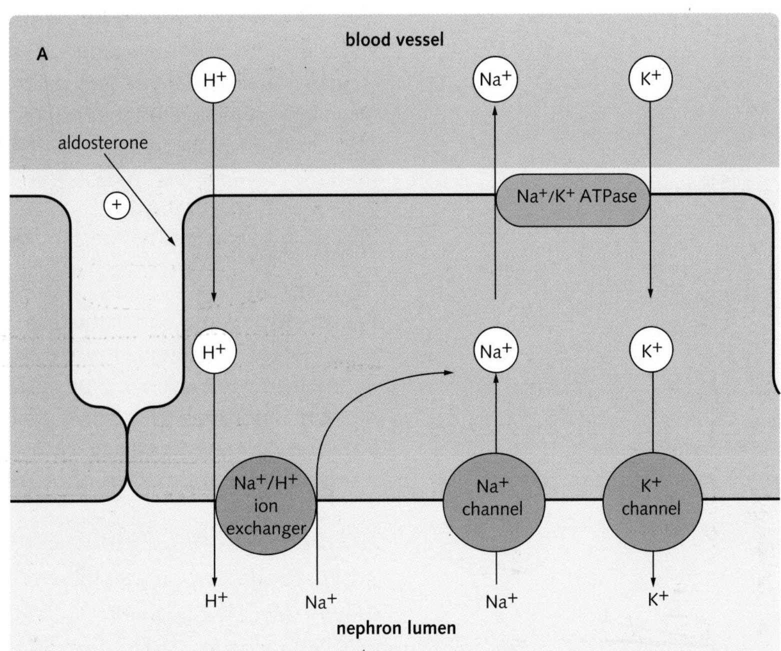

Fig. 4.7B Effects of proteins induced by aldosterone in the nephron

Protein	Location	Action	Physiological response
Na^+/K^+ ATPase	Cell membrane on the side of the blood supply	Active pump that increases cell potassium and lowers cell sodium levels	Creates an ion gradient that drives the other proteins
Na^+ channel	Cell membrane on the side of the nephron	Reabsorbs sodium from the nephron lumen	Increases plasma sodium and water to increase blood volume
K^+ channel	Cell membrane on the side of the nephron	Excretes potassium into the nephron lumen	Decreases plasma potassium
Na^+/H^+ ion exchanger	Cell membrane on the side of the nephron	Reabsorbs sodium in exchange for hydrogen ions	Makes the plasma more alkaline

Fig. 4.7 Intracellular and physiological actions of aldosterone in the nephron. Aldosterone acts to increase the levels of the four proteins shown (A) causing the physiological responses (B).

Intracellular actions of cortisol

Like all steroid hormones, cortisol acts via intracellular receptors to regulate gene expression. The receptor and genes vary between cells, and this accounts for the wide range of actions. The anti-inflammatory actions are produced by inhibiting phospholipase A_2, an enzyme that is essential for the production of prostaglandins from arachidonic acid.

Most cortisol (95%) is transported round the body bound to plasma proteins:

- 80% bound to cortisol-binding protein.
- 15% bound to albumin.
- 5% free and active.

Cortisol is inactivated in the liver by conjugation and then excreted from the kidney. About 1% of cortisol is excreted into the urine without metabolism. This can be detected by 24-hour urine collection to estimate blood cortisol levels.

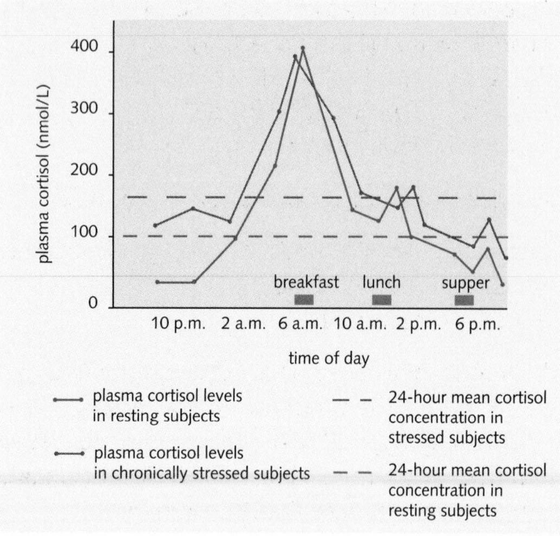

Fig. 4.8 Circadian variation in plasma cortisol in resting and chronically stressed subjects.

The immunosuppressive properties of synthetic corticosteroids ('steroids', e.g. prednisolone) are commonly employed in the treatment of autoimmune conditions and inflammatory disorders.

Androgens

Androgens are sex steroids, i.e. hormones involved in the growth and function of the male and female genital tract. They also stimulate muscle growth (anabolism), hence their use as an illicit drug in sport. Androgens are made in the adrenal gland in both males and females. However, in males they account for only a small proportion of total androgen production.

Actions of adrenal androgens

Adrenal androgens are synthesized in the zona reticularis of the adrenal gland; the main adrenal androgens are:

Fig. 4.9 Physiological effects of cortisol and the symptoms of Cushing's syndrome

Process/system affected	Effect of cortisol	Related pathology in Cushing's syndrome
Carbohydrate metabolism	Raises blood glucose by stimulating gluconeogenesis and preventing glucose uptake	Hyperglycaemia and diabetes
Protein metabolism	Increases breakdown of proteins in skeletal muscle, skin and bone to release amino acids	Muscle weakness and wasting; thin easily bruising skin
Fat metabolism	Stimulates lipolysis and increases fatty acid levels in the blood	Fat redistributed to the face and trunk causing a moon face, buffalo hump, and abdominal stretch marks
Immune system	Suppresses the action and production of immune cells; inhibits the production of cytokines and antibodies	Infections, poor healing, peptic ulceration
Endocrine system	Suppresses the secretion of anterior pituitary hormones: ACTH, LH, FSH, TSH and GH	Suppression of growth in children
Nervous system	Influences fetal and neonatal neuron development; influences behaviour and cognitive function; augments the actions of the sympathetic system	Depression, insomnia, psychosis and confusion
Water metabolism	Has weak mineralocorticoid actions: raises sodium and water retention	Hypertension and heart failure
Calcium metabolism	Decreases calcium absorption from the gut; increases calcium excretion in the kidneys; increases calcium resorption from bones	Osteoporosis

ACTH, adrenocorticotrophic hormone; FSH, follicle-stimulating hormone; GH, growth hormone; LH, luteinizing hormone; TSH, thyroid-stimulating hormone.

- Dehydroepiandrosterone (DHEA).
- Androstenedione.

Androgens secreted by the adrenal glands have weak biological activity, but they are converted to more active androgens, such as testosterone, by aromatase and other enzymes in peripheral tissues.

Adrenarche

The initiation of androgen secretion from the adrenal glands is called adrenarche. It occurs a few years before puberty (about 7–9 years of age), and it is marked by maturation of the zona reticularis and a rise in plasma DHEA.

In males, the early development of the male sex organs may result from adrenal androgens released after adrenarche. In male adult life adrenal androgens account for only 5% of total activity, so they are physiologically negligible. Androgens are discussed in greater detail in Chapter 14.

In the female, adrenal androgens are responsible for about 50% of total androgen activity from adrenarche to the end of life. These hormones help to promote the growth of female pubic and axillary hair.

DISORDERS OF THE ADRENAL CORTEX

The main diseases of the adrenal cortex are caused by an excess or deficiency of mineralocorticoids or glucocorticoids. There are four named diseases affecting the adrenal cortex hormones, however, they are rare diseases:

- Cushing's syndrome—chronic excessive cortisol production.
- Cushing's disease—ACTH-secreting tumour.
- Conn's syndrome—aldosterone-secreting tumour.
- Addison's disease—deficiency of cortisol and aldosterone.

Both Cushing's and Conn's are important endocrine causes of hypertension.

Hyperaldosteronism

Excess aldosterone production causes sodium ion and water retention with increased excretion of potassium and hydrogen ions. The main symptoms and signs (Fig. 4.10) are:

- Hypertension (high blood pressure).
- Hypokalaemia (low potassium).
- Alkalosis (raised blood pH).
- Polyuria and polydipsia (thirst).
- Muscle weakness and spasm.

A number of blood tests are used for diagnosis:

- Urea and electrolytes (U + Es) for hypokalaemia.
- Aldosterone levels (raised).
- Renin levels (variable).

Aldosterone increases blood volume, which inhibits renin secretion. If renin levels are low then the disorder is primary hyperaldosteronism, i.e. the disease originates in the adrenal glands. The adrenal glands can then be imaged by CT/MRI scanning.

Renin stimulates aldosterone release via angiotensin II, so high renin levels suggest secondary hyperaldosteronism. This disorder is external to the adrenal glands; it is a common response to heart failure and renal disease.

Primary hyperaldosteronism and Conn's syndrome

Primary hyperaldosteronism is a rare disease that is responsible for about 1% of patients with hypertension. The vast majority of primary hyperaldosteronism is caused by Conn's syndrome, in which the patients have an adenoma of the zona glomerulosa. This is discussed later in the chapter.

> The triad of hypertension, hypokalaemia and alkalosis should raise the suspicion of Conn's syndrome. Conn's syndrome is the result of an adrenocortical adenoma causing primary hyperaldosteronism. Hyperaldosteronism can also been seen as part of congenital adrenal hyperplasia due to the presence of excess ACTH. Patients with Conn's syndrome have a high plasma aldosterone. They also have low plasma renin due to the effects of chronic water/salt retention. Renal artery stenosis can also cause this pattern of symptoms, but these patients have a high plasma renin.

Secondary hyperaldosteronism

Secondary hyperaldosteronism is a very common problem caused by activation of the renin–angiotensin system. The most common cause is excessive diuretic therapy, but it is also a feature of:

Fig. 4.10 Clinical symptoms of hyperaldosteronism and hypoaldosteronism

Action of aldosterone	Hyperaldosteronism	Hypoaldosteronism
Increases plasma Na^+	Hypernatraemia rarely occurs because of other mechanisms regulating fluid volume	Loss of Na^+ is accompanied by loss of water, so plasma Na^+ concentration does not change
Decreases plasma K^+	Hypokalaemia	Hyperkalaemia
Decreases plasma H^+	Metabolic alkalosis	Mild metabolic acidosis
Maintains extracellular fluid volume	Hypertension	Volume depletion and postural hypotension

- Congestive heart failure.
- Renal artery stenosis.
- Nephritic syndrome.
- Cirrhosis with ascites.

All these conditions result in decreased renal perfusion, which stimulates renin release.

Excess cortisol

Cushing's syndrome

Cushing's syndrome is a rare condition caused by a chronic excess of glucocorticoids. The disorder can be in the anterior pituitary gland or the adrenal cortex, or it may result from excess medication. It has a five-year mortality of about 50% if it is not treated. The symptoms and signs of Cushing's syndrome are shown in Figs 4.9 and 4.11; it is most common in adult women.

Diagnosing excess cortisol is complicated by the circadian variation in cortisol secretion. Two main tests are employed to overcome this problem:

- 24-hour urinary free cortisol: 1% of free cortisol is excreted unmetabolized, and this can be measured to give an accurate reflection of plasma cortisol.
- Overnight dexamethasone suppression test: plasma cortisol is measured before an oral dexamethasone (a synthetic glucocorticoid) dose and then at 8 a.m. the next morning. In a normal person plasma cortisol would be suppressed.

Treatment with glucocorticoids

Glucocorticoids (often simply called 'steroids') are used to treat a wide range of medical conditions, usually to reduce immune reactions. These conditions include asthma, inflammatory bowel disease, rheumatoid arthritis and post-transplantation. Patients are treated with the lowest dose that will control their condition because prolonged use can cause the features of Cushing's syndrome. Inhaled steroids are used in asthma to reduce the systemic dose, especially in children, in whom growth retardation may occur.

Cushing's disease

Most Cushing's syndrome is caused by Cushing's disease. Cushing's disease refers to the specific condition of excess corticosteroids as a result of pituitary adenomas. This stimulates the adrenal cortex to secrete excess cortisol, leading to bilateral enlargement of the cortex. The negative feedback that normally prevents excess ACTH release is absent in the tumour.

This type of tumour causes Cushing's syndrome with the additional sign of pigmented skin. This is due to the melanocyte-stimulating action of ACTH on the receptors for the structurally similar melanocyte-stimulating hormone (α-MSH)—formed by the same gene (POMC) that makes ACTH. Cushing's disease occurs most frequently in young adult women.

Cushing's disease is treated by surgical removal of the pituitary adenoma. This may result in panhypopituitarism (see Chapter 2 for more details).

Ectopic adrenocorticotrophic hormone production

Ectopic ACTH can be secreted by the rare, but highly malignant, small-cell anaplastic carcinoma of the lung (also called oat-cell carcinoma). This carcinoma displays the characteristics of a neuroendocrine cell despite developing from bronchial epithelium. Even more rarely, tumours of the thymus, ovary, pancreas

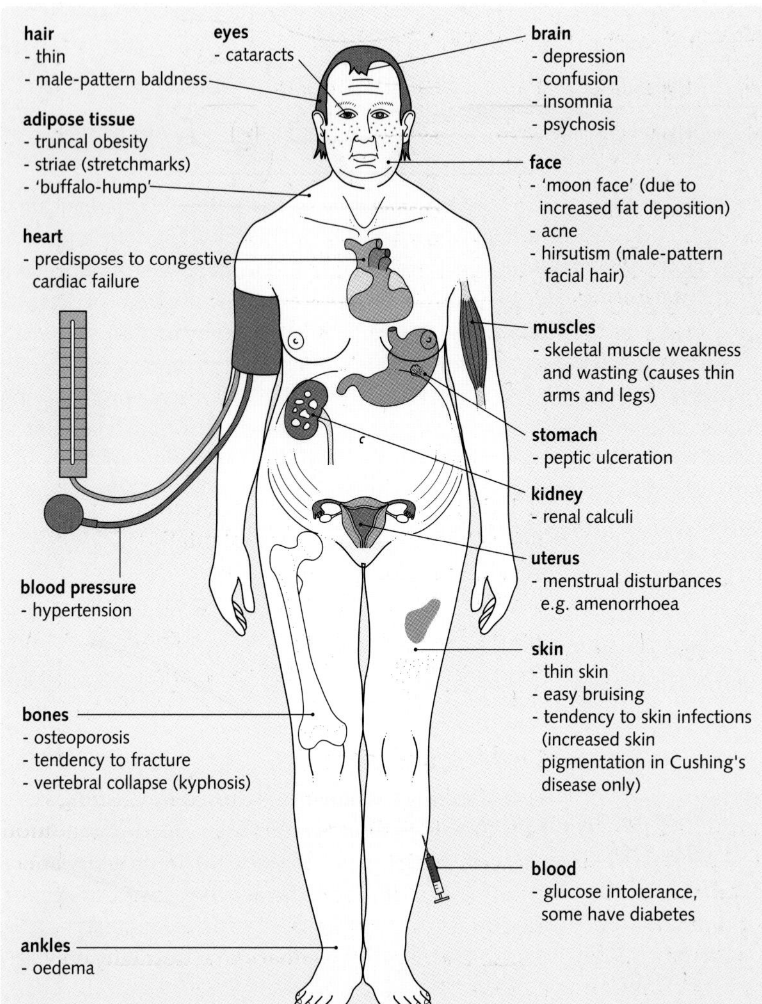

Fig. 4.11 Symptoms and signs of Cushing's syndrome.

and carcinoid tumors can secrete ACTH or CRH. The excess production is so dramatic that patients rarely exhibit features of Cushing's syndrome before death. Ectopic hormones are discussed in Chapter 10.

Neoplasia of the adrenal cortex

Benign adenoma of the adrenal cortex is relatively common, but only a small proportion secrete hormones. If cortisol is secreted, then Cushing's syndrome develops; aldosterone-secreting adenomas cause Conn's syndrome.

Adrenal adenomas are the most common cause of Cushing's syndrome in children, but they account for only 10% of adult disease. In Conn's syndrome, adenomas of the adrenal cortex are the most common cause of primary hyperaldosteronism in all age groups. Adenomas associated with either syndrome are removed surgically, but cortisol replacement is necessary due to long-term ACTH inhibition.

Carcinoma of the adrenal cortex is a very rare condition. Such carcinomas secrete vast excesses of glucocorticoids and androgens. The patient usually dies before the physical features of Cushing's syndrome develop.

Deficiency of cortisol and aldosterone

Congenital adrenal hyperplasia (CAH)

ACTH controls the production of all the hormones in the zona fasciculata and the zona reticularis. Cortisol is solely responsible for negative feedback on ACTH production. Therefore, any deficiency in cortisol relieves the suppression of ACTH release and glucocorticoid, mineralocortcoid and androgen production are perturbed. The gland tends to get larger under the trophic influence of ACTH, and the condition is referred to as congenital adrenal hyperplasia (CAH).

One cause of CAH is an autosomal recessive deficiency of 21-hydroxylase. This enzyme is required for the synthesis of aldosterone and cortisol, and both hormones are deficient. Low cortisol triggers ACTH release resulting in hyperplasia of the adrenal cortex. Low aldosterone results in salt loss and neonatal shock in some babies. The enlarged adrenal cortex secretes excess androgens, causing adrenogenital syndrome. This presents differently in each sex. It causes ambiguous genitalia in both males and females. In males, it causes early (precocious) pseudopuberty; signs of secondary sexual development can be found by 6 months of age, but the child is not fertile. Early bone epiphyseal fusion causes short adult height.

In females, androgen excess causes masculinization (also called virilization). The symptoms are similar to those found in polycystic ovarian syndrome as described in Chapter 13. They include:

- Masculine body shape.
- Balding of temporal skull.
- Increased muscle bulk.
- Deepening of the voice.
- Enlargement of the clitoris.

> Precocious puberty, salt-losing crisis or ambiguous genitalia all indicate a possible diagnosis of CAH. Plasma levels of 17-hydroxy progesterone, which are raised in CAH, are used as a screen. Treatment focuses on determining the baby's gender by karotyping and replacing glucocorticoids and mineralocorticoids.

Adrenal cortex insufficiency

Adrenal cortex insufficiency tends to affect the whole adrenal cortex rather than specific layers. Accordingly, deficiency of glucocorticoids, mineralocorticoids and androgens occur together, although clinical effects are due to cortisol and aldosterone deficiency. These effects are shown in Fig. 4.12. Hydrocortisone (cortisol) and fludrocortisone (a mineralocorticoid) therapy must be initiated before the underlying disease process is treated.

Suspected adrenal cortex insufficiency is investigated using the ACTH stimulation test. A synthetic ACTH analogue is injected and plasma cortisol levels are measured every 30 minutes. If the cortisol levels do not rise sufficiently, then the disease is of the adrenal cortex (i.e. Addison's disease).

Addison's disease

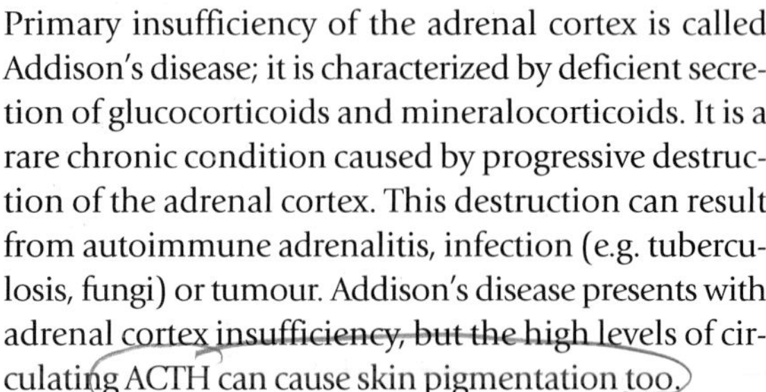

Primary insufficiency of the adrenal cortex is called Addison's disease; it is characterized by deficient secretion of glucocorticoids and mineralocorticoids. It is a rare chronic condition caused by progressive destruction of the adrenal cortex. This destruction can result from autoimmune adrenalitis, infection (e.g. tuberculosis, fungi) or tumour. Addison's disease presents with adrenal cortex insufficiency, but the high levels of circulating ACTH can cause skin pigmentation too.

An acute exacerbation of Addison's disease is called an adrenal crisis. It is a life-threatening emergency caused by stressful events such as infection. Its presentation is the same as acute adrenal cortical failure.

Acute adrenal cortical failure

Acute adrenal cortex failure is a life-threatening condition characterized by:

- Hypotensive shock.
- Hypovolaemic shock.
- Hypoglycaemia.

> The inhibitory action of cortisol on ACTH release is important clinically. Patients treated with long-term 'steroids' cannot simply stop because ACTH release, and therefore cortisol production, would also stop. Instead, the dose must be lowered over a number of months.

The adrenal cortex can be destroyed acutely by bilateral haemorrhagic necrosis following disseminated intravascular coagulation. Essentially, blood clots block the venous drainage of the adrenal cortex, causing cell death. These clots can form following severe septicaemia. Meningococcal septicemia is the most common cause and this is called Waterhouse–Friderichsen syndrome.

A similar situation can occur if long-term high-dose steroid treatment is stopped abruptly. The prolonged treatment chronically suppresses ACTH release from the anterior pituitary gland so that no cortisol is secreted from the adrenal cortex for a number of weeks.

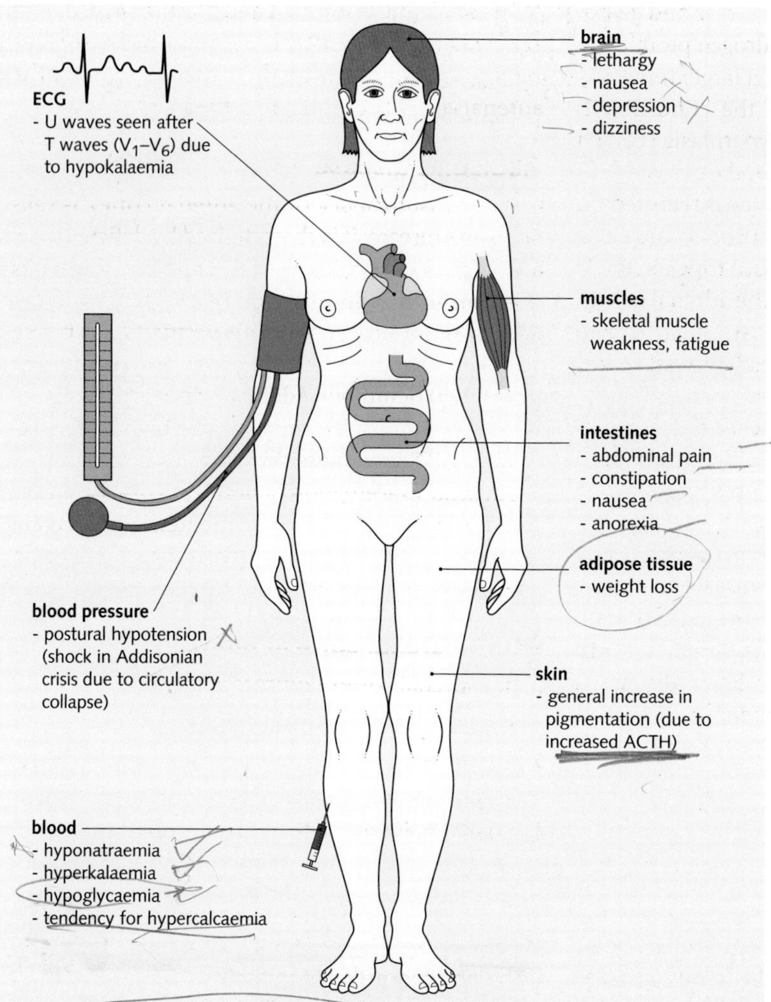

Fig. 4.12 Symptoms and signs of Addison's disease. (ACTH, adrenocorticotrophic hormone.)

Secondary adrenocortical insufficiency

Disorders of the hypothalamus and anterior pituitary gland can also cause deficiency of adrenal cortex steroid hormones. Any condition that causes a reduction in CRH or ACTH release will prevent the synthesis of glucocorticoids especially. These conditions are described in more detail in Chapter 2.

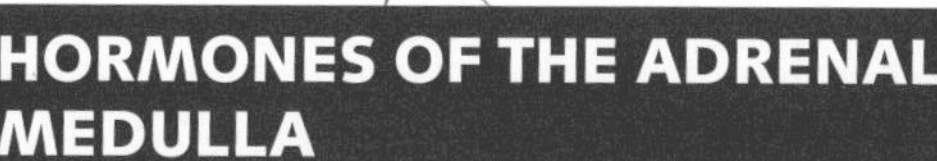

HORMONES OF THE ADRENAL MEDULLA

The adrenal medulla secretes two hormones: noradrenaline and adrenaline, which are catecholamines (Fig. 4.13). Eighty per cent of catecholamine released from the adrenal glands is adrenaline. The remainder of catecholamines are released at sympathetic nerve synapses.

> Once cortisol excess has been confirmed, further tests using higher doses of dexamethasone and measuring ACTH levels can locate the source. If a 24-hour suppression test is positive and ACTH is undetectable, this suggests an adrenaloma. If the 24-hour test is positive and ACTH is high, this suggests either pituitary tumour, which can be suppressed with 48-hour suppression test or ectopic ACTH, which cannot be suppressed with 48-hour suppression test. CT scans are used once a source has been identified.

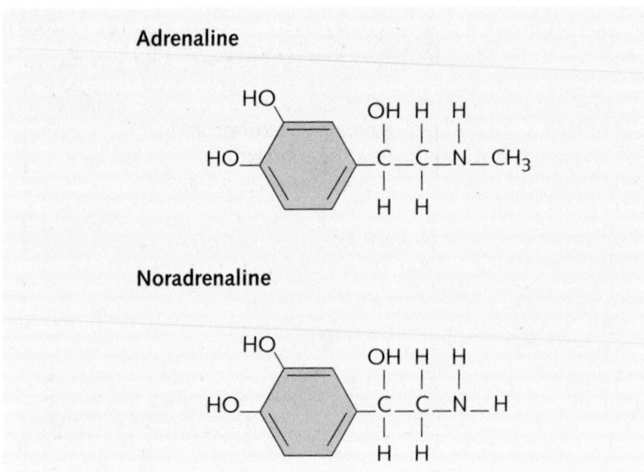

Fig. 4.13 Structure of adrenaline and noradrenaline.

Regulation

Catecholamines are released in response to stress (e.g. exercise, pain, shock, hypoglycaemia and imminent exams). Stress stimulates an area of the hypothalamus that activates both the adrenocortical and sympatheticoadrenal systems. It receives no direct regulation from the pituitary gland. Catecholamines exert their effects over a shorter time course than cortisol.

Actions

Catecholamines from the adrenal medulla perform similar functions to direct sympathetic neuronal connections, in that they prepare the body for fight or flight. Their effects last longer than the neuronal signals, so they help to minimize the harm caused by repeated stress. Adrenaline and noradrenaline have similar effects to each other.

Their main actions are described in Fig. 4.14. (for more detail on the sympathetic nervous system, see *Crash Course Nervous System*).

Intracellular actions

Adrenal catecholamines bind to receptors in a similar manner to neuronal signals. These extracellular receptors are linked to intracellular G-proteins that initiate a signal cascade. The effect of the signal depends on the receptor present and the cell type, which are classified into alpha- and beta-adrenergic receptors.

Synthesis

Noradrenaline is synthesized from the amino acid tyrosine, which is then converted to adrenaline in response to cortisol from the adrenal cortex.

The medullary cells store catecholamines in cytoplasmic granules. They are released into blood sinusoids by exocytosis in response to acetylcholine from preganglionic sympathetic neurons.

Breakdown

Catecholamines circulate bound to albumin. They are degraded by two enzymes in the liver:

- Monoamine oxidase (MAO).
- Catechol-O-methyl transferase (COMT).

Adrenaline and noradrenaline are converted to vanillyl mandelic acid (VMA or HMMA), which is released into the urine. Urinary VMA levels are measured to detect phaeochromocytomas, a rare tumour of the adrenal medulla that is discussed below.

DISORDERS OF THE ADRENAL MEDULLA

Phaeochromocytomas

Phaeochromocytomas are very rare tumours of the catecholamine-producing cells in the adrenal medulla. They are usually benign and present in only one gland (unilateral). Adrenaline and noradrenaline are secreted in large quantities, causing severe, sporadic (paroxysmal) hypertension that can produce headaches. With time, the hypertension can become constant, leading to heart failure.

The first choice test for diagnosing this tumour is plasma free metanephrines. Other tests include the detection of high levels of catecholamine breakdown products in the urine, e.g. VMA. It is treated by surgical excision. The surgery has a high perioperative mortality due to the unstable blood pressure.

Catecholamine-producing tumours can also develop in sympathetic ganglia. These usually occur beside the abdominal aorta, near the bifurcation.

Multiple endocrine neoplasia syndromes

A very rare autosomal dominant mutation causes inheritable phaeochromocytoma. These tumours can also develop in both glands (bilaterally) as a component of multiple endocrine neoplasia syndromes (MEN type II), described in Chapter 10.

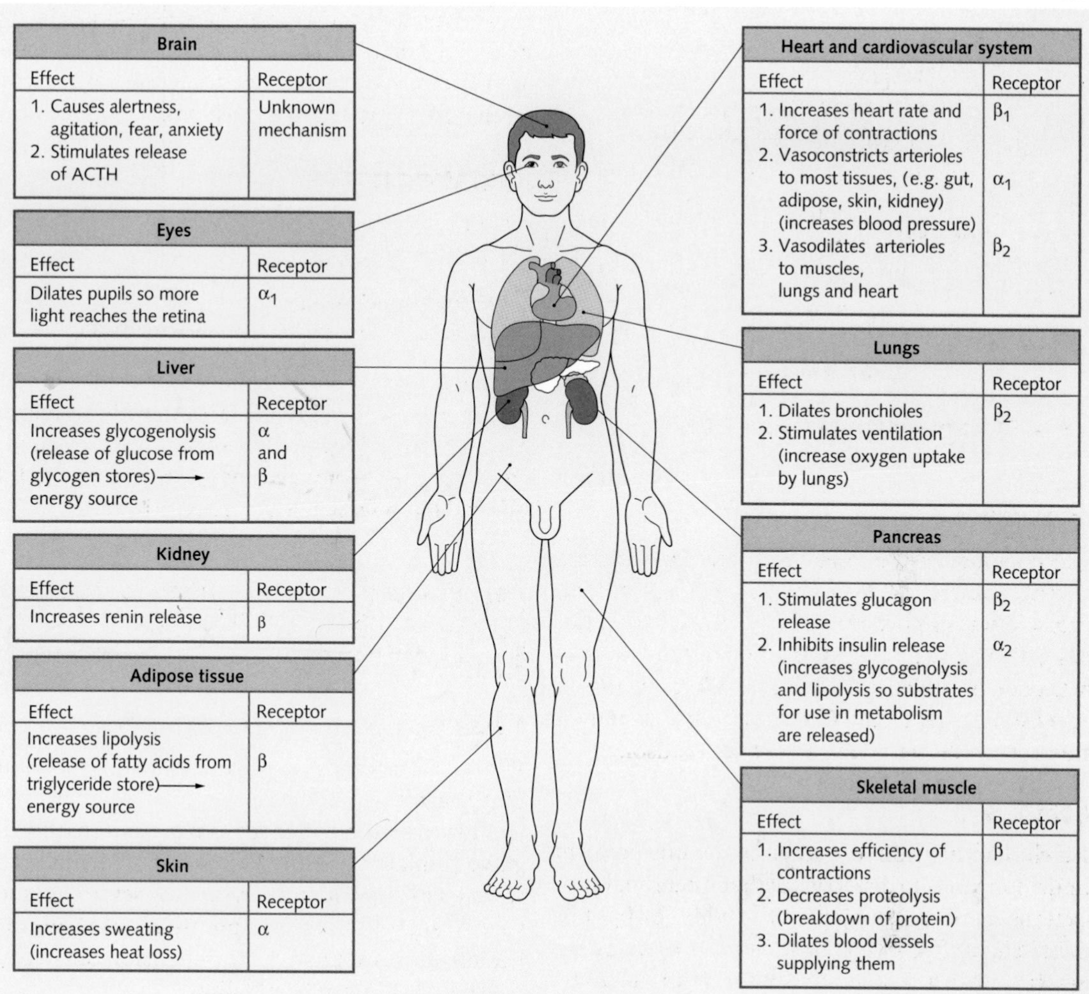

Fig. 4.14 Physiological effects of adrenaline and noradrenaline and the receptors present in each tissue/organ. (ACTH, adrenocorticotrophic hormone.)

A + N ⟶ VMA or HMMA

5 The pancreas and diabetes

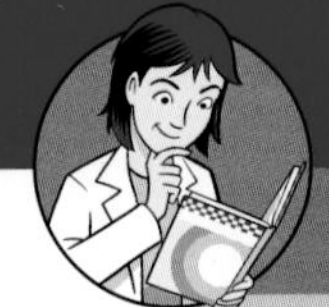

Objectives

By the end of this chapter you should be able to:

- Describe the anatomical location of the pancreas.
- Describe how the endocrine cells are arranged within the pancreas.
- List the hormones secreted by the pancreas, along with the cell type responsible.
- Describe the development of the pancreas.
- Discuss how the hormone insulin is synthesized.
- Describe insulin receptors and how they function.
- Explain why a basal level of insulin is always secreted.
- State the dietary principles that should be followed by all diabetics.
- Describe the intracellular mechanism that allows high glucose levels to trigger insulin secretion.
- Describe the action of insulin on glucose uptake and metabolism.
- Describe the action of insulin on amino-acid and fatty-acid metabolism, including the processes it inhibits.
- List the actions of glucagon and the factors that stimulate its secretion.
- List three hormones that can raise blood glucose levels.
- Compare the two types of diabetes mellitus.
- Explain how ketoacidosis develops in IDDM and why this does not occur in NIDDM.
- List the symptoms caused by hyperglycaemia and starvation; explain how dehydration develops.
- Describe the complications of diabetes mellitus, along with preventive screening.
- Discuss how diabetes mellitus is diagnosed and monitored.
- List the symptoms of hypoglycaemia and explain how this can be prevented.
- Briefly describe the tumours that can develop in the endocrine cells of the pancreas.

The pancreas has both exocrine and endocrine functions. This chapter will focus on the endocrine component, which consists of hormone-producing cells distributed throughout the pancreas in 'islets'. The hormonal products of these cells, insulin and glucagon, are essential in the regulation of plasma glucose levels. Unlike many other hormones operating via feedback to the pituitary, insulin production is regulated directly by the glucose acting on the pancreas.

The pancreas is a retroperitoneal organ found between the duodenum and the spleen. The endocrine cells are arranged within the pancreas in clusters called the islets of Langerhans. These clusters contain four types of cell, the most important and numerous of which are the insulin-producing β-cells. After a meal, glucose enters the blood from the gastrointestinal (GI) tract. Insulin is released from the pancreas to promote the uptake and use of glucose by cells and to keep blood glucose within tightly controlled limits. When blood glucose levels drop, insulin secretion is inhibited in favour of another pancreatic hormone called glucagon. This hormone opposes many of the actions of insulin and primarily initiates the breakdown of stored metabolic fuels. Fig. 5.1 shows how these hormones regulate blood glucose.

Insulin deficiency or insulin resistance causes diabetes mellitus. Diabetes is the most common endocrine disorder and projections estimate that 300 million people will be affected by 2025. A deficiency in insulin function causes a rise in blood glucose (hyperglycaemia) and glucose is excreted in the urine (glycosuria). Water follows the movement of glucose, so the patient produces excess urine and becomes dehydrated.

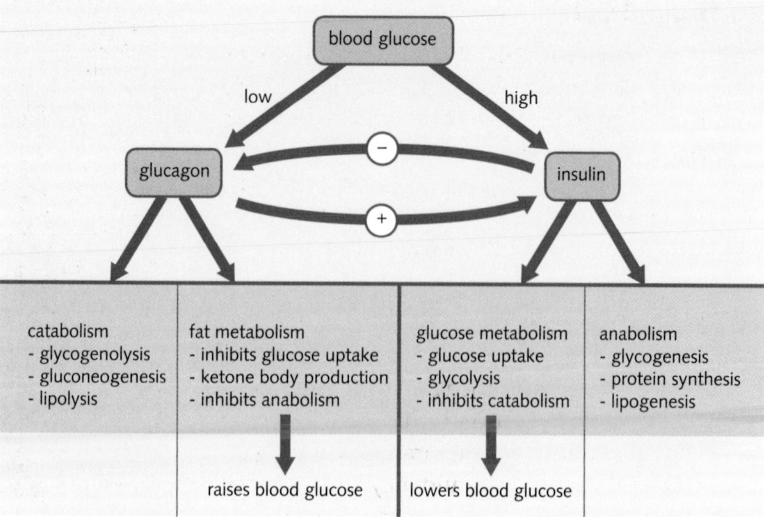

Fig. 5.1 Hormonal regulation of blood glucose and metabolism by insulin and glucagon.

Important words:
Anabolism: processes that build large molecules
Catabolism: processes that break down large molecules
Glycosuria: glucose in the urine
Polyuria: large volume of urine

There are two types of diabetes mellitus. Type 1 (insulin-dependent diabetes mellitus; IDDM) is more common in the young and always requires insulin injections. Type 2 (non-insulin-dependent diabetes mellitus; NIDDM) is very common in the elderly, and can sometimes be controlled through diet alone. Poor control of diabetes causes a number of serious and potentially life-threatening complications.

LOCATION AND ANATOMY

The pancreas is a long, flat organ that lies on the posterior of the abdominal wall, anterior to the vertebral bodies, aorta, and inferior vena cava. It is a retroperitoneal structure situated between the duodenum and spleen. For descriptive purposes, it is divided into four sections (Fig. 5.2):

- Head.
- Uncinate process.
- Body.
- Tail.

Head and uncinate process

The head lies within the curve of the duodenum with the uncinate process located posteriorly and inferiorly. The uncinate process is separated from the head by the superior mesenteric vessels. The inferior vena cava and bile duct lie posteriorly; a clinical consequence of this is that the bile duct can be obstructed by masses in the head of the pancreas.

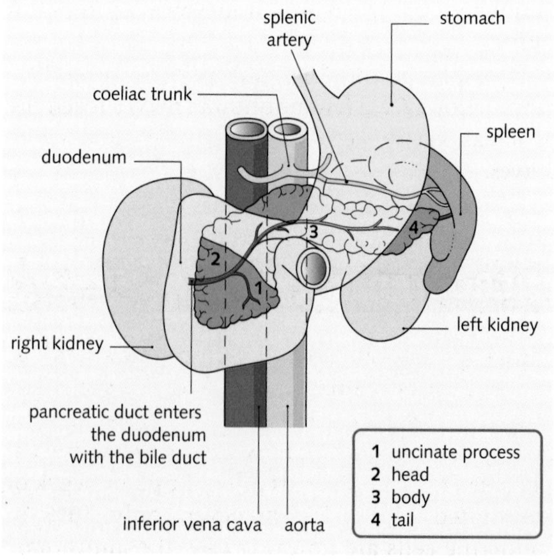

Fig. 5.2 Location of the pancreas in the retroperitoneal abdomen.

Body and tail

The body of the pancreas passes over the aorta and the left kidney, while the stomach lies in front. The body slopes upwards as it passes from right to left. The coeliac trunk (a large branch of the aorta) is a superior relation, giving rise to the splenic artery that runs along the upper pancreatic border. The tail crosses the left kidney to touch the hilum of the spleen.

Pancreatic duct

The exocrine secretions of the pancreas, which are rich in digestive enzymes, are carried in the pancreatic duct to the duodenum. The main duct runs from the tail to the head with numerous small branches joining on the way. It joins the bile duct and they open into the duodenum at the major duodenal papilla (ampulla of Vater). In some individuals a smaller accessory duct drains the superior part of the head of the pancreas (the accessory duct of Santorini). It opens into the duodenum separately, at the minor duodenal papilla, about 2 cm proximal to the main papilla.

Blood, lymphatics and nerves

The pancreas is supplied with blood from branches of the splenic artery (a branch of the coeliac trunk) and from the superior and inferior pancreaticoduodenal arteries from the coeliac and superior mesenteric arteries, respectively. Blood drains into the splenic vein and the superior mesenteric vein parts of the portal vein to the liver. Both splenic vessels lie along the upper border of the body and tail. Lymph drains to preaortic lymph nodes via a number of routes.

The main control of the endocrine pancreas is hormonal; however, a few autonomic nerves reach the pancreas via the coeliac plexus and splanchnic nerves.

MICROSTRUCTURE

The pancreas contains exocrine (enzyme secreting) and endocrine (hormone secreting) tissue. The endocrine cells are arranged in spherical clusters called islets of Langerhans within the exocrine tissue (see Fig. 5.3). Each islet has a rich network of fenestrated capillaries, however, only 10% of endocrine cells are innervated by the autonomic nervous system.

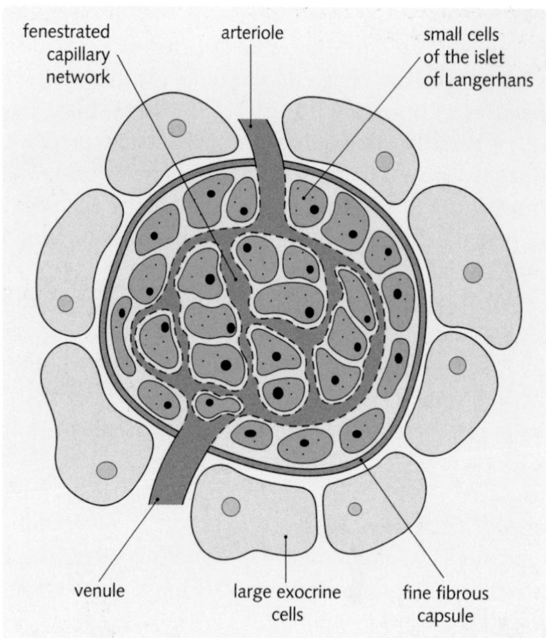

Fig. 5.3 Microstructure of the pancreas showing an islet of Langerhans surrounded by exocrine tissue.

The islets are made up of endocrine cells containing dense secretory granules. These cells are APUD (amine precursor uptake and decarboxylation) cells (see Chapter 6). There are four types of endocrine cell:

- Glucagon-secreting α-cells (20%).
- Insulin-secreting β-cells (70%).
- Somatostatin-secreting δ-cells (8%).
- Pancreatic polypeptide-secreting F-cells (2%).

Insulin and glucagon help regulate blood glucose levels. Somatostatin inhibits the release of insulin and glucagon. Pancreatic polypeptide inhibits the exocrine (i.e. non-endocrine) functions of the pancreas.

DEVELOPMENT

The pancreas is an endodermal structure that develops from two buds derived from the foregut:

- Dorsal bud—the larger bud that forms the majority of the gland.
- Ventral bud—the smaller bud from the right side near the bile duct.

The ventral bud rotates behind the duodenum, along with the bile duct, to lie posterior to the dorsal bud. This smaller ventral bud forms the uncinate process as it fuses with the larger dorsal bud. The ducts usually fuse so that the end of the pancreatic duct is formed from the smaller ventral bud. The duct of the dorsal bud may persist as the accessory pancreatic duct. This sequence of events is shown in Fig. 5.4.

All the pancreatic cells are thought to arise from a single endodermal precursor. *Notch*, *TGF-beta* and *sonic hedgehog* are key genes in determining whether endodermal cells become pancreatic precursors, whether these cells differentiate into exocrine or endocrine cells and, finally, which islet cell lineage is followed. Other factors, including cell adhesion molecules (integrins and NCAMS) and proteolytic enzymes (i.e. matrix metalloproteinases), determine how the precursor cells migrate through the developing pancreas.

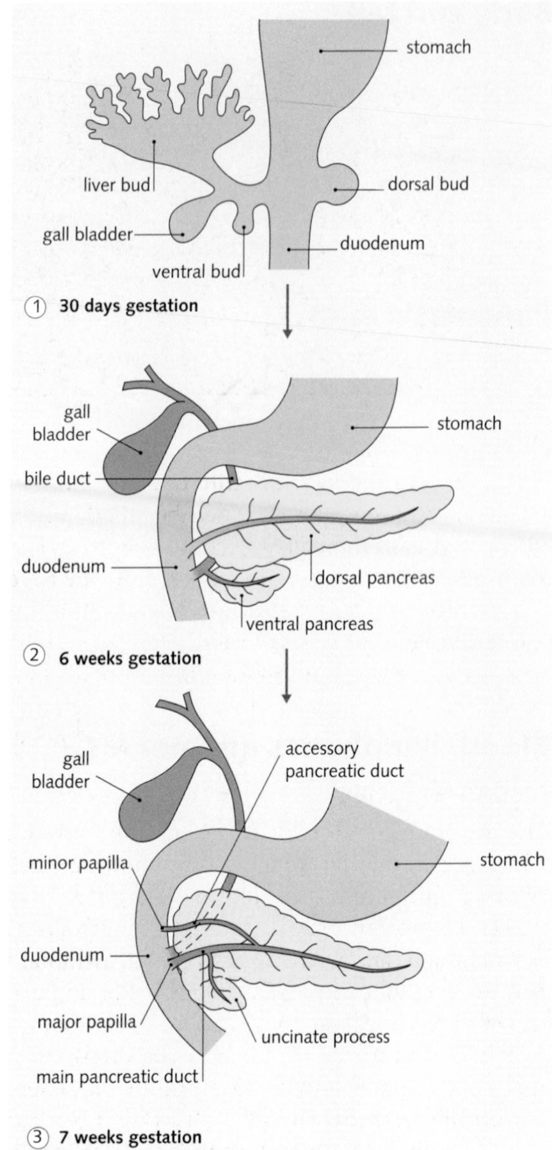

Fig. 5.4 Embryological development of the pancreas.

HORMONES

Insulin

Insulin is a hormone that promotes the uptake, storage and use of glucose. The beta islet cells secrete insulin when they detect high blood glucose levels. As glucose levels fall a few hours after a meal, insulin secretion is reduced. The stored glucose can then be released to maintain blood levels. Insulin secretion never ceases completely; there is always a basal level of insulin in the blood.

Synthesis

Insulin is a polypeptide hormone consisting of two short chains (A and B) linked by disulphide bonds. A single gene controls the production of pre-pro-insulin, which is broken down to form proinsulin. Further cleavage occurs within the secretory vesicles resulting in two molecules: insulin and C peptide.

Since equimolar insulin and C peptide are produced, C peptide acts as a useful marker for β-cell activity in diabetics who receive insulin treatment.

Control of insulin secretion

Glucose diffuses into the beta islet cells. Insulin secretion is increased by high blood glucose. The pancreatic cells detect this stimulus directly because it raises ATP production. Other metabolites (energy molecules such as amino acids and triglycerides, i.e. fat) have a similar but weaker effect. The raised intracellular ATP levels inhibit membrane-bound potassium channels, causing the β-cell to depolarize. The depolarization opens voltage-sensitive calcium channels, raising intracellular calcium, which promotes the secretion of preformed insulin secretory granules by exocytosis. Adults normally produce 45–50 units of insulin each day. This pathway is shown in Fig. 5.5.

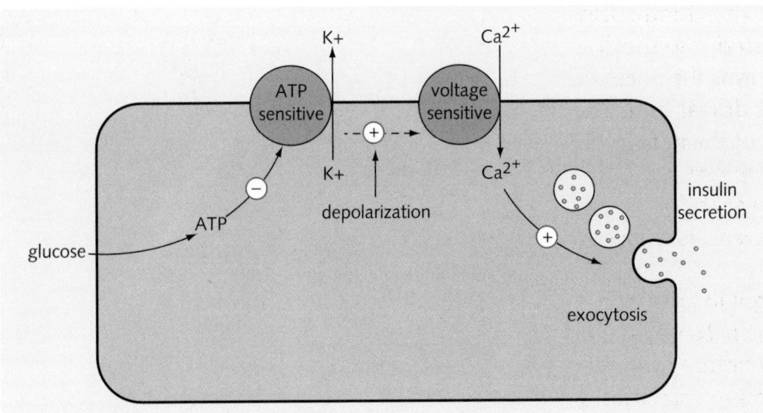

Fig. 5.5 Intracellular stimulation of insulin secretion by glucose.

Although metabolite concentrations are the main regulators of insulin release, a number of other stimuli can also affect this pathway. These stimuli can have an inhibitory or stimulatory effect but can never reduce plasma insulin levels completely. The hormone glucagon, which is released when metabolite levels fall, acts as an important inhibitor of insulin's action; however, it stimulates insulin secretion. Fig. 5.6 shows the main factors that control secretion.

Insulin receptors

The insulin receptor consists of an alpha subunit, which is extracellular, and an intracytoplasmic beta subunit, which has tyrosine kinase activity. It must act via cell-surface receptors because it is a polypeptide hormone and cannot readily cross the cell membrane. Insulin receptors are present in most cells, and they can be sequestered into the cell to inactivate them.

When insulin binds to the tyrosine kinase receptors, it causes phosphorylation of tyrosine side chains within the receptor. The phosphorylated receptor forms a complex with and phosphorylates insulin receptor substrate 1 (IRS-1). This activated molecule then initiates a cascade of phosphorylation and aggregation of other proteins to bring about the intracellular effects of insulin.

Actions of insulin

Insulin has an anabolic effect; it promotes the synthesis of larger molecules. The stimulation of insulin receptors regulates many enzymes concerned with metabolites. The specific enzymes vary between cells (Fig. 5.7), but the overall effects are:

- Increased uptake of metabolites.
- Conversion of metabolites to stored forms (this is an anabolic effect).
- Decreased breakdown of stored metabolites.
- Recruitment of glucose channels to the cell membrane (e.g. GLUT 4).
- Use of glucose for energy over other metabolites.

Breakdown of insulin

Circulatory insulin has a half-life of 4 hours and is broken down by insulinases in the liver, kidney and placenta.

Glucagon

Glucagon is released when blood levels of metabolites are low, causing the release of stored metabolites. In many respects, glucagon has the opposite effect of insulin and functions to ensure there is an adequate supply of energy between meals. Its secretion from α cells is stimulated by a number of factors, of which falling blood glucose is the most important. The main factors are shown in Fig. 5.6.

Synthesis and actions

Glucagon is a single-chain polypeptide hormone formed from a larger precursor in a similar manner to insulin. The precursor is pre-proglucagon, which is cleaved in the storage vesicles to yield proglucagon and, finally, glucagon and the glucagon-like peptides.

Glucagon is a catabolic hormone; it promotes the breakdown of large molecules. Glucagon binds to a G-protein-coupled receptor on the cell membrane, and cAMP acts as a second messenger to initiate a cascade effect. Its effects vary between tissues (Fig. 5.8) but broadly its actions are:

- Inhibition of glucose and amino acid uptake.
- Breakdown of stored metabolites into useable metabolites (catabolism).

Fig. 5.6 Factors controlling insulin and glucagon secretion

	Insulin		Glucagon	
	Stimulants	**Inhibitors**	**Stimulants**	**Inhibitors**
Blood glucose	High	Low	Low	High
Metabolites	Amino acids, fatty acids and ketones	–	Amino acids	Fatty acids and ketones
Hormones	Glucagon, some gastrointestinal tract peptides, growth hormone, adrenocorticotrophic hormone (ACTH), thyroid-stimulating hormone (TSH)	Adrenaline, somatostatin	Adrenaline, some gastrointestinal tract peptides	Insulin, somatostatin
Innervation	Parasympathetic	Sympathetic	Parasympathetic and sympathetic	–
Other	–	Hypocalcaemia	–	–

Fig. 5.7 Metabolic effects of insulin on target cells

Target cells	Action of insulin
Muscle cells and many other cells	Stimulates glucose uptake
	Stimulates glycogenesis (glucose→glycogen)
	Stimulates glycolysis (glucose→energy)
	Stimulates amino-acid uptake and protein synthesis
	Inhibits glycogenolysis (glycogen→glucose)
	Inhibits proteolysis (protein→amino acids)
Adipose cells	Stimulates glucose uptake
	Stimulates lipogenesis (glucose→fatty acids)
	Inhibits lipolysis (fatty acids→energy)
Liver cells	Stimulates glycogenesis (glucose→glycogen)
	Inhibits glycogenolysis (glycogen→glucose)
	Inhibits gluconeogenesis (amino acids→glucose)
Hypothalamus	May stimulate satiety (fullness)

Fig. 5.8 Metabolic effects of glucagon on target cells

Target cells	Action of glucagon
Muscle cells and many other cells	Stimulates glycogenolysis (glycogen→glucose)
	Inhibits glucose uptake
	Inhibits glycolysis (glucose→energy)
	Inhibits amino-acid uptake and protein synthesis
Adipose cells	Stimulates lipolysis (fatty acids→energy)
Liver cells	Stimulates glycogenolysis (glycogen→glucose)
	Stimulates gluconeogenesis (amino acids→glucose)
	Stimulates ketogenesis (fatty acids→ketone bodies)

- Use of fatty acids for energy over other metabolites.
- Promotes hepatic output of ketone bodies.

ENDOCRINE CONTROL OF GLUCOSE HOMEOSTASIS

All cells in the body are capable of using glucose as an energy source by the process of glycolysis. Most cells can also use fatty acids with two important exceptions:

- Neurons (particularly in the CNS), although they can adapt to use ketone bodies.
- Blood cells.

If blood glucose levels drop too low (hypoglycaemia) then the brain is starved of energy. If levels rise too high (hyperglycaemia) then glucose can become toxic. Blood glucose is tightly controlled within narrow limits to prevent either scenario. Fasting glucose levels are normally 3.5–5.5 mmol/L.

For glucose levels to be maintained (glucose homeostasis), the body must be able to increase or decrease these levels in response to changes. There are a number of ways that the body can respond (Fig. 5.9). The liver is especially important in raising blood glucose.

Insulin and glucagon

Glucose homeostasis is maintained by the interplay between insulin and glucagon. These two hormones act as antagonists of each other. Their blood concentrations mirror each other because they are secreted under opposing conditions (Fig. 5.10).

- Insulin lowers blood glucose by stimulating uptake, metabolism and anabolism. It also inhibits the actions of glucagon.
- Glucagon raises blood glucose by simulating gluconeogenesis (synthesis of glucose from amino acids) and glycogenolysis (breakdown of glycogen to release glucose). It also inhibits the actions of insulin but stimulates insulin secretion.

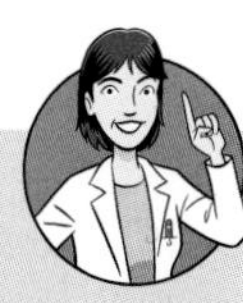

Insulin is the only hormone that lowers blood glucose levels but a number of hormones, including glucagon and adrenaline, can raise them.

Other hormones

Three non-pancreatic hormones also significantly increase blood glucose:

- Adrenaline—released in response to stress; it inhibits insulin.
- Cortisol—released in response to stress; it reduces sensitivity to insulin, which explains the diabetes seen in Cushing's patients
- Growth hormone—released at night; it reduces sensitivity to insulin.

All three hormones can stimulate glycogenolysis and gluconeogenesis to raise blood glucose levels directly. Neural signals and other hormones can cause less significant rises in blood glucose.

Fig. 5.9 Responses that alter blood glucose levels

Responses that raise blood glucose	Responses that lower blood glucose
Ingestion of glucose in the diet	Increased uptake in cells
Gluconeogenesis—the irreversible conversion of amino acids to glucose (liver)	Metabolism to produce energy
Glycogenolysis—the reversible breakdown of glycogen to release glucose (liver)	Glycogenesis—the reversible conversion of glucose to glycogen
	Lipogenesis, the irreversible conversion of glucose to fatty acids

Hyperglycaemia

Hyperglycaemia is an excess of glucose in the blood; it is defined as a fasting concentration >7.8 mmol/L. This can occur in:

- Diabetes mellitus—a common disease caused by insulin deficiency or insulin resistance (reduced sensitivity).
- Glucagonoma—a very rare tumour of the α cells that secrete glucagon.

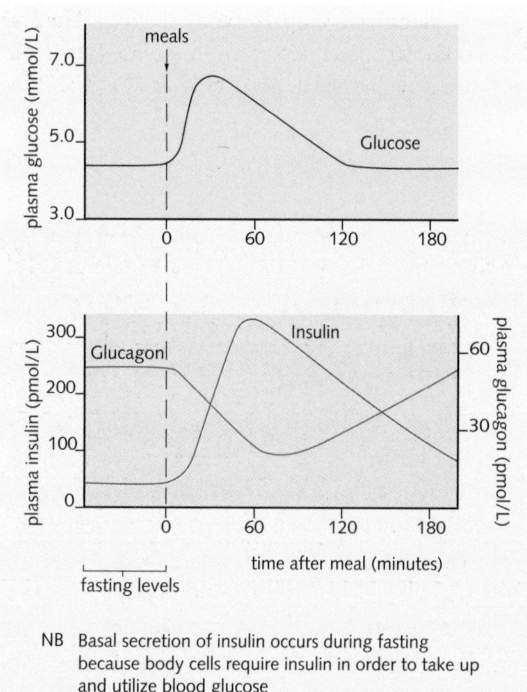

Fig. 5.10 Changes in blood levels of glucose, insulin and glucagon after a carbohydrate-rich meal.

Hypoglycaemia

Hypoglycaemia is a deficiency of blood glucose; it is defined as a concentration <2.5 mmol/L. It can be caused by:

- Overtreatment of diabetes mellitus, either excess insulin or β-cell stimulating drugs.
- Non-diabetic disorder causing fasting hypoglycaemia.
- Idiopathic excessive insulin secretion causing hypoglycaemia after glucose ingestion.
- Insulinoma, with hypersecretion of insulin

DISORDERS

Diabetes mellitus

Types of diabetes mellitus

Diabetes mellitus (DM) is caused by insulin deficiency or insulin resistance (reduced sensitivity). These abnormalities result in chronic hyperglycaemia (excess blood glucose) and metabolic disturbance. It is a very common disease affecting about 2% of the population. There are two types:

- Type 1—[old name: insulin-dependent DM (IDDM)] caused by insulin deficiency.
- Type 2—[old name: non-insulin-dependent DM (NIDDM)] caused by insulin deficiency and/or resistance.

Type 1 diabetes

Type 1 diabetes is caused by autoimmune destruction of the β-islet cells and insulin deficiency. Autoantibodies can be detected in the blood. It is most common in the young, but it can occur at any age. There is a genetic component of about 30% mostly due to human leucocyte antigen (HLA) genes.

Type 2 diabetes

Type 2 diabetes is usually a disease of the elderly, especially those who are obese, and it accounts for 90% of diabetes cases worldwide. It can be caused by insulin deficiency, insulin resistance or a combination of both. Family history is very important, since there is almost 100% concordance in identical twins. 'Metabolic syndrome' is the constellation of Type 2 diabetes alongside obesity, hypertension and hyperlipidaemia (excess fatty acids in the blood)

Type 2 diabetes can develop in young people, in whom it is called maturity-onset diabetes in the young (MODY). This is becoming more common with rising juvenile obesity.

Other causes of diabetes mellitus

Diabetes can also develop secondary to a number of conditions. These include pancreatitis, prolonged corticosteroid use (Cushing's syndrome), acromegaly and thyrotoxicosis.

Symptoms and presentation

Insulin has many important effects on the regulation of glucose and metabolism. Accordingly, the effects of diabetes can appear quite complicated. The effects make more sense if they are thought of in four categories:

- Symptoms of **hyperglycaemia** in both Type 1 and Type 2 diabetes.
- Symptoms of **starvation** particularly in Type 1 diabetes.
- Symptoms of **ketoacidosis** in Type 1 diabetes.
- Symptoms of chronic **complications** in Type 2 and Type 1 diabetes.

Symptoms of hyperglycaemia

Hyperglycaemia causes dehydration because glucose is an osmotically active substance, i.e. it draws water towards it. In hyperglycaemia, glucose concentration is high in the blood and low in the cells so the cells become dehydrated. The excess glucose is also excreted in the kidney and again water follows this movement. Excess water is lost from the body along with electrolytes. The resulting symptoms are shown in Fig. 5.11.

Symptoms of starvation

In Type 1 diabetes, the body enters a state of starvation because cells cannot use the excess glucose; this is caused by the high levels of glucagon. The lack of insulin prevents glucose entering cells and being metabolized. Muscle protein and adipose tissue are broken down to release metabolites and this causes the symptoms shown in Fig. 5.11.

Symptoms of diabetic ketoacidosis (DKA)

Ketoacidosis only develops in Type 1 diabetes. Lipolysis (fat breakdown) is a major component of Type 1 diabetes resulting in raised blood fatty acid levels. These

Fig. 5.11 Symptoms of diabetes mellitus

Symptoms due to hyperglycaemia	Symptoms due to starvation	Symptoms due to ketoacidosis	Symptoms due to chronic complications
Polyuria (increased urine volume)	Weight loss	Vomiting	Decreased visual acuity
Glycosuria (glucose in the urine)	Wasting	Acetone smell on the breath	Reduced sensation in the limbs
Polydipsia (thirst)	Weakness	Ketonuria, polyuria and dehydration	Proteinuria
Tiredness		Hyperventilation	Oedema
Tendency to infections		Reduced consciousness	Intermittent claudication
Dehydration (loose skin, hypotension and tachycardia)		Convulsions	Ischaemic heart disease
Coma		Coma	Hypertension

fatty acids are converted to acetyl coenzyme A (acetyl CoA), an excess of which can overload the tricarboxylic acid (TCA) or Krebs cycle, so the liver uses the excess to synthesize ketone bodies. These are synthesized more quickly than they are metabolized by peripheral tissues so they build up in the blood.

The excess ketone bodies are osmotically active, so they compound the dehydration caused by glucose. Since they are acidic, they can cause a metabolic acidosis (ketoacidosis), which causes severe symptoms (see Fig. 5.11).

Presentation of Type 1 diabetes

Type 1 diabetes presents with a short history of polyuria, tiredness and weight loss followed by dehydration and ketoacidosis (Fig. 5.12). The onset is relatively quick (over a number of weeks) so complications have not developed by the time it presents. Diabetes should be suspected in young patients complaining of tiredness or with frequent skin infections (e.g. boils). Failure to treat a Type 1 patient with insulin can result in rapid death from cerebral oedema following ketoacidosis.

Presentation of Type 2 diabetes

The onset of Type 2 diabetes is much slower than that of Type 1 diabetes, with hyperglycaemia developing over a number of years. By the time of presentation, the patient has often been exposed to excess glucose for so long that complications are already present; in

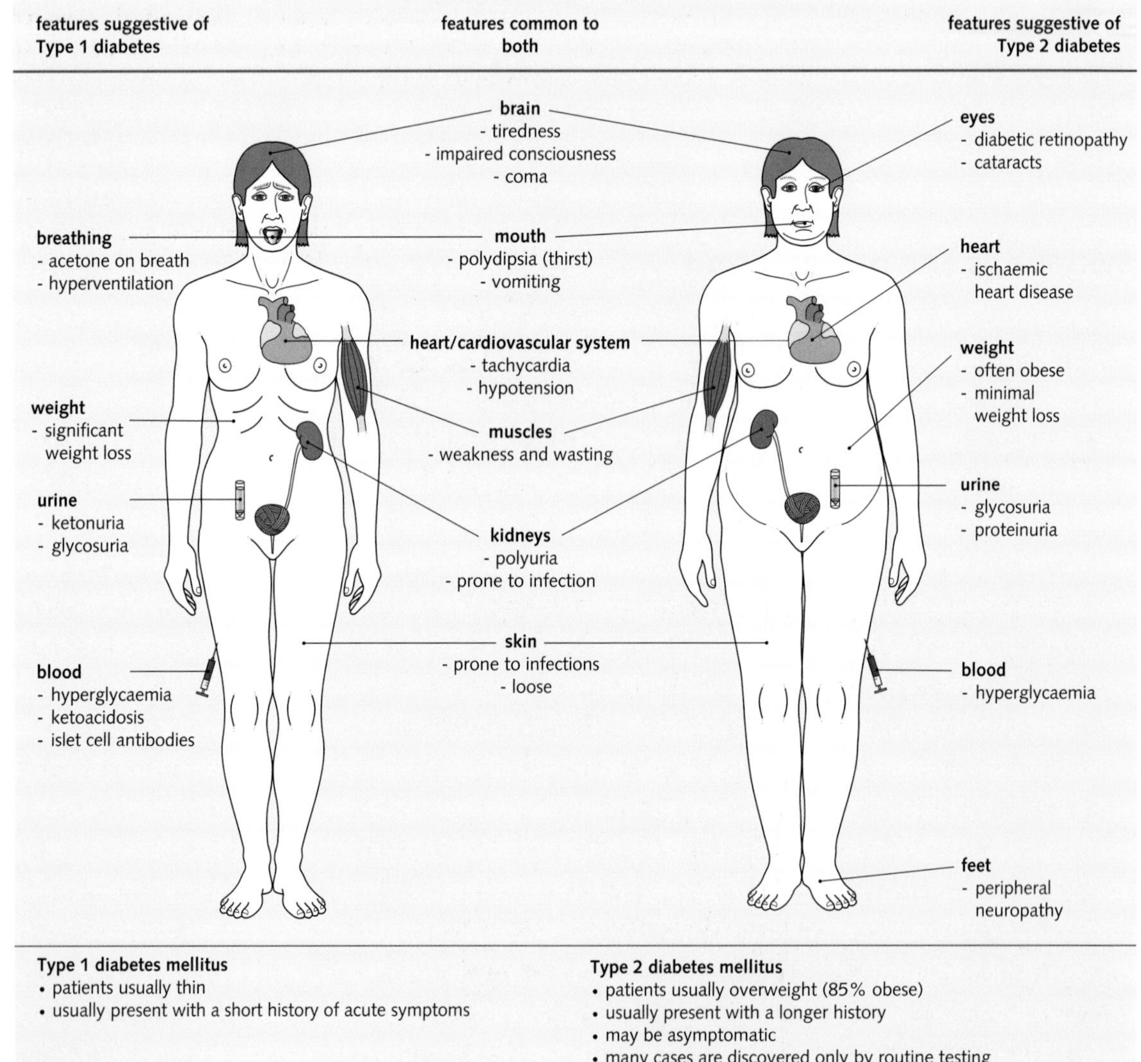

Fig. 5.12 Presentation of Type 1 (insulin-dependent diabetes mellitus; IDDM) and Type 2 (non-insulin-dependent diabetes mellitus; NIDDM).

fact, they may be the presenting feature (see Fig. 5.12). The earliest complications are retinopathy and peripheral neuropathy. Type 2 diabetes patients can present in a coma due to dehydration instead of ketoacidosis. Severe hypoglycaemia and dehydration can result in hypovolaemic (low blood volume) shock. In the worst cases, this can result in a **H**yper**O**smolar **N**on-**K**etotic coma (HONK coma).

Ketoacidosis never occurs in Type 2 diabetes, because some insulin activity is maintained:

- Anabolic actions (glucose uptake and metabolism) require high levels of insulin.
- Anticatabolic actions (inhibition of lipolysis and protein breakdown) only require low levels of insulin.

In Type 2 diabetes, insulin deficiency or resistance does not fall below this lower level so the lipolysis and excess fatty-acid release that cause ketoacidosis do not occur.

Complications

Both types of diabetes can produce complications despite treatment; however, good glucose control lowers the risk of most complications. Chronic complications are grouped according to the size of blood vessel they affect:

- Macrovascular—large vessel disease due to accelerated atherosclerosis.
- Microvascular—small vessel disease due to hyaline arteriolosclerosis.

Macrovascular complications

Diabetes causes accelerated atherosclerosis due to chronically raised fatty-acid levels (hyperlipidaemia) following low insulin levels. Atheroma develops more rapidly and more severely than in non-diabetics, and it can block arteries causing ischaemia and a high risk of infarction. The major sites of macrovascular disease are shown in Fig. 5.13.

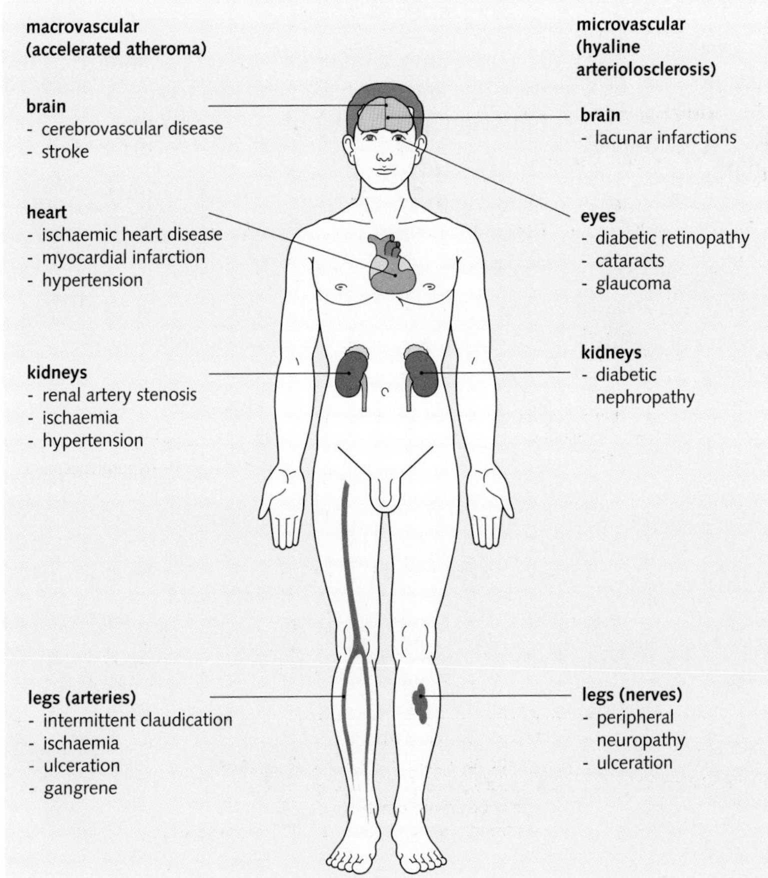

Fig. 5.13 Chronic complications of diabetes mellitus.

Microvascular complications

While atherosclerosis develops in major arteries, the smaller arterioles and capillaries are at risk of hyaline arteriolosclerosis. This is characterized by thickening of the vessel wall and basement membrane. The vessel lumen is reduced, causing localized ischaemia. Futhermore, the vessel also becomes 'leaky', which may be a direct reaction to excess glucose. There are four main patterns of microvascular disease (Figs 5.13 and 5.14). Diabetic retinopathy is the most common cause of blindness in the 30–65 year age group.

Diagnosis

Blood glucose levels are normally 3.5–5.5 mmol/L after an overnight fast. Diabetes is diagnosed if this fasting blood glucose is above 7.8 mmol/L on two occasions. Since NIDDM can develop gradually, a spectrum of disease is seen between normal blood glucose and diabetic blood glucose. A number of markers suggest the need for further observation:

- Glycosuria (glucose in urine).
- Fasting blood glucose of 6–7 mmol/L.
- Random blood glucose of >11.1 mmol/L.

To clarify the diagnosis, a glucose tolerance test is sometimes used. The fasting blood glucose is measured as normal, and the patient is then given a drink containing 75 g glucose. Blood glucose is measured 2 hours later and diabetes is diagnosed if this second measurement is above 11.1 mmol/L.

Treatment

The treatment of diabetes aims to lower blood glucose and normalize metabolism with the least possible interference. Treatment of diabetes should also involve management of obesity, hypertension and dyslipidaemia if these are present. Patient education is essential; ideally patients will regulate their own medication according to their lifestyle. There are three types of treatment:

- Diet alone (Type 2).
- Diet and oral hypoglycaemic agents (Type 2).
- Diet and insulin (Types 1 and 2).

All patients with Type 1 and many with Type 2 diabetes are treated with subcutaneous insulin injections to reduce acute and chronic complications.

Diet

Regulation of diet is essential in all diabetics to help maintain blood glucose levels. Four principles govern this treatment:

- Avoid carbohydrates that can be rapidly absorbed (e.g. glucose) to prevent hyperglycaemia.
- Eat regular, small meals to prevent hypoglycaemia.
- Control calorie intake to lose/stabilize weight (especially Type 2).
- Eat a low-fat, healthy diet to reduce atherosclerosis.

In reality, more than 50% of patients fail to follow their diet and very few manage to achieve long-standing weight loss.

Oral hypoglycaemic agents

Type 2 diabetes can be treated with oral medication to lower blood glucose. A number of medications are available:

- Sulfonylureas (e.g. gliclazide) stimulate β-cells by inhibiting the membrane-bound K^+ channel; the resulting depolarization causes insulin release

Fig. 5.14 Progressive changes caused by complications of diabetes mellitus

Condition	Early changes	Late changes	End result
Retinopathy	Microaneurysms, haemorrhages,hard exudates	Soft exudates, neovascularization	Blindness
Nephropathy	Proteinuria, oedema	Decline of glomerular filtration rate	Renal failure and death
Peripheral neuropathy	Reduced reflexes, reduced sensation (glove and stocking pattern)	Burning or aching sensation, joint deformity	Ulceration and amputation
Lacunar infarcts	Microinfarcts in the brain, asymptomatic	Progressive neurological deficits	Dementia and parkinsonism

(see Fig. 5.5). Side effects include weight gain and hypoglycaemia.

- Biguanides (e.g. metformin) increase peripheral glucose uptake and reduce glucose output from the liver. Their mechanism of action is not understood. Side effects include nausea, diarrhoea and lactic acidosis.
- Acarbose inhibits intestinal enzymes, preventing the digestion of starch; blood glucose rises more slowly after a meal as a result. Side effects include flatulence and diarrhoea.
- Thiazolidinediones (e.g. pioglitazone) are drugs that promote insulin sensitivity, and they are usually used in combination with other drugs. They may have a risk of heart failure and liver toxicity.

Subcutaneous insulin injections

Insulin must be injected because it is inactivated by digestion if taken orally. Subcutaneous injections of insulin are used to treat all Type 1 patients and some with Type 2. It is usually injected into the thigh, upper arm or abdomen. Intensive monitored therapy to maintain low blood glucose has been proven to reduce long-term complications.

Many different types of insulin are available. In the past, porcine (from pigs) insulin was used, but recombinant human insulin is now favoured, since it reduces immunological reactions.

> Preparations of insulin vary in their duration of action and regimes are adapted according to the patient's lifestyle and requirements. Typically, long-acting insulin (Lente) is given in the morning and at night to provide basal insulin requirements and short-acting insulin is administered 15 minutes prior to a meal to cope with the postprandial hyperglycaemia. If control is poor in the morning on this regime then night time insulin (Lente) is adjusted. Insulin Lispro is a very rapidly acting insulin preparation that can be used before a meal.

Monitoring glucose control

Diabetics use monitoring to assess current blood glucose levels and long-term control. The following tests are available:

- Urine testing for glucose: this can be performed at home, but it is unreliable.

> Patients with Type 2 diabetes are often treated with insulin in a similar manner to those with Type 1. This does not mean that they have developed Type 1. Insulin treatment helps to control blood glucose, which has been proven to reduce complications.

- Capillary blood spot testing: this simple test gives an instant digital reading of blood glucose, it can be performed at home and is used to determine insulin or sugar doses.
- Glycosylated haemoglobin (HbA1C): glucose binds directly and irreversibly to haemoglobin to form HbA_{1C}. The proportion of HbA_{1C} in the blood gives a measure of glucose control over the previous 2 months. It is used very commonly in clinical practice.
- Fructosamine: this is formed when glucose binds to serum albumin. It gives a measure of glucose control in the last 2 weeks but is rarely used in clinical practice.

Hypoglycaemia

Individuals with diabetes mellitus can experience hypoglycaemia in a number of situations:

- Low carbohydrate intake (e.g. missed meal).
- Unexpected exercise.
- Insulin overdose.
- Malabsorption.

Symptoms

Diabetics must know the symptoms of their hypoglycaemic attacks, and they should always carry a sugary snack in case they feel a 'hypo' coming on. If action is not taken to prevent it, then recognizing the symptoms and signs of hypoglycaemia can be life saving; they are shown in Fig. 5.15. These symptoms are caused by raised adrenaline secretion and low cerebral glucose. Severe hypoglycaemia can result in a coma. This is treated with intravenous infusion of 50 mL 50% dextrose, and sugary drinks once the patient regains consciousness. Glucagon pens are now available for intramuscular injection in the event of a 'hypo'.

Screening to prevent complications

Along with preventing short-term hypo/hyperglycaemia, diabetic clinics aim to minimize the long-

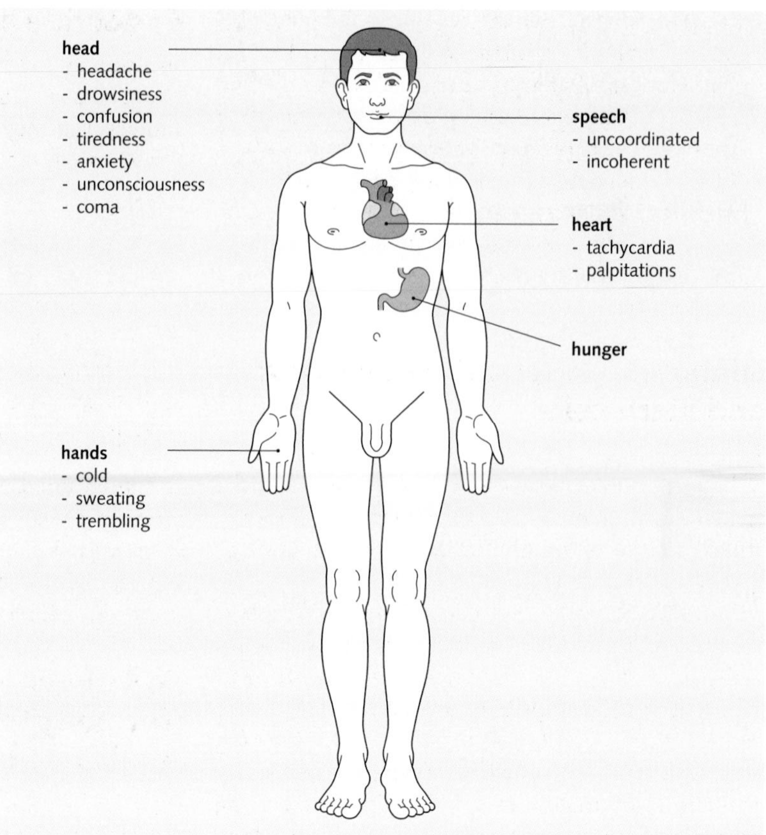

Fig. 5.15 Symptoms of hypoglycaemia.

term complications. Many of these complications are treatable if they are detected in their early stages, i.e. before symptoms develop.

Eyes

Retinopathy is a very common cause of blindness, and the early stages are completely treatable by laser photocoagulation. The eyes of diabetics should be tested and inspected regularly for signs of deterioration or retinopathy.

Kidneys

Urine samples should be checked regularly for microalbuminuria caused by early nephropathy (kidney damage). If present, then blood glucose should be regulated more aggressively. An angiotensin-converting enzyme (ACE) inhibitor can be used to prevent the resulting hypertension and to slow the progression to end-stage renal failure.

Feet

The feet of elderly or immobile diabetics should be examined regularly by chiropodists. The combination of peripheral neuropathy and peripheral vascular disease can lead to injury, ulceration, infection and, eventually, gangrene. Poorly perfused gangrenous feet may need to be amputated. This can be prevented by early treatment and dressing or vascular surgery in severe cases.

Hypoglycaemia in non-diabetic patients

Most people should be able to tolerate fasting for several days without developing hypoglycaemia. If a patient is unable to do so then the mnemonic 'EXPLAIN' lists the possible causes:

- EXogenous drugs (e.g. alcohol and insulin).
- Pituitary insufficiency, growth hormone deficiency.
- Liver failure or defective liver enzymes.
- Addison's disease—deficiency of cortisol that raises blood glucose levels (also Autoimmune causes).
- Insulinomas—a type of islet-cell tumour (see below).
- Non-pancreatic tumour—by ectopic insulin secretion or simply consuming glucose.

Endogenous insulin is formed by the cleavage of proinsulin to insulin and c-peptide. If a patient experiences hypoglycaemia in the presence of high insulin levels, c-peptide measurements help to distinguish between excess endogenous insulin (e.g. insulinoma) and excess exogenous insulin (e.g. overdose or Munchausen by proxy)

Diabetes, pancreatic transplants and stem cells

Type 1 diabetes results from autoimmune destruction of beta islet cells and 95% of Type 2 diabetes is the result of insulin resistance, which manifests clinically when the islet cells can no longer produce enough insulin to compensate for the resistance.

Understanding the molecular biology of pancreatic development may offer new therapeutic options for diabetes. Islet cell transplant is becoming established as a treatment for Type 1 diabetes but the supply of tissue is short. As the factors (e.g. *Notch, sonic hedgehog* and *TGF-beta*) that control development are discovered it is hoped that they can be used to stimulate the expansion or regeneration of islet cells in vivo, which would overcome the tissue shortage and the immunological complications of transplantation. Alternatively, this knowledge might be used to drive beta islet cell stem-cell differentiation in vitro (Fig. 5.16).

Endocrine pancreatic neoplasia

Tumours of the endocrine cells in the pancreas are called islet-cell tumours; they are usually benign and solitary, but they often secrete a specific hormone. Tumours are named according to the hormone they secrete:

- Insulinomas are the most common type of islet-cell tumour. The excess insulin that they secrete causes severe hypoglycaemic attacks, which can lead to coma.
- Glucagonomas are very rare tumours that secrete glucagon. They are often asymptomatic, but they may cause diabetes mellitus.

Extremely infrequently, islet-cell tumours can secrete other hormones, such as gastrin in Zollinger–Ellison syndrome. Other rare tumours can produce vasoactive intestinal polypeptide (VIP) or adrenocorticotrophic hormone (ACTH).

The metabolic syndrome (formerly insulin resistance syndrome or syndrome X)

Type 2 diabetes is often associated with hyperglycaemia, hyperinsulinaemia, dyslipidaemia, hypertension and central obesity (adipose tissue in an abdominal distribution). This collection of problems is collectively referred to as the metabolic syndrome and is associated with an increased risk of stroke and

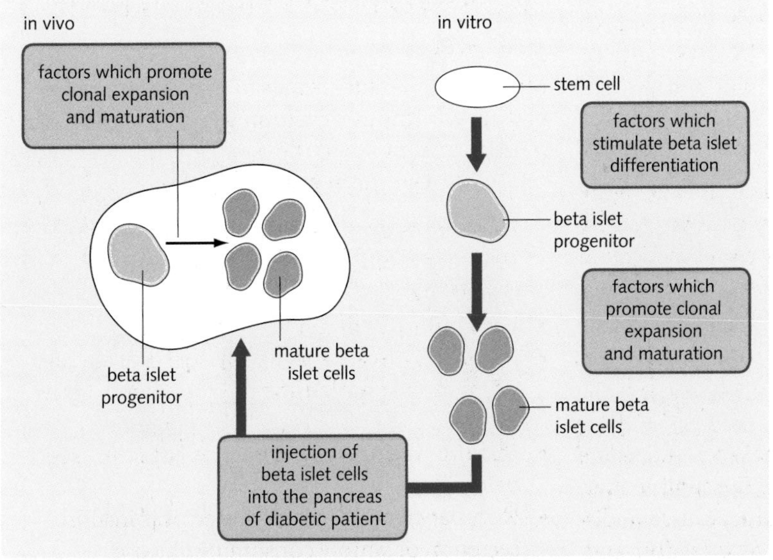

Fig. 5.16 The action of leptin on fertility. (FSH, follicle-stimulating hormone; GnRH, gonadotrophin-releasing hormone; LH, luteinizing hormone.)

coronary heart disease, which may be the result of hypertriglyceridaemia or hyperinsulinaemia. There are several theories about why these factors cluster. Some suggest that it is simple genetic linkage, whilst others think that insulin resistance is the initiating event, as it drives the synthesis of triglycerides and very-low-density lipoproteins (VLDL), which in turn lead to obesity and coronary vascular disease. Alternatively, as adipose tissue produces several hormones that mediate insulin sensitivity, it may be obesity itself which creates the metabolic syndrome. Growing adipocytes produce tissue necrosis factor α (TNF-α), which increases insulin resistance. Adiponectin is produced by adipose tissue and decreases insulin resistance but its levels decrease with obesity. Whilst the identification of a single underlying cause remains elusive, the metabolic syndrome serves to highlight the importance of treating other cardiac risk factors in diabetes patients.

Endocrine role of adipose tissue and appetite

Adipose tissue is an endocrine tissue that secretes a polypeptide hormone called leptin as well as adiponectin. The levels of leptin correlate well with the percentage of adipose tissue, creating an endocrine indicator of energy stores. This signal is transported across the blood–brain barrier, where it binds to leptin receptors in the hypothalamus that stimulate Janus kinases (JAKs). These activate signal transducer and activators of transcription (STAT) proteins, which promote transcription of leptin genes. The end result of this signalling pathway is an increase in the release of anorexigenic (appetite reducing) peptides (e.g. α-melanocyte-stimulating hormone) and a decrease in the release of orexigenic (hunger inducing) peptides [e.g. neuropeptide Y (NPY)]. Leptin has two main effects:

- Appetite reduction.
- Stimulation of gonadotrophin-releasing hormone (GnRH) production.

Leptin resistance caused by the blood–brain barrier may prevent remarkable weight loss. It has been suggested that only a fixed amount of leptin can be transported across this barrier so that excess leptin in the blood does not increase leptin in the CNS above a fixed level. Disorders in this barrier may also account for some cases of obesity. Inherited leptin deficiency is an incredibly rare recessive disorder that causes gross obesity and infertility.

The action of leptin on GnRH release (Fig. 5.17) explains the infertility of underweight women. This is a protective response to prevent pregnancy in the undernourished. Leptin is also secreted prepubertally and it plays a role in the onset of puberty. Body weight is a better predictor of the onset of menstruation than age.

> The leptin gene was cloned from transgenic obese mice after it was discovered that they lacked a circulating satiety factor. In humans with a genetic leptin deficit, exogenous leptin has proven effective in the treatment of obesity. However in obese patients capable of producing leptin, exogenous leptin administration has been only moderately effective. Attention is now being focused on many of the other appetite regulators, including ghrelin and its antagonist obestatin.

Ghrelin

Ghrelin is a gut peptide that increases circulating growth hormone, increases gastric motility, enhances carbohydrate use and stimulates appetite. Ghrelin rises before a meal, which suggests a role in meal initiation.

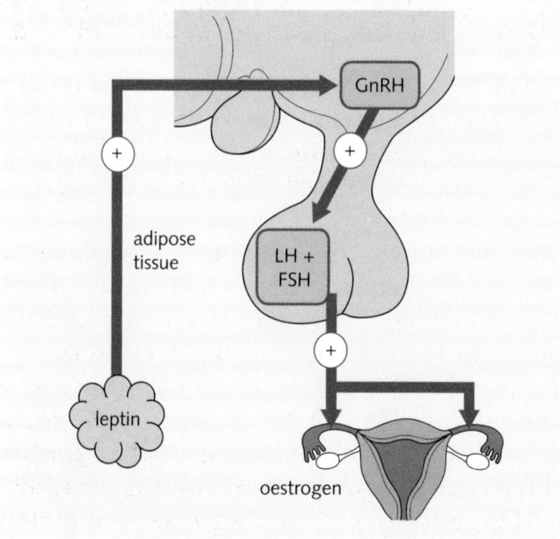

Fig. 5.17 The action of leptin on fertility. (FSH, follicle-stimulating hormone; GnRH, gonadotrophin-releasing hormone; LH, luteinizing hormone.)

Up and coming hormones

6

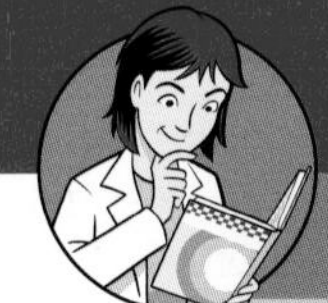

Objectives

By the end of this chapter you should be able to:

- Define APUD, describe a cell and list three examples, with the hormones they secrete.
- Describe the actions of gastrin, cholecystokinin and secretin.
- Describe the anatomical location of the pineal gland and explain what types of cell are present.
- Describe melatonin and how it is synthesized.
- Recognize the signals that trigger the release of melatonin.
- Describe the function of the suprachiasmatic nucleus (SCN) and explain how it is affected by melatonin.
- Describe jet-lag from an endocrine point of view.

This chapter describes several tissues whose endocrine functions are still being realized:

- Gastrointestinal (GI) tract—secretes many hormones that regulate digestive function. Some act on distant organs by travelling through the blood, while others act locally as mediators.
- Pineal gland—secretes melatonin, which regulates circadian rhythms.

ENDOCRINE CELLS IN THE GASTROINTESTINAL TRACT

Enteroendocrine cells are the product of one of the four stem-cell lineages that exist within intestinal epithelium and are considered to be part of the 'diffuse endocrine system'. They secrete a host of peptides, in various combinations, in response to stimuli reflecting nutrient consumption (e.g. intestinal distension or chemical stimuli) both within and outside the intestine. They potentiate or inhibit the release and action of each other and therefore form a complex network capable of coordinating the absorption and digestion of food at the level of the intestine and at the level of the CNS with respect to the regulation of appetite—the 'gut–brain axis'. The main peptides will be considered individually below but the role of these peptides in concert is just beginning to emerge and this complex system will probably require computer modelling before it becomes more useful clinically.

Some GI-tract peptides, e.g. vasoactive intestinal peptide (VIP), cholecystokinin (CCK) and gastrin, also act as neurotransmitters in the CNS and the neurons that innervate the GI tract (called the enteric nervous system). This overlap demonstrates the close relationship and common origin of the endocrine and nervous systems. The following functions are regulated in the CNS by these peptide neurotransmitters:

- Biological rhythms—VIP.
- Satiety (fullness after food)—CCK.
- Thermoregulation—bombesin.
- Growth—somatostatin.

The APUD concept

APUD cells are a group of endocrine cells that secrete small peptide hormones in many tissues throughout the body. The name 'APUD' (amine precursor uptake and decarboxylation) reflects the conversion of actively absorbed amine precursors into amino acids, which are used to make peptides hormones. These cells are linked by three features:

- Appearance under an electron microscope (e.g. neurosecretory granules).
- Biochemical pathway for amine or peptide hormone synthesis.
- Embryological origin is from neural crest cells, which migrate to foregut and other locations.

They are also called neuroendocrine cells, due to their secretion of both neurotransmitters and 'hormones'. The following cells are examples of APUD cells:

- Islets of Langerhans cells that secrete insulin and glucagon.
- Enteroendocrine cells (see below).
- Parafollicular cells that secrete calcitonin; they are found in the thyroid gland.
- Juxtaglomerular complex that secretes renin; found in the kidneys.
- Neuroendocrine cells of the respiratory tract that secrete 5-hydroxytryptamine (5-HT; serotonin) and calcitonin.

Gastrointestinal tract peptides

The major peptides secreted by the enteroendocrine cells of the GI tract are described below. Figs 6.1 and 6.2 show the location of GI-tract peptide release and the major actions of four GI-tract hormones. The actions of other peptides are shown in Fig. 6.3.

Delivery

GI-tract peptides reach their target cells by two means:

- Endocrine, via the blood.
- Paracrine, act locally to affect nearby cells.

Some peptides have both endocrine and paracrine functions, e.g. somatostatin.

Gastrin

Gastrin is predominantly secreted by enteroendocrine cells (G-cells) in the pylorus of the stomach after a meal. It is secreted in response to:

- Peptides or amino acids in the stomach.
- Vagal stimulation (i.e. parasympathetic).
- Distension of the stomach.

It acts to increase protein breakdown, specifically by:

- Stimulating enterochromaffin-like cells to release histamine. This acts on the histamine-2 (H_2) receptors of parietal cells in the stomach to promote the release of hydrochloric acid and intrinsic factor.
- Stimulating the release of hydrochoric acid directly through its action on the CCK receptors of parietal cells.
- Stimulating the chief cells of the stomach to secrete pepsin.
- Increasing gastric motility.
- Relaxing the pyloric and ileocaecal sphincters.

Patient presenting with recurrent peptic ulcers, especially if there is a family history of endocrine cancers, should be investigated for Zollinger–Ellison syndrome. These patients have gastrin-producing pancreatic adenomas or islet hyperplasia, which causes excessive release of gastrin, over-stimulation of the parietal cells, acidification of the stomach contents and destruction and ulceration of the stomach mucosa.

Secretin

Secretin is secreted by the duodenum and the rest of the small intestine in response to acid secreted by the stomach and other luminal contents, including ethanol. It neutralizes the acid produced by gastrin release by:

- Stimulating pancreatic and liver secretion of bicarbonate.
- Inhibiting acid secretion from the parietal cells of the stomach.

Cholecystokinin

CCK is secreted in the duodenum in the presence of fat or amino acids. It increases the breakdown of fat by:

- Causing contraction of the gall bladder and release of bile into the duodenum.
- Stimulating pancreatic enzyme secretion (e.g. lipase).
- Causing some bicarbonate release from the pancreas.
- Shifting gastric contractions from proximal to antral.
- Producing a sensation of fullness.

Ghrelin

A gut-derived peptide that stimulates appetite and growth hormone release from the anterior pituitary. Ghrelin increases hunger through its action on hypothalamic feeding centres. It also stimulates gastric emptying.

Glucose-dependent insulinotrophic peptide

Glucose-dependent insulinotrophic peptide (GIP), formerly called gastric inhibitory peptide (also GIP), is secreted by the enteroendocrine K cells of the duodenum in response to fats and carbohydrates. It acts to:

- Stimulate insulin secretion if blood glucose is high.
- Inhibit gastric acid production and gastric motility.

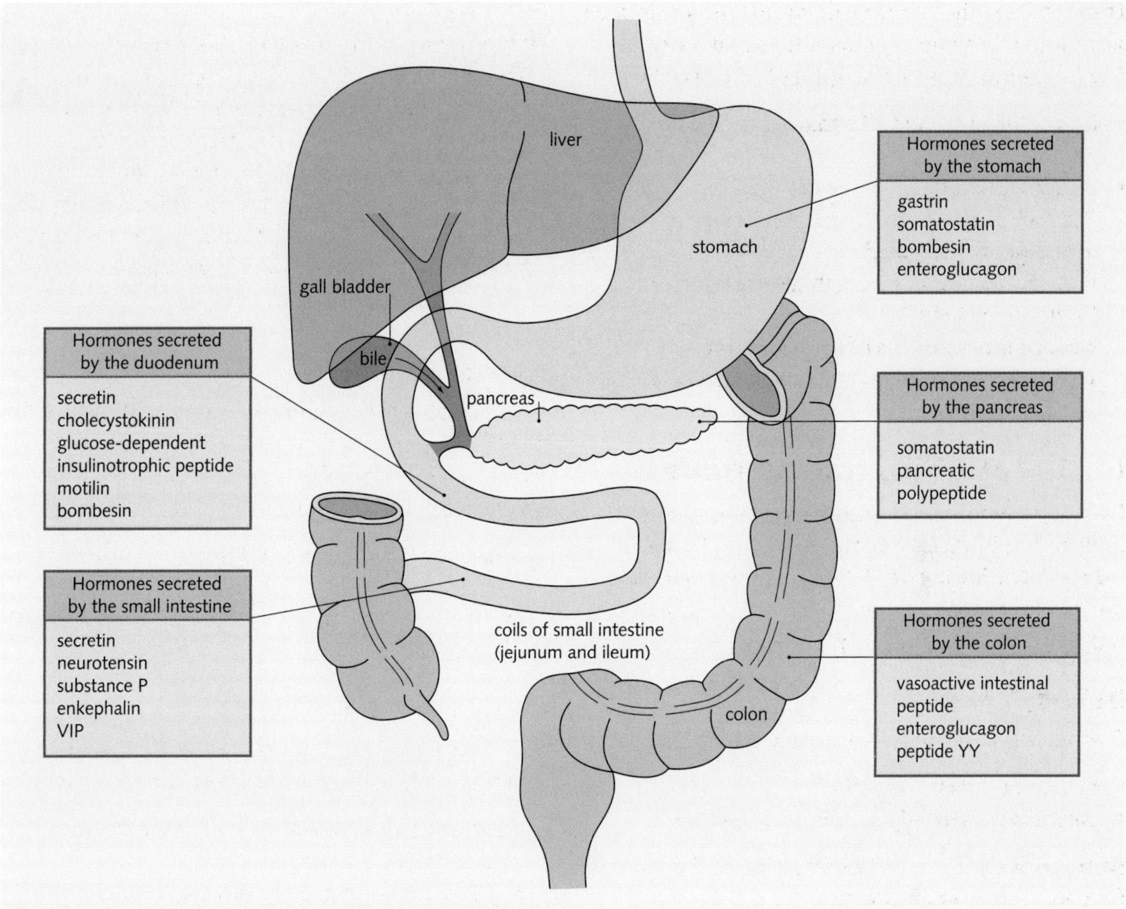

liver
stomach
gall bladder
bile
pancreas
Hormones secreted by the stomach
gastrin
somatostatin
bombesin
enteroglucagon
Hormones secreted by the duodenum
secretin
cholecystokinin
glucose-dependent insulinotrophic peptide
motilin
bombesin
Hormones secreted by the pancreas
somatostatin
pancreatic polypeptide
Hormones secreted by the small intestine
secretin
neurotensin
substance P
enkephalin
VIP
coils of small intestine (jejunum and ileum)
Hormones secreted by the colon
vasoactive intestinal peptide
enteroglucagon
peptide YY
colon

Fig. 6.1 Sites at which the gastrointestinal tract peptides are secreted.

liver
stomach
HCO_3^-
secretin
gastrin
gastric acid
bile
secretin
CCK
HCO_3^-
insulin
pancreas
duodenum
GIP

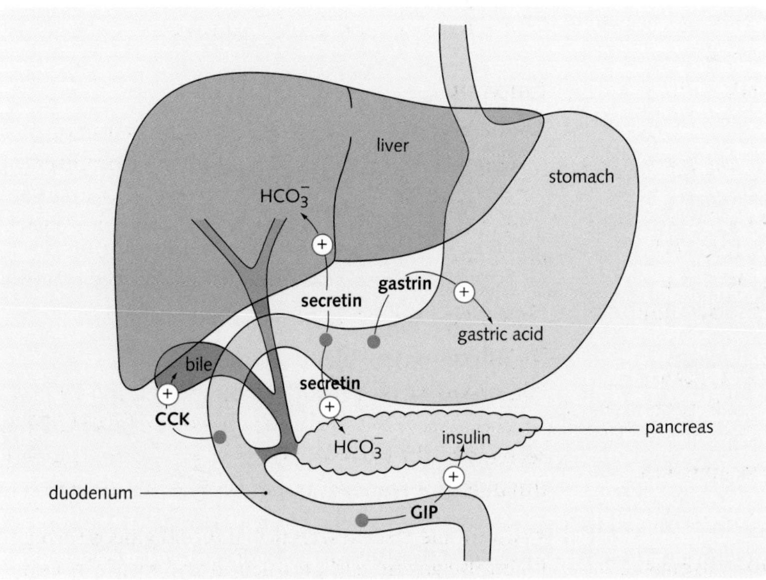

Fig. 6.2 Major actions of four gastrointestinal tract hormones. (CCK, cholecystokinin; GIP, glucose-dependent insulinotrophic peptide.)

Fig. 6.3 The sites of secretion, stimuli for secretion and actions of the minor gut peptides

Gut peptide	Site of secretion	Stimulus for secretion	Action of peptide
Enteroglucagon	A cells in the stomach and L cells in the colon	Presence of glucose and fat in the stomach	Reduces gastric-acid secretion and gut motility
Bombesin	P cells in the stomach and duodenum	Fasting	Stimulates gastrin release
Motilin	EC cells in the duodenum	Absence of food in the duodenum	Speeds gastric emptying and stimulates colonic motility
Vasoactive intestinal polypeptide (VIP)	D1 cells and neurons in the small intestine and colon	Gut distension	Stimulates local gut secretion, motility and blood flow
Peptide YY (related to pancreatic polypeptide)	PYY cells of the colon	Presence of intestinal fat	Inhibits gastric motility and acid secretion (peptide YY is elevated in coeliac disease and cystic fibrosis)
Substance P	Enteric neurons in the small intestine	Cholecystokinin (CCK), 5-hydroxytryptamine (5-HT)	Stimulates gut motility, secretion and immune response; may have a role in inflammatory bowel disease
Enkephalin	Enteric neurons in the small intestine	Unknown	Inhibits gut motility and secretion
Neurotensin	N cells of the small intestine	Presence of intestinal fat	Stimulates local gut motility, secretion and immune response

Somatostatin

Somatostatin is secreted mainly by the δ-cells of the islets of Langerhans in the pancreas, but also by the stomach and GI-tract neurons. It is also secreted by the hypothalamus, where it is called growth hormone inhibiting hormone (GHIH), and it inhibits the release of growth hormone and TSH. In the intestine secretion is stimulated by:

- Acidity and amino acids in the stomach.
- High blood glucose.
- CCK.

Somatostatin acts to slow down digestion by inhibiting:

- Secretion of gastrin, insulin and glucagon.
- Secretion of pancreatic enzymes and bile.
- Gastric motility.

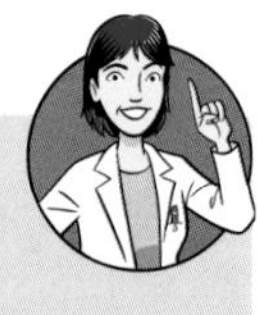

Patients with the rare somatostatinoma (a somatostatin-producing tumour) present with a triad of diabetes, gall bladder disease and diarrhoea.

Pancreatic polypeptide

Pancreatic polypeptide is secreted by the F-cells of the islets of Langerhans in the pancreas, in response to protein in the stomach or low blood glucose. Its actions remain unclear but it slows the absorption of food by:

- Inhibiting gall bladder contraction.
- Inhibiting pancreatic enzyme secretion.

Insulin and glucagon

Insulin and glucagon are both peptides secreted by enteroendocrine cells in the pancreas. The important functions they perform are described in Chapter 5

PINEAL GLAND

Structure

Macrostructure

The pineal gland coordinates circadian (daily) rhythms of dark-light (day-night) cycles by secreting the hormone melatonin. Darkness stimulates its release.

It is a small gland found at the posterior end of the corpus callosum, forming a section of the roof in the posterior wall of the third ventricle (Fig. 6.4).

The pineal gland begins to calcify after puberty, making it a useful midline marker in X-rays and computed tomography (CT) scans.

Microstructure

The pineal gland is composed of two types of neural cell:

- Pinealocytes—specialized secretory neurons.
- Glial support cells.

In keeping with all endocrine organs, it has a very rich blood supply that forms a network of capillaries surrounded by the pinealocytes. It receives innervation from many parts of the brain, but the main connections are with the:

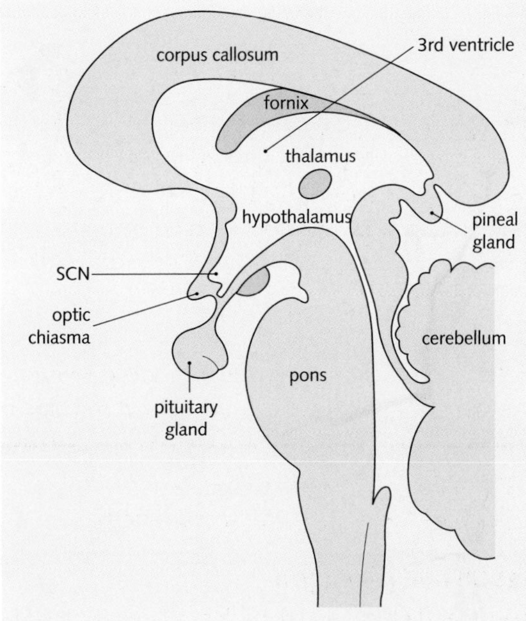

Fig. 6.4 Median section of the mid-brain and brainstem showing the anatomical location of the pineal gland and suprachiasmatic nucleus (SCN).

- Suprachiasmatic nucleus (SCN).
- Retina.
- Sympathetic system.
- Parasympathetic system.

Function

The pineal gland synthesizes and secretes the hormone melatonin (NB not melanin, the brown skin pigment). Melatonin is a modified form of the amino acid tryptophan, which is first converted to 5-HT then to melatonin.

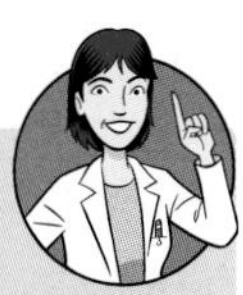

There is evidence that reprogramming the pineal gland may help in the treatment of seasonal affective disorder.

Regulation

In the absence of light signals, circadian rhythms still exist but are not synchronized with the day–night cycle. The suprachiasmic nucleus (SCN) in the hypothalamus serves as an 'intrinsic clock', which interacts with an external rhythm stimulus (or *Zeitgeber*), in this case light, to coordinate melatonin release with the external day–night cycle. This system allows the conversion of inhibitory light stimuli into a hormonal stimulus that can regulate:

- Day and night (circadian rhythm).
- Seasonal breeding rhythms (e.g. deer, birds).

Effects of melatonin

Melatonin has three main effects:

- It induces sleep (hypnotic effect).
- It resets the SCN.
- It influences the hypothalamus, especially the reproductive functions.

Circadian rhythms influence almost every cell in the body. Hormones are secreted from the hypothalamus, pituitary gland and gonads with a circadian rhythm, e.g. secretion of corticotrophin-releasing hormone (CRH) and adrenocorticotrophic hormone (ACTH) peak early in the morning. These variation in hormone levels throughout the day are thought to be determined by the actions of the SCN and the pineal gland. The regulation and actions of melatonin are shown in Fig. 6.5.

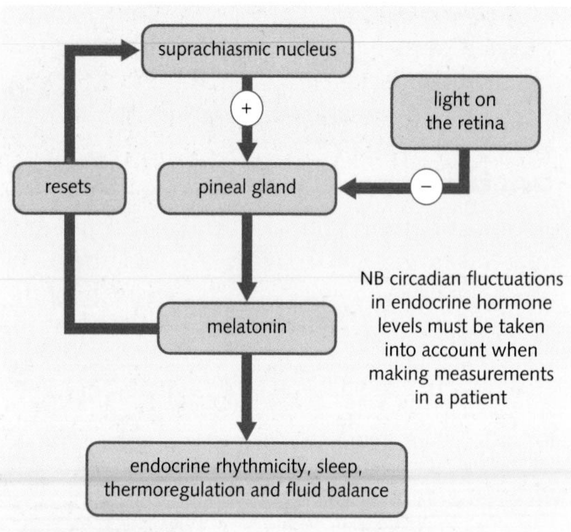

Fig. 6.5 Regulation of melatonin and its actions.

Jet lag and melatonin treatment

The pineal gland has evolved to allow adaptation to changing day length (i.e. seasons). However, resetting of the SCN is best demonstrated by a jet flight in the following way:

- When a person leaves his or her home country the SCN and pineal gland are synchronized: at night, darkness and SCN activation stimulate melatonin production, inducing sleep.
- If the person flies across time zones, the SCN continues to oscillate in accordance with the previous time zone, which means that the timing of melatonin production (and, therefore, tiredness) does not change.
- At a rate of adjustment of a couple of hours a day, the SCN adapts to the new time zone.

Taking oral melatonin can shorten the period of jet lag. Melatonin should be taken at the times of darkness in the new time zone whilst on the plane and for several days at the destination. For shift work, the melatonin should be taken during the period of desired sleep. The SCN is reset more quickly and the body becomes resynchronized.

7 Endocrine control of fluid balance

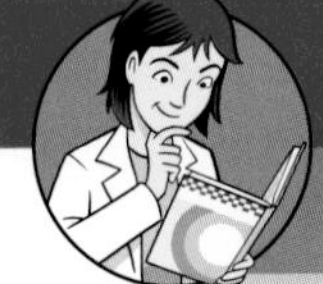

Objectives

You should be able to:

- Describe the processes by which water can be lost or gained from the body.
- Understand how blood volume and peripheral resistance influence blood pressure.
- Explain the regulation, secretion and actions of ADH.
- Describe the regulation and secretion of renin and angiotensin.
- Understand how ACE inhibitors act.
- Describe the actions of renin and angiotensin II.
- Explain the regulation and action of aldosterone.
- Name three peptides that affect fluid balance, along with their actions.
- Describe the physiological changes underlying dehydration.
- List the common causes of dehydration and the signs and symptoms that result.
- List the common causes of water retention and the signs and symptoms that result.

Fluid balance is important in maintaining appropriate perfusion of vital organs, in determining electrolyte concentrations and in meeting the body's demand for water. Humans have evolved to consume and store an excess of water at meal times, rather than being subject to constant thirst. Using this supply of water, the body is able to adapt to demand by regulating renal water excretion. Changes in plasma osmolality and plasma volume stimulate the release of various hormones. These hormones can differentially regulate renal sodium and water reabsorption and serve to restore plasma osmolality and volume to equilibrium. As blood pressure is affected by fluid balance, many of these hormones are also vasoactive. The main hormones involved in regulating fluid balance are:

- Antidiuretic hormone (ADH)—from the posterior pituitary gland (Fig. 7.1).
- Renin from the kidney (Fig. 7.2).
- Aldosterone—from the adrenal cortex (Fig. 7.2).

An understanding of fluid balance is essential in medicine, whether it be in the management of dehydration, hyponatraemia, hypernatraemia, hypertension or shock.

FLUID BALANCE

The importance of water

Water is needed for thermoregulation, metabolism, joint lubrication, toxin transport and many other processes. In an average 70-kg man, there are 42 litres of water, of which 28 litres are in the extracellular compartment and 14 litres are in the intracellular compartment (3 litres of which is plasma).

The importance of sodium

Fluid balance is intimately linked to sodium balance. Sodium ions are osmotically active (they attract water across membranes) and they are present in large quantities within the body. Water tends to passively follow movements of sodium ions. The normal plasma concentration of sodium ions is 135–145 mmol/L. In the kidney, water reabsorption is enabled by a high concentration of sodium ions in the renal medulla and can be regulated by controlling the reabsorption of sodium or by allowing water to move more freely.

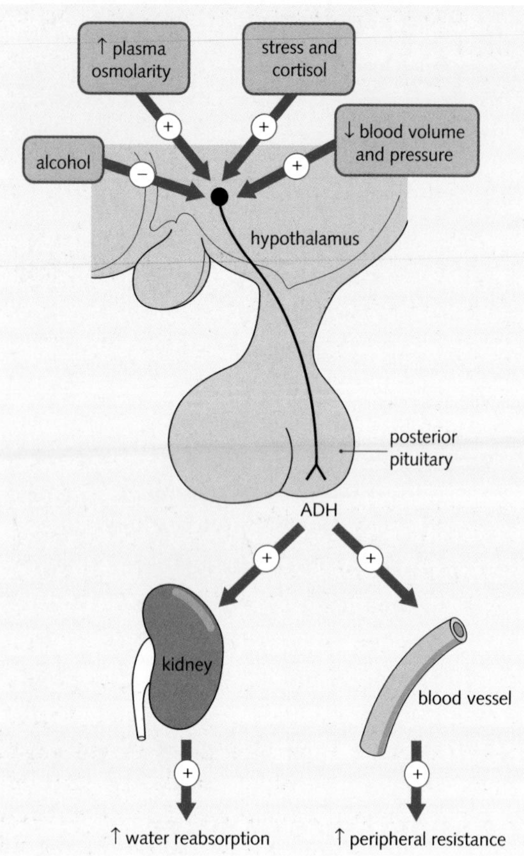

Fig. 7.1 Hormonal regulation of plasma osmolality by antidiuretic hormone (ADH).

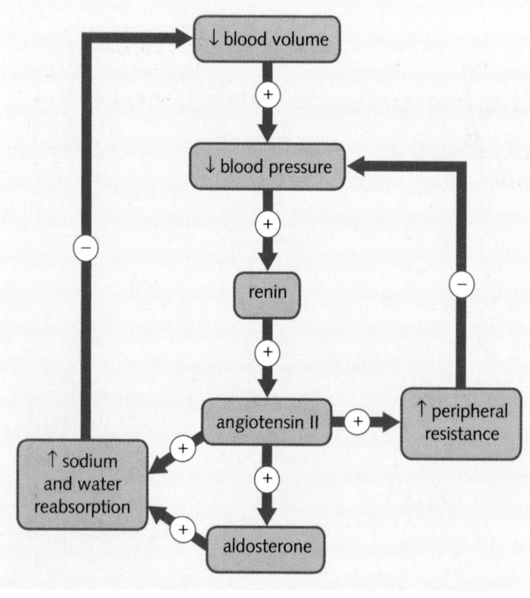

Fig. 7.2 Hormonal regulation of blood volume by renin, angiotensin II and aldosterone.

The importance of fluid volume

In addition to the maintenance of an adequate water supply, fluid balance, in particular fluid volume, is a key determinant of blood pressure. In order to ensure organs are appropriately perfused, the body is able to adapt to changes in fluid volume by adjustings:

- Cardiac output (i.e. stroke volume and rate).
- Peripheral resistance (i.e. vasodilatation or vasoconstriction).

Determinants of fluid balance

Water excretion

Water excretion is controlled mainly by the kidney. The kidney filters the entire blood volume once every 5 minutes. Water and sodium are filtered into the kidney tubules by the glomeruli but most is reabsorbed back into the blood. Sodium ions are actively reabsorbed, while water passively follows the sodium by osmosis. Any sodium or water that is not reabsorbed is excreted in the urine.

Fluid balance can be regulated in the kidneys by altering two factors:

- Sodium reabsorption.
- Permeability of the tubules to water.

Water is also lost by the processes shown in Fig. 7.3, but these losses are less significant than the actions of the kidney.

Water homeostasis

Water is largely acquired without immediate need by eating and drinking at meal times (Fig. 7.3). However, under conditions of drought when the kidneys reduce urine volume to a minimum, a small obligate urine loss remains and insensible water losses continue. In response, osmoreceptors in the hypothalamus detect rising plasma osmolality or in extreme cases falling plasma volume, and stimulate thirst. The threshold osmolality for thirst stimulation is higher than that for vasopressin release to conserve water. In evolutionary terms, this has allowed us to move away from watering holes as we can adjust plasma water content without constant thirst. Some hormones involved in fluid balance, including angiotensin II, can also stimulate thirst directly.

Factors that regulate fluid balance

Fluid balance is regulated by controlling the intake and excretion of water and sodium. Hormones regulate this balance by acting on:

Fig. 7.3 Expected intake and output of water over a 24-hour period

Water intake (mL)	Water loss (mL)
Drinking: 1500 Food: 500 Metabolism: 400	Urine: 1500 Respiration: 400 Skin evaporation: 400 Faeces: 100
Total: 2400	Total: 2400

- Thirst—stimulated in the hypothalamus.
- Volume and concentration of water excreted in the urine.
- Peripheral resistance, which affects blood pressure.

There are four main hormones that regulate fluid balance; their sites and actions on the kidney nephron are shown in Fig. 7.4:

- Antidiuretic hormone (ADH; vasopressin)—conserves water.
- Renin—stimulates angiotensin II synthesis, effects an increase in peripheral resistance in response to hypovolaemia and stimulates aldosterone release.
- Angiotensin II—conserves sodium and, therefore, water.
- Aldosterone—conserves sodium and, therefore, water.

The response to these hormones can be altered in different contexts, such as fear or cardiac overload, and this contextual information is relayed by other hormones, nerves and chemical factors, including:

- Atrial natriuretic factor (ANF).
- Renal sympathetic nerves and catecholamines.
- Kinins.
- Prostaglandins.
- Dopamine.

HORMONES INVOLVED IN FLUID BALANCE

Antidiuretic hormone

ADH (or vasopressin) acts on the kidney to conserve water. It increases the permeability of the collecting ducts so that more water is reabsorbed, resulting in the production of more concentrated urine. ADH also induces a rise in peripheral resistance by stimulating arteriolar constriction—hence vasopressin, the old name for this hormone. ADH regulates fluid balance

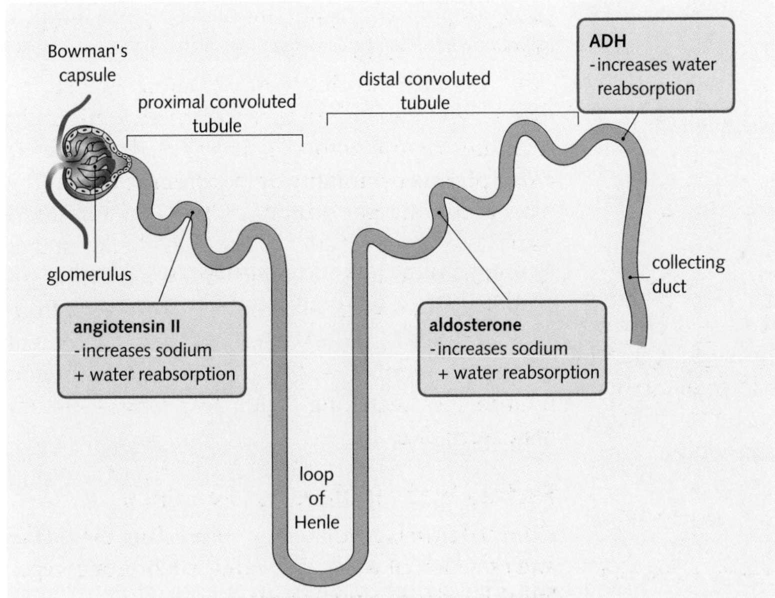

Fig. 7.4 Location and type of action by the three major hormones in the kidney nephron. (ADH, antidiuretic hormone.)

by influencing the movement of water directly, not through sodium movement. Although it does cause some fluid retention its main role is in maintaining water balance and not plasma volume. The regulation and actions of ADH are shown in Fig. 7.1.

Synthesis and secretion

ADH is a polypeptide hormone synthesized by neurosecretory cells in the supraoptic nucleus of the hypothalamus. It is transported along their axons to the posterior pituitary gland, where it is stored in vesicles. This process is described in more detail in Chapter 2.

ADH is secreted by the posterior pituitary gland in response to stimuli which reflect a loss of intravascular water:

- High plasma osmolality (concentrated blood).
- Low blood volume.

ADH is rapidly degraded by the liver and kidney enabling tight control of water balance.

Intracellular actions

ADH acts on G-protein-linked vasopressin receptors (V receptors) found on the cell surface of target cells. These target cells are found in two tissue types:

- Kidney—ADH acts on V_2 receptors, which use cAMP as a second messenger to cause recruitment of aquaporins (water channels) to the apical membrane. These channels increase uptake of water from the collecting duct to the renal medulla.
- Blood vessels—ADH acts on V_1 receptors causing smooth muscle contraction (i.e. vasoconstriction). Inositol triphosphate (IP_3) acts as a second messenger causing calcium levels to rise and ultimately resulting in vasoconstriction.

Effects

On the kidneys

ADH is secreted in response to high blood osmolality. It increases the reabsorption of water at the kidney by increasing the permeability of the collecting duct. This allows a disproportionate reabsorption of water relative to sodium such that blood osmolality decreases and concentrated urine is produced.

On the blood vessels

ADH is also secreted in response to low blood volume. It causes arteriolar vasoconstriction, which increases peripheral resistance and raises blood pressure. This action is not usually involved in the regulation of physiological blood pressures, but it is an important response to the reduction of blood volume associated with severe haemorrhage.

Deficiency and excess

ADH deficiency causes diabetes insipidus, in which excess dilute urine is produced causing fluid loss, dehydration, and high plasma osmolarity due to hypernatraemia.

ADH excess is called the 'syndrome of inappropriate ADH secretion (SIADH)', and results in water retention.

Both of these conditions are described in more detail in Chapter 2.

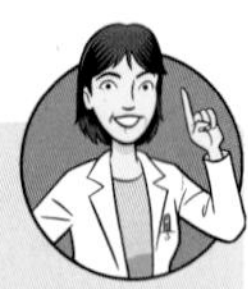

ADH secretion is inhibited by alcohol, causing large volumes of dilute urine to be excreted, resulting in dehydration the next morning.

The renin–angiotensin system

The main hormones involved in pressure-volume regulation form the renin–angiotensin II system. Renin forms part of an autoregulatory feedback loop, as it is secreted in response to low tubular sodium content or low perfusion pressure and its downstream effectors act on the kidney to conserve sodium and water. The principal downstream effector is angiotensin II, which increases reabsorption of sodium and therefore water in the proximal tubules of the kidney. Angiotensin II also increases peripheral resistance and aldosterone release. The regulation and actions of renin and angiotensin II are shown in Fig. 7.4.

Synthesis and secretion of renin

Renin is a small peptide enzyme secreted by the cells of the juxtaglomerular complex. This structure is made of three cell types (Fig. 7.5):

- Macula densa—part of the distal tubule of the nephron that detects sodium.
- Juxtaglomerular cells—part of the afferent and efferent glomerular arterioles that releases renin.
- Extraglomerular mesangial or lacis cells.

The function of this structure is complex; however, it can detect both sodium in the distal convoluted

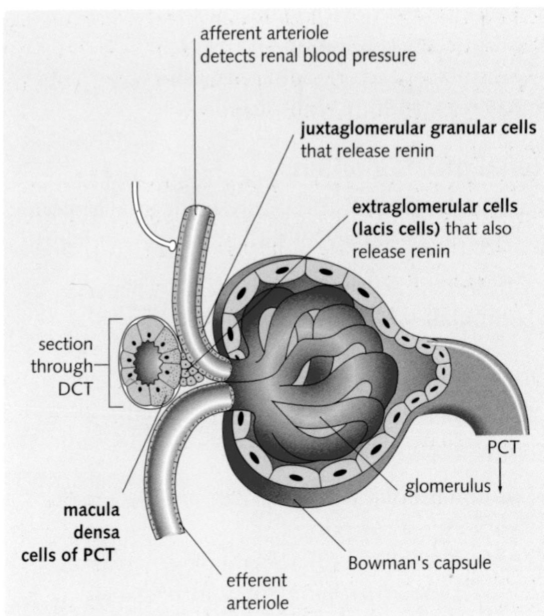

Fig. 7.5 Structure of the juxtaglomerular complex. (DCT, distal convoluted tubule, lying very close to the afferent and efferent arterioles; PCT, proximal convoluted tubule.)

tubule and blood pressure. The juxtaglomerular cells secrete renin in response to low blood pressure.

Effects of renin

Renin is an enzyme that acts on a plasma protein called angiotensinogen, synthesized by the liver. It cleaves this protein to form angiotensin I, which is then rapidly converted to angiotensin II by the action of angiotensin-converting enzyme (ACE) in the blood. ACE is a major site of action for the ACE inhibitor class of antihypertensive drugs.

Haemorrhage, dehydration, salt loss and renal artery stenosis all generate a stimulus for the juxtaglomerular cells to secrete renin. In most cases, this is a useful response to conserve water. However, in renal artery stenosis, the response is maladaptive and results in inappropriate sodium and water retention. Prostaglandins are involved in regulating the tone of the renal arterioles. Non-steroidal anti-inflammatory (NSAID) drugs, such as ibuprofen, inhibit prostaglandins which can lead to renin release and resultant sodium and water retention.

Effects of angiotensin II

Angiotensin II has four important actions, which serve to increase blood volume and pressure to appropriate levels:

- Stimulating aldosterone release from the adrenal cortex which activates pumps in the proximal tubule to increase sodium reabsorption, thereby increasing water reabsorption.
- Peripheral vasoconstriction to raise blood pressure.
- Stimulating sensation of thirst in the hypothalamus.
- Inhibiting renin release (negative feedback).

Thus, angiotensin II conserves sodium and water and raises the blood pressure.

ACE inhibitors inhibit production of angiotensin II, causing lower blood volume and reduced peripheral resistance. Both actions decrease blood pressure, so these drugs are used to treat hypertension and heart failure. ACE inhibitors also act on other substrates, including kinins, which are thought to contribute to the hypotensive effect. Angiotensin receptor blockers (ARBs), which do not reduce kinin levels are also used in the treatment of hypertension.

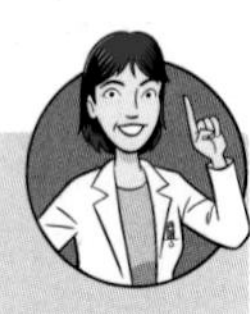

The main site of ACE action and angiotensin II synthesis is the endothelium of the capillaries in the lung.

Aldosterone

Aldosterone is a mineralocorticoid steroid hormone synthesized by the zona glomerulosa cells of the adrenal cortex. The main stimulus for secretion is angiotensin II, so it is often considered part of the renin–angiotensin II system. Other factors that inhibit the synthesis of aldosterone include heparin, atrial natriuretic factor (ANF) and dopamine. Aldosterone causes the conservation of sodium and water. See Chapter 4 for a complete description of aldosterone and the associated disorders. The regulation and actions of aldosterone are shown in Figs 7.2 and 7.4.

Intracellular actions

Aldosterone acts on intracellular receptors in the distal convoluted tube of the kidney. It causes sodium to be reabsorbed in exchange for potassium. Water follows the movement of sodium as the internal concentration increases, and is reabsorbed.

Effects

Aldosterone is secreted in response to high potassium or reduced blood volume through the action of renin and angiotensin II. It acts to conserve sodium and water, thereby restoring to equilibrium those parameters that stimulate its release.

Other hormones involved in the regulation of fluid balance

Natriuretic factors

Natriuresis is the excretion of an excessive amount of sodium in the urine and diuresis is the production of large quantity of urine. Natriuretic factors have a diuretic effect, the opposite effect of ADH, angiotensin II and aldosterone. They increase sodium excretion, resulting in concomitant water excretion. This causes blood volume to decrease and blood pressure to drop. Natriuretic factors act as an 'escape mechanism' to prevent excess water retention. Inappropriate natriuresis leads to a salt-losing syndrome entailing dehydration, hypotension and even sudden death.

Atrial natriuretic factor (ANF)

ANF is a polypeptide hormone synthesized and stored in atrial myocytes and released in response to cardiac muscle distension. ANF levels therefore correlate with hypervolaemic states and are emerging as an important prognostic marker in heart failure.

The main actions of ANF are to stimulate natriuresis and diuresis and to reduce blood pressure by:

- Decreasing sodium and water reabsorption by kidneys.
- Inhibiting renin, vasopressin and aldosterone secretion.
- Stimulating vasodilatation.

Kinins

Kinins are potent vasoactive polypeptides formed in the blood vessels by the action of the enzyme kallikrein on the precursor kininogen. They act in the kidney to:

- Inhibit the action of ADH.
- Stimulate vasodilation.
- Stimulate prostaglandin synthesis.
- Decrease sodium reabsorption.

Renal prostaglandins

Renal prostaglandins are locally acting lipid molecules synthesized by kidney cells. They act in the kidney to:

- Inhibit the action of ADH and aldosterone.
- Stimulate vasodilatation in the kidney.

Dopamine

Dopamine is an amine synthesized in the proximal tubule cells. It acts in the kidneys to:

- Inhibit tubular Na^+/K^+-ATPase and decrease sodium reabsorption.
- Induce renal vasodilation thereby increasing renal blood flow, glomerular filtration rate, natriuresis and diuresis.

DISORDERS OF FLUID BALANCE

A deficiency of water is called dehydration; it may or may not be accompanied by sodium deficiency. The causes and effects of dehydration are shown in Fig. 7.6.

An excess of water is called fluid retention; it may or may not be accompanied by an excess of sodium. The causes and effects of fluid retention are shown in Fig. 7.7.

Intravenous fluid replacement in patients otherwise unable to acquire fluids is essential. Normal daily fluid requirements (2400 mL) must be maintained and in addition extraordinary losses from haemorrhage, vomit or other causes must be restored. The principal fluid categories are crystalloids, colloids and blood products. Crystalloids include normal saline (0.9%), which is used to replace water and sodium but long-term use results in a drop in oncotic pressure and interstitial fluid accumulation (oedema).

Fig. 7.6 Causes and effects of dehydration

		Deficient sodium and water	Deficient water
Cause	Deficient input	Decreased ingestion, e.g. unconscious	Unable to find water, hypothalamic thirst disorder
	Excess output	Diarrhoea, vomiting, burns, haemorrhage, aldosterone deficiency	Diabetes insipidus and mellitus
Effect	Plasma osmolarity	No change	Raised
	Symptoms	Thirst, postural dizziness, weakness, collapse, headache, apathy, confusion, coma	
	Signs	Hypotension, tachycardia, slow capillary refill, reduced skin turgor, cool peripheries, sunken eyes, dry membranes, weight loss	

Fig. 7.7 Causes and effects of fluid retention

		Excess sodium and water	Excess water
Cause	Excess input	Excess fluid transfusion	Excess drinking, e.g. psychological
	Deficient output	Cardiac or renal failure	Acute renal failure or SIADH
Effect	Plasma osmolarity	No change, causes oedema	Decreased, no oedema
	Symptoms	Nausea, vomiting, anorexia, muscle weakness, headache, apathy, confusion, fits, coma	
	Signs	Hypertension, raised JVP, displaced apex beat	

JVP, jugular venous pressure.

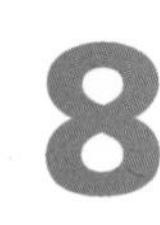

Endocrine control of calcium homeostasis

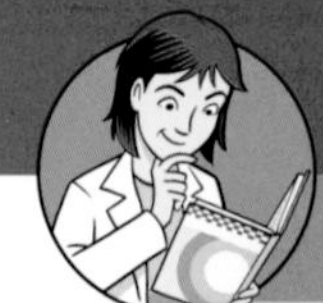

Objectives

By the end of this chapter you should be able to:

- Explain what happens when blood calcium levels rise.
- Explain what happens when blood calcium levels fall.
- Describe the action of parathyroid hormone on the kidneys, bones and intestines.
- Describe the action of vitamin D on the kidneys, bones and intestines.
- Recall how vitamin D is activated and which hormone controls this process.
- Describe the action of calcitonin on the kidneys, bones and intestines.
- Describe the difference between primary, secondary and tertiary hyperparathyroidism and recall the disorders that commonly cause these conditions.
- List the symptoms caused by primary hyperparathyroidism; do calcium levels rise or fall?
- List the symptoms caused by secondary hyperparathyroidism; do calcium levels rise or fall?
- List the symptoms and causes of hypoparathyroidism.

Hormones play an important role in the regulation of several mineral ions, notably calcium, phosphate and magnesium. Calcium is a cofactor for enzymatic reactions, a common intracellular signalling molecule and is essential for nerve conduction and skeletal, cardiac and smooth muscle contraction. Serum calcium levels must be tightly regulated to maintain these processes and prevent complications such as cardiac arrest. Hormones serve to maintain calcium homeostasis through their actions on the uptake of calcium in the intestines, release of calcium from the bone and excretion of calcium through the kidneys.

Blood calcium levels are regulated by three hormones (Fig. 8.1):

- Parathyroid hormone (PTH)—raises blood calcium levels.
- Vitamin D—raises calcium intake from the gastrointestinal tract.
- Calcitonin—raises calcium excretion and lowers blood levels.

PTH is the most important of these hormones. Calcium-sensing receptors on the parathyroid cells monitor serum calcium and release PTH in response to increased serum calcium. PTH, in turn, acts on the intestine, bone and kidneys to increase serum calcium. An excess or deficiency of this hormone can cause hyper- and hypocalcaemia, respectively.

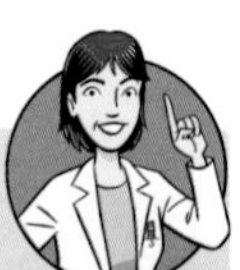

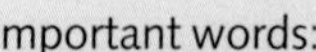

Important words:
Hyperparathyroidism: an excess of parathyroid hormone
Osteoclast: a cell that breaks down bone, releasing calcium
Osteoblast: a cell that lays down bone using calcium
Reabsorption: when substances are reclaimed from the kidney tubule after being filtered out of the blood.

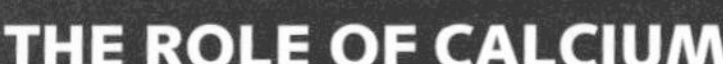

THE ROLE OF CALCIUM

Calcium is a mineral obtained from the diet and excreted by the kidneys. Ninety-nine per cent of the total body calcium is in bone. The remaining 1% can be exchanged freely between plasma and the extracellular and intracellular compartments. Forty per cent of serum calcium is bound to albumin, a further 10% is bound to other proteins and the rest is in an unbound ionized form. Calcium is essential for:

- Bone mineralization acting in concert with phosphate ions (PO_4^-).
- Skeletal, cardiac and smooth muscle contraction.
- All processes that involve exocytosis, including synaptic transmission and hormone release.

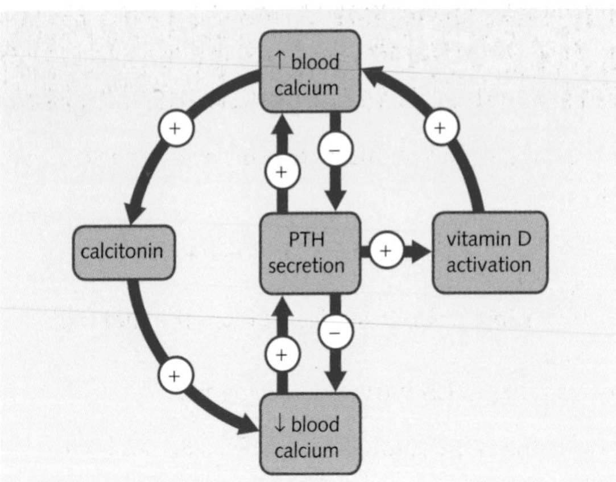

Fig. 8.1 Hormonal regulation of blood calcium by parathyroid hormone (PTH), vitamin D and calcitonin.

- Enzymatic reactions.
- Intracellular signalling.

The processes requiring calcium are described in Fig. 8.2.

MECHANISMS INVOLVED IN CALCIUM HOMEOSTASIS

Calcium intake

The recommended daily allowance (RDA) of calcium is 1 g for normal adults, 1.2 g for pregnant women. If an individual is effectively maintaining the calcium balance, only 20% of the dietary calcium is absorbed. Absorption is influenced by:

- Diet—lactose in milk increases absorption, phytic acid in brown bread decreases absorption.
- Age—absorption is increased in the young and decreased in the elderly.
- Hormones—vitamin D increases absorption.
- Pregnancy and lactation—both increase absorption.

Calcium balance

Calcium balance is calculated as absorbed calcium minus excreted calcium. This balance is affected by age and some diseases:

- Children usually have a positive calcium balance; this allows bones to grow.
- In adults, input and output should be the same.
- Postmenopausal women tend to have a negative calcium balance (i.e. calcium is lost).

Calcium in the blood

Calcium levels must be maintained within tight limits and the normal range of total serum calcium is 2.12–2.65 mmol/L. Dietary intake is variable, so the body must be able to adapt to increased or reduced plasma calcium. Calcium regulation involves the loss or gain of calcium via three tissues: kidneys, intestines and bones.

Fig. 8.2 Processes that require calcium

System	Rde of calcium
Bone formation	Calcium is a vital mineral component of bone; it makes the bone strong and rigid
Blood clotting	Many clotting factors are activated by calcium
Muscle contraction	Calcium binds to troponin, which allows myosin to bind to actin
Intracellular signalling	Calcium regulates the activity of a number of intracellular proteins in response to the second messenger IP_3
Nervous system	Calcium is essential for membrane potential and depolarization; synapses use calcium to release neurotransmitters
Endocrine system	All processes that involve exocytosis (e.g. hormone secretion) require calcium
Cardiovascular system	Calcium regulates the membrane potential and contraction of muscle cells

The movements and distribution of calcium in the body are shown in Fig. 8.3. The movements are regulated by the three hormones discussed below.

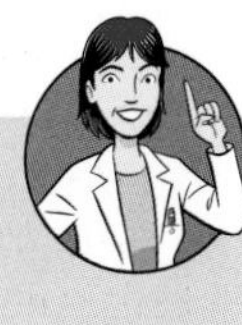

Bones structures are dynamic and bone is constantly being broken down and remodelled.

Forty per cent of plasma calcium is bound to albumin. Diseases that lower plasma albumin (e.g. cirrhosis or myeloma) can increase unbound (i.e. active) calcium levels, causing symptoms of hypercalcaemia. When measuring plasma calcium levels, it is total blood calcium that is measured. Albumin levels must be taken into account to calculate unbound, corrected calcium levels.

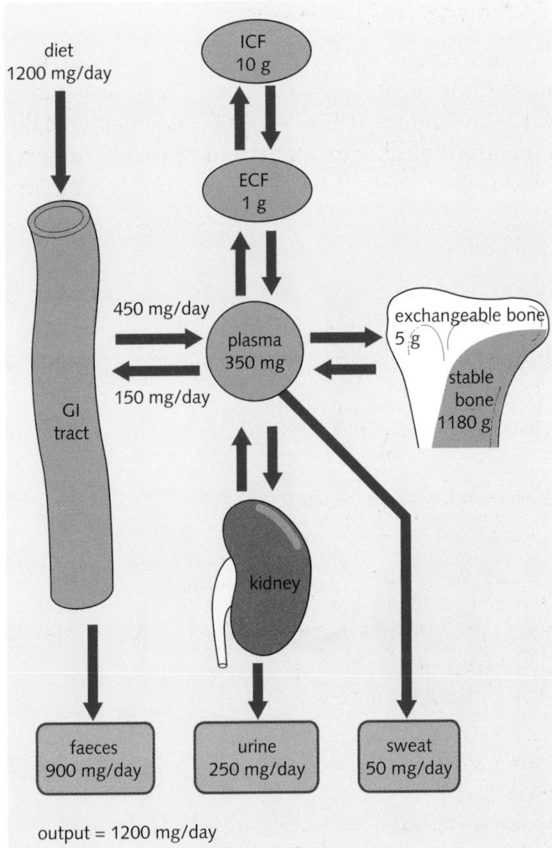

Fig. 8.3 Normal distribution and movements of calcium in the body. (ECF, extracellular fluid; GI, gastrointestinal; ICF, intracellular fluid.)

HORMONES INVOLVED IN CALCIUM HOMEOSTASIS

Three hormones regulate calcium levels in the blood and tissues:

- Parathyroid hormone from the parathyroid gland.
- Vitamin D (cholecalciferol) from the diet and skin.
- Calcitonin from the thyroid gland.

Their effects are summarized in Figs 8.1 and 8.4.

Parathyroid hormone and the parathyroid glands

PTH is essential for life and is synthesized by the chief cells in the parathyroid glands. The four small glands are found behind the thyroid gland in the neck. The principal effects of PTH are to increase serum calcium and reduce serum phosphate.

PTH is released in response to low blood calcium. Its actions are aimed at raising calcium levels back to their normal physiological concentration. Once blood calcium levels are restored, PTH production is inhibited.

Parathyroid glands

Blood supply, nerves and lymphatics

The parathyroid glands are four oval-shaped structures about 5 mm across; they are embedded in the thyroid capsule behind both lateral lobes. These glands are described as superior and inferior pairs. The number of parathyroid glands often varies between 2 and 6 and the location of the inferior pair differs widely. They are supplied by branches of the inferior thyroid artery.

Microstructure

There are three cell types in the parathyroid glands:

- Chief cells—synthesize parathyroid hormone (PTH).
- Oxyphil cells—are inactive endocrinologically, but they can form Hurthle cell carcinomas.
- Adipocytes—contain fat and their numbers also increase with age.

Development

The parathyroid glands are endodermal structures that develop from the pharyngeal pouches. The inferior parathyroid glands are formed by the dorsal portion of the 3rd pouch while the dorsal portion of the 4th pouch forms the superior parathyroid glands.

Fig. 8.4 Summary of the actions of parathyroid hormone (PTH), calcitonin, and vitamin D on calcium regulation

	PTH	Vitamin D	Calcitonin
Secreted/activated in response to:	Low blood calcium	PTH	High blood calcium
Kidneys	Calcium reabsorbed; vitamin D activated	Calcium reabsorbed	Calcium excreted
Bones	Calcium released	Calcium trapped	Calcium trapped
Intestines	Negligible	Calcium absorbed	Negligible

Parathyroid hormone

Synthesis and receptors

PTH is a polypeptide hormone synthesized as pre-pro-parathyroid hormone. Two cleavage reactions leave PTH, a protein of 84 amino acid residues. Low plasma calcium triggers the release of PTH from vesicles, upregulation of PTH transcription and, under conditions of chronic hypocalcaemia, can stimulate the chief cells to proliferate. Under normal conditions, calcium inhibits PTH release at near maximal capacity. The system is therefore well suited to adapt to a sudden fall more than a sudden rise in plasma calcium.

PTH acts via G-protein linked receptors on the cell surface. These receptors are found on osteoblasts, renal tubule cells and cells in the intestinal epithelium. The receptors use cyclic AMP (cAMP) as a second messenger to regulate the phosphorylation of intracellular proteins. These proteins are either activated or deactivated as a result; this brings about the effects of PTH.

Actions

PTH is the most important regulator of blood calcium levels. The actions of PTH on calcium regulation are shown in Fig. 8.5.

On the kidneys

PTH has three major effects:

- Increase of calcium ion reabsorption by stimulating active uptake in the distal convoluted tubule.
- Increase of phosphate ion excretion by inhibiting uptake in the proximal and distal convoluted tubules.
- Stimulation of 1α-hydroxylase, an enzyme that activates vitamin D.

On the bones

PTH causes the release of calcium from the bone. PTH stimulates osteoblast proliferation and differentiation and therefore increases bone production. PTH receptors are not found on osteoclasts but these cells are stimulated indirectly by factors released by the activated osteoblasts. Upregulation of osteoclastic activity causes increased bone breakdown. The resultant increase in bone turnover can have different effects on net bone mass but always results in increased serum calcium. The actions are:

- Direct inhibition of osteoblast collagen synthesis.
- Indirect stimulation of osteoclast bone erosion.
- Increased collagenase synthesis to erode the bone.
- Increased hydrogen ion release to create an acidic environment to enhance bone erosion.

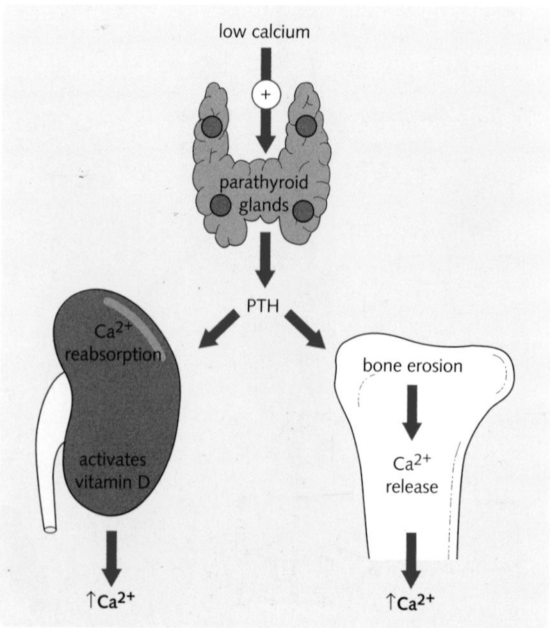

Fig. 8.5 Actions of parathyroid hormone (PTH) on the kidney and bone.

On the intestines

PTH may have a direct action on calcium absorption in the upper small intestine, but this is unproven. The major effects are indirect, through the activation of vitamin D.

Vitamin D

Vitamin D is absorbed by the small intestine as part of the diet (e.g. dairy food) or is synthesized from cholesterol in the skin. Vitamin D synthesis requires ultraviolet (UV) light, usually derived from the sun. Vitamin D is the major determinant of intestinal calcium and phosphate reabsorption.

Activation

Human vitamin D is an inactive steroid called cholecalciferol (or vitamin D_3); this fat-soluble steroid is stored in adipose tissue. Two reactions must take place in different organs to activate vitamin D; they are shown in Fig. 8.6.

The activated vitamin D (1,25-dihydroxy cholecalciferol) molecule is shown in Fig. 8.7. It can be inactivated by 24-hydroxylase found in the kidney. This enzyme catalyses the formation of 1,24,25-trihydroxycholecalciferol, which is rapidly excreted.

All forms of vitamin D are transported in the blood by a specific plasma protein or within chylomicrons. Vitamin D is fat soluble, so it can cross cell membranes. It acts via specific intracellular receptors that are found in the same locations as PTH receptors.

Actions

The actions of vitamin D on calcium regulation are shown in Fig. 8.8.

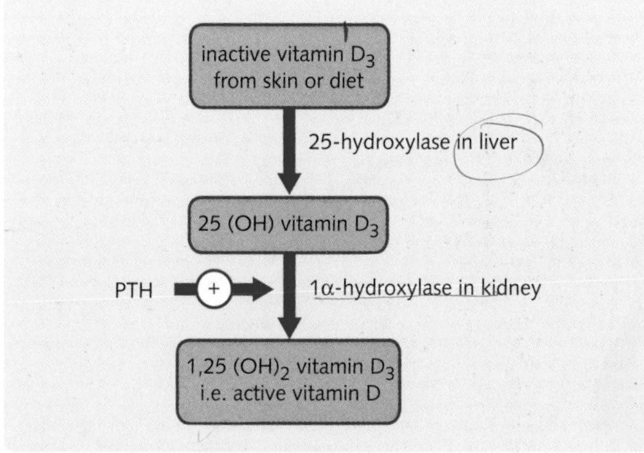

Fig. 8.6 Activation of vitamin D. (25 (OH) vitamin D_3, 25-hydroxyvitamin D_3; 1,25 $(OH)_2$ vitamin D_3, 1,25-dihydroxyvitamin D_3.)

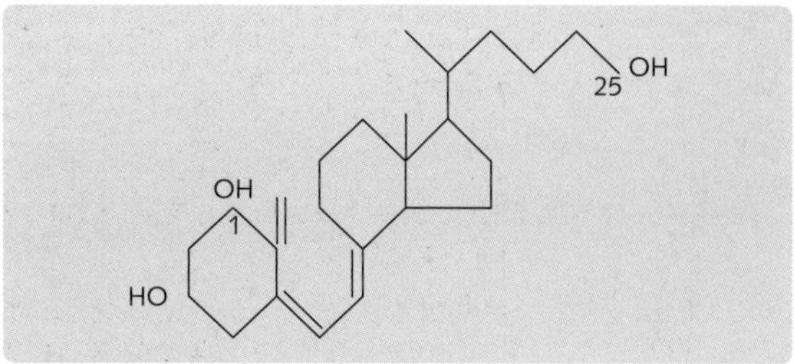

Fig. 8.7 Structure of 1,25-dihydroxyvitamin D_3, the active form of vitamin D.

On the kidney

Activated vitamin D has three effects:

- Increase of calcium reabsorption in the proximal and distal convoluted tubule.
- Increase of phosphate reabsorption in the proximal convoluted tubule.
- Inhibition of 1α-hydroxylase activity. This is a form of negative feedback.

On the bones

Vitamin D affects bone remodelling by modulating calcium levels and by directly stimulating osteoblast activity to increase bone mass and calcification. Disorders of vitamin D absorption or activation can results in inadequate mineralization of bones (rickets in children or osteomalacia in adults) If this is due to kidney disease, it is called renal osteodystrophy (discussed later).

On the intestines

The main action of vitamin D is stimulation of active calcium and phosphate absorption in the duodenum and jejunum. The exact mechanism is unclear, but vitamin D increases the synthesis of calcium-binding proteins in the intestinal cells. This action on the intestines takes a long time to produce an effect, so it does not raise calcium levels acutely.

Calcitonin

Calcitonin is secreted by the parafollicular cells (C cells) in the thyroid gland. The development and anatomy of this gland is described in Chapter 3. Calcitonin is secreted in response to high blood calcium, and it lowers calcium levels. It is not essential to life, but it acts to fine tune blood calcium levels.

Synthesis and receptors

Calcitonin is a polypeptide hormone that is formed by the breakdown of a larger prohormone. Calcitonin is stored in secretory vesicles, from which it is released

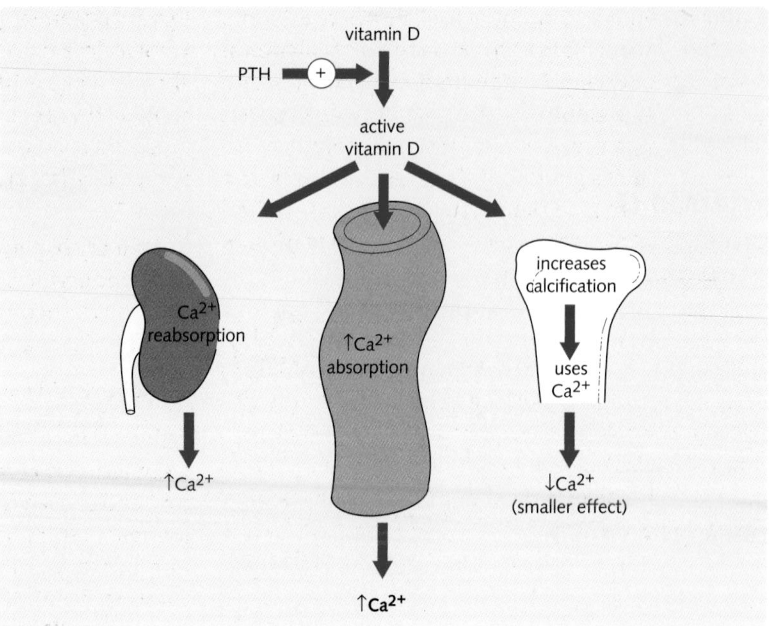

Fig. 8.8 Actions of vitamin D on the gastrointestinal tract, bone (PTH, parathyroid hormone.) and kidney.

when blood calcium levels rise. Rising calcium is detected by the same calcium-sensing receptor which is present on parathyroid cells.

Calcitonin acts on G-protein coupled receptors that release cAMP to bring about cellular effects.

Actions

The actions of calcitonin on calcium regulation are shown in Fig. 8.9.

On the kidney

Calcitonin inhibits the reabsorption of calcium and phosphate. These ions are excreted as a result.

On the bones

Calcitonin acts primarily on osteoclasts in the bone. It inhibits these cells to prevent all stages of bone erosion. This prevents calcium and phosphate release into the blood, so their levels are lowered.

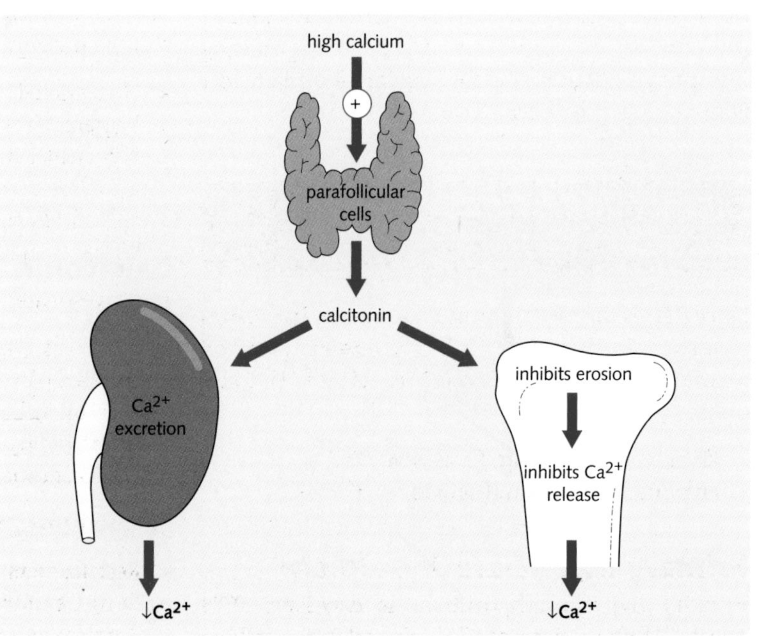

Fig. 8.9 Actions of calcitonin on the kidney and bone.

Calcitonin is not essential for calcium regulation, and there are no clinical consequences of calcitonin deficiency or excess. Neither removal of the thyroid gland with its parafollicular cells at thyroidectomy nor calcitonin-secreting medullary cell malignancy affect calcium balance significantly. Calcitonin is used therapeutically to reduce pain associated with vertebral fractures and to treat Paget's disease (a condition of excessive bone resorption).

Never give the antibiotic tetracycline to young children, as it binds to calcium in their teeth, making them yellow. In adults, milk should not be used to swallow tablets of tetracycline.

Phosphate

Calcium and phosphate are regulated by similar processes and together they constitute 65% of the weight of bone. They form hydroxyapatite crystals, which mineralize the bone and give it strength. Phosphate is also an essential component of nucleic acids, phospholipid membranes, ATP and signalling molecules. PTH-induced bone resorption causes the release of phosphate. However, phosphate lowers ionized calcium levels and therefore antagonizes the calcium-raising ability of PTH. This potential antagonism is overcome by PTH concomitantly exerting a strong phosphaturic action, thereby keeping phosphate low whilst trying to raise serum calcium.

DISORDERS OF CALCIUM REGULATION

Since PTH is the most important hormone in calcium homeostasis, disorders of this system are grouped according to their effect on PTH release. The two groups are:

- Hyperparathyroidism (excess of PTH).
- Hypoparathyroidism (deficiency of PTH).

Primary hyperparathyroidism

Primary hyperparathyroidism is excessive PTH release. All the actions of PTH raise calcium levels so hypercalcaemia (excess blood calcium) results. Hypercalcaemia and excess PTH cause the symptoms shown in Fig. 8.10. Prolonged hyperparathyroidism causes bone demineralization and softening, called osteomalacia in adults and rickets in children. The symptoms and signs of these diseases are shown in Fig. 8.11.

Primary hyperparathyroidism is a relatively common endocrine disorder (about 1 in 1000 people), and it is especially common in postmenopausal women. The main causes are:

- Parathyroid gland adenoma (80%).
- Diffuse parathyroid gland hyperplasia (15%).

Neoplastic chief cells are not inhibited by high calcium, and consequently PTH secretion is unregulated. Malignant tumours of the parathyroid gland are very rare, but they can be associated with other endocrine tumours in multiple endocrine neoplasia (MEN) syndromes. These are discussed in Chapter 10.

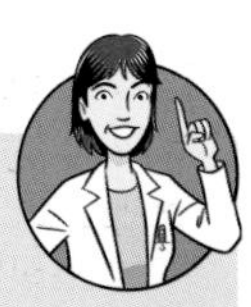

When clerking a patient with suspected hypercalcaemia, remember: 'Bones, stones, abdominal groans and psychic moans'.

Diagnosis and treatment

Primary hyperparathyroidism is usually detected on routine testing and is suspected if a patient has:

- Unexpected bone weakness.
- Hypercalcaemia symptoms and signs.
- Hypercalcaemia on a blood test with low phosphate levels.
- Dehydration.
- Severe thirst.

It is investigated by:

- Blood test (increased plasma calcium and reduced plasma phosphate).
- Measuring blood PTH (increased).
- Radiography to show bone reabsorption.
- Radioisotope scanning of the parathyroid glands.

There are three treatment options:

- Restrict dietary calcium.
- Drug treatment (e.g. calcitonin).
- Surgical removal of the parathyroid gland(s).

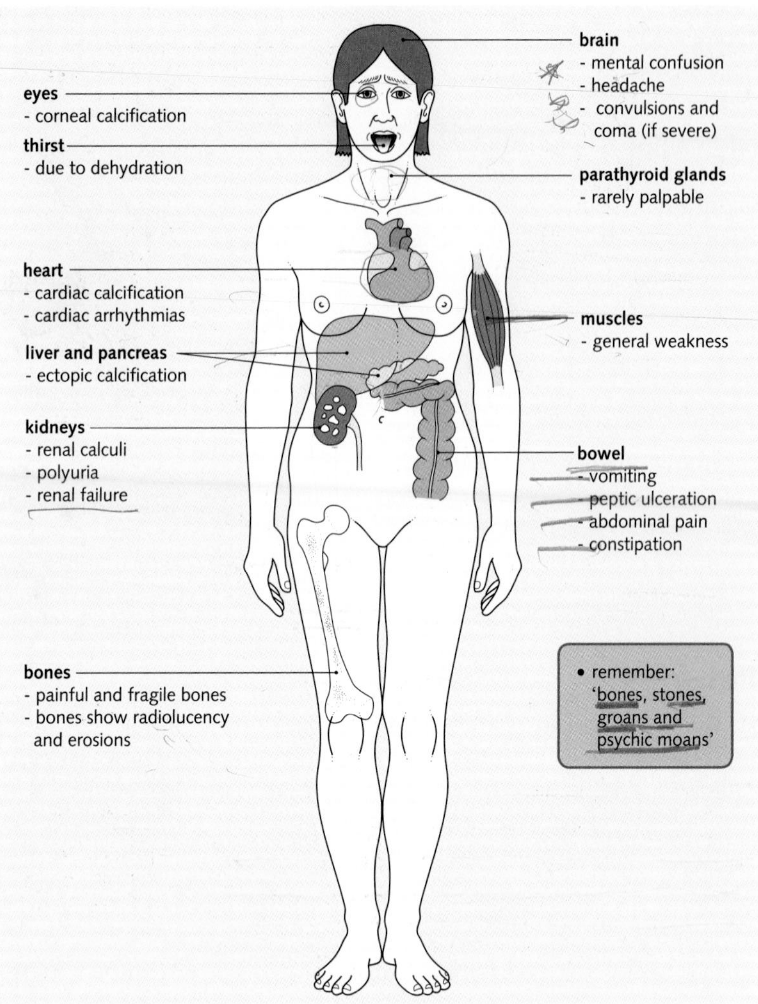

Fig. 8.10 Symptoms and signs of hypercalcaemia.

Fig. 8.11 Signs and symptoms caused by rickets and osteomalacia

Rickets (childhood)	Osteomalacia (adulthood)
'Knock-knees' or 'bow-legs' caused by bending of the long bones	Bone pain
Chest deformities, back deformities (e.g. kyphosis) and protruding forehead	Bones appear 'thin' on X-ray, with localized lucencies (called Looser's zones)
Features of hypocalcaemia	Fractures (common in the neck of the femur)
	Features of hypocalcaemia (e.g. proximal myopathy causes waddling gait)

Secondary hyperparathyroidism

Many diseases can cause hypocalcaemia (e.g. chronic renal failure), which stimulates PTH secretion as a compensatory response. If hypocalcaemia is prolonged, the parathyroid glands can enlarge by hyperplasia to secrete excess PTH. This is called secondary hyperparathyroidism.

Osteomalacia is also a feature of secondary hyperparathyroidism because of the excess PTH. Hypocalcaemia and excess PTH cause the symptoms shown in Fig. 8.12.

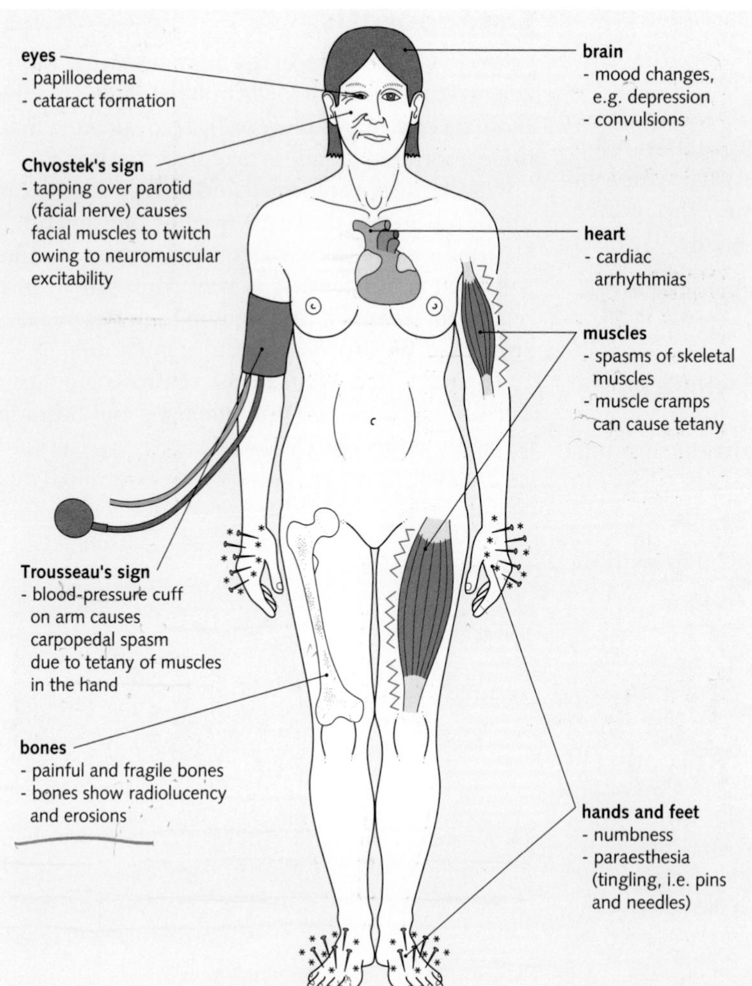

Fig. 8.12 Symptoms and signs of hypocalcaemia.

Causes of secondary hyperparathyroidism

Hypocalcaemia can be caused by:

- Chronic renal failure.
- Vitamin D deficiency.

In chronic renal failure, the kidneys fail to reabsorb calcium. Renal osteodystrophy can also develop as a result of impaired 1α-hydroxylase activity. Reduced filtration causes hyperphosphataemia, which in turn causes reduced production of $1,25(OH)_2D_3$. Reduced $1,25(OH)_2D_3$ stimulates PTH, which causes calcium release and bone turnover. The bones become demineralized as a consequence of PTH activity. Furthermore, metastatic calcification (calcification in inappropriate places) occurs due to the combination of high serum calcium and phosphate.

Vitamin D deficiency can occur if the diet is deficient in vitamin D or the skin does not receive sunlight (e.g. elderly people who stay indoors and only see the sun through glass, or women in cultures who cover their skin). Deficiency of activated vitamin D causes hypocalcaemia as a result of impaired calcium absorption in the intestines. There is a normal amount of bone but it does not mineralize fully—osteomalacia.

Tertiary hyperparathyroidism

Tertiary hyperparathyroidism is a complication of secondary hyperparathyroidism. Very rarely, an adenoma can develop in the hyperplastic parathyroid glands caused by prolonged hypocalcaemia. If the underlying cause of hypocalcaemia is corrected, then hypercalcaemia can develop due to excess PTH secretion. This complication is diagnosed and treated as a primary parathyroid adenoma.

Hypoparathyroidism

Hypoparathyroidism is the deficiency of PTH resulting in hypocalcaemia. It causes the usual symptoms of hypocalcaemia (see Fig. 8.12) but without osteomalacia. The main causes are listed below:

- Complication of thyroid or parathyroid surgery.
- Idiopathic hypoparathyroidism—an autoimmune disorder.
- Pseudohypoparathyroidism—congenital PTH resistance.
- Investigations reveal reduced serum calcium and increased serum phosphate.

Pseudohypoparathyroidism is the result of resistance to PTH and the patients have raised PTH with the symptoms of hypoparathyroidism.

> Hypocalcaemia may cause carpopedal spasm, which can be elicited by occluding the brachial artery with a blood-pressure cuff (Trousseau's sign). Hypocalacemia can also be demonstrated clinically by the twitching of facial muscles in response to a tap of the facial nerve (Chvostek's sign). If hypocalcaemia is suspected on clinical examination the common causes can be recalled using the mnemonic HARVARD: **H**ypoparathyroidism (also hyperphosphataemia and hypomagnesaemia), **A**cute pancreatitis, **R**enal failure, **V**itamin D_3 deficiency, **A**lkalosis, **R**habdomyolysis, **D**rugs (e.g. bisphosphonates).

Osteoporosis

Osteoporosis is the most common bone disease. It is characterized by inadequate bone mass and fragility. It can be caused by failure to reach peak bone mass, bone resorption or failure to replace lost bone.

New bone is not formed and microfractures cannot be repaired so the bones become thin and brittle. Osteoporosis is associated with deficiencies of androgens and oestrogens. It is very common in postmenopausal women, and signs of bone degeneration are seen in 100% of 80-year-old women.

The main treatments of osteoporosis are dietary calcium and vitamin D supplements and hormone replacement therapy (HRT; see Chapter 13). Calcitonin can be used; however, it is very expensive and it must be injected subcutaneously.

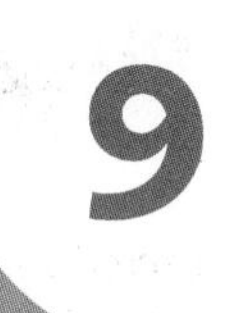

9 Endocrine control of growth

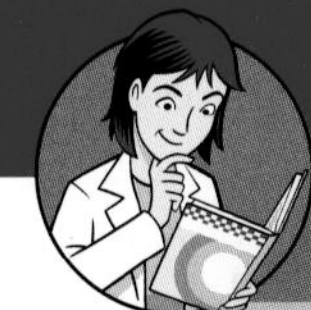

Objectives

By the end of this chapter you should be able to:

- Describe the regulation of growth hormone and IGF secretion.
- State the factors that stimulate the secretion of growth hormone.
- Describe the actions of IGFs on cells.
- Describe the actions of IGFs on the growth plate of bones.
- Name other factors that affect growth.
- Name four peptide growth factors, the tissue that secretes them, and where they have an effect.
- Understand how height is determined.
- Understand how the mean parental height is calculated, and what the boundaries of 'normal' height are from the MPH?
- List the symptoms of acromegaly.
- Understand how acromegaly is diagnosed.

Growth hormone (GH) is often described as a pituitary hormone that acts directly on tissues instead of stimulating peripheral endocrine tissues like other anterior pituitary hormones. This view has been challenged by the discovery of insulin-like growth factors (IGFs) secreted by the liver in response to GH. The regulation of growth, therefore, follows the conventional pattern starting in the hypothalamus (described in Chapter 2).

Growth is a process that takes place at many levels. It can be defined as an increase in:

- Anabolism (e.g. protein synthesis).
- Cell size and number.
- Cell maturation and maintenance.
- Organ size.
- Body size or weight.

Acting through IGFs, GH stimulates all the processes listed above. By promoting anabolic processes, the cell increases in size. This promotes cell division and maturation, causing the organ to grow. The cellular actions of GH begin before birth and continue throughout life, though the rate varies. The fastest rate of growth is in the fetus and neonate; however, a growth spurt also occurs during puberty.

The growth of the body is limited by the epiphyses (growth plates) at the ends of the long bones. GH stimulates these plates to grow, causing the bones to lengthen and body height to increase. It also stimulates fusion of these growth plates preventing further growth.

Important words:
Anabolism: the process of building large molecules from smaller ones
Epiphysis: the end of a long bone (plural, epiphyses)
Epiphyseal growth plate: an area of cartilage between the epiphysis and shaft of the bone that proliferates during childhood, resulting in elongation of the bone
Growth factor: any chemical that stimulates cellular growth
Cell maturation: when a cell differentiates to reach its final form

DIRECT CONTROL OF GROWTH

Growth hormone (GH)

GH (also called somatotrophin) is a polypeptide that is secreted by the somatotroph cells in the anterior pituitary gland. Like many pituitary hormones, it is synthesized as a precursor molecule (pre-progrowth hormone). Two cleavages release the active hormone. For more information about the anterior pituitary, see Chapter 2.

Regulation of secretion

GH secretion is regulated by two hypothalamic releasing factors:

- Growth-hormone releasing hormone (GHRH).
- Somatostatin (also called growth-hormone inhibiting hormone or GHIH).

GHRH is released in a pulsatile manner, especially during deep sleep or hypoglycaemia, and GH release follows this pattern. Secretion of GH from the anterior pituitary gland is also regulated by the negative feedback of IGF-1 and other growth factors (Fig. 9.1).

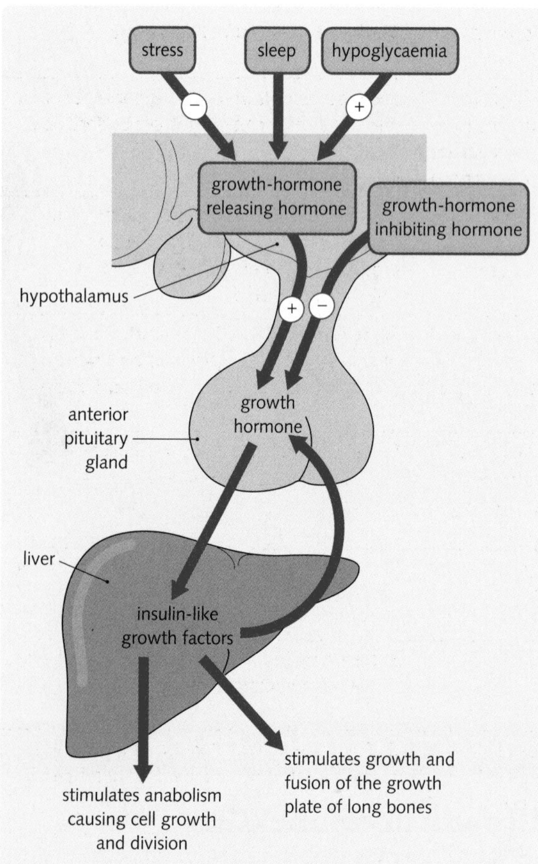

Fig. 9.1 Hormonal regulation of growth hormone.

Effects

GH promotes the growth and maintenance of most cells. It exerts most of its effects by:

- Stimulating the uptake of amino acids.
- Stimulating the synthesis of proteins.

GH exerts most of its effects via IGFs. GH promotes their synthesis, mainly in the liver but also in other tissues.

GH is transported in the blood bound to GH-binding protein. It acts via G-protein and Janus kinase (JAK) receptors on the cell surface of target cells.

Insulin-like growth factors

Insulin-like growth factors (IGFs or somatomedins) are polypeptide hormones that exist in two forms: IGF-1 and IGF-2. They resemble insulin in structure and they act through similar receptors. IGF-1 is more important as a stimulator of growth.

IGFs are transported in the blood by a number of IGF-binding proteins.

Metabolic actions

Both IGF hormones have some insulin-like actions, e.g. increasing amino-acid uptake and protein synthesis. However, they also oppose the actions of insulin on glucose by preventing glucose uptake and causing glycogen breakdown to raise blood glucose.

Growth actions

The increase in protein synthesis caused by the metabolic effects of IGF hormones causes cells to grow. This stimulates cell division and maturation, causing organs and soft tissues to enlarge.

The growth of the long bones depends on the state of the epiphyseal growth plate. This plate is a layer of chondrocytes (cartilage cells) located between the end (epiphysis) and shaft (diaphysis) of the bone (Fig. 9.2). Before puberty, IGFs stimulate these chondrocytes to grow, divide and mature into osteocytes (bone cells), allowing the bone to lengthen whilst maintaining a population of chondrocytes in the plate for further growth. During puberty, IGFs and sex steroids stimulate the chondrocytes within the plate to mature into osteocytes so that the epiphysis and diaphysis become fused together. The bone is no longer able to lengthen with further IGF stimulation so final adult height is reached.

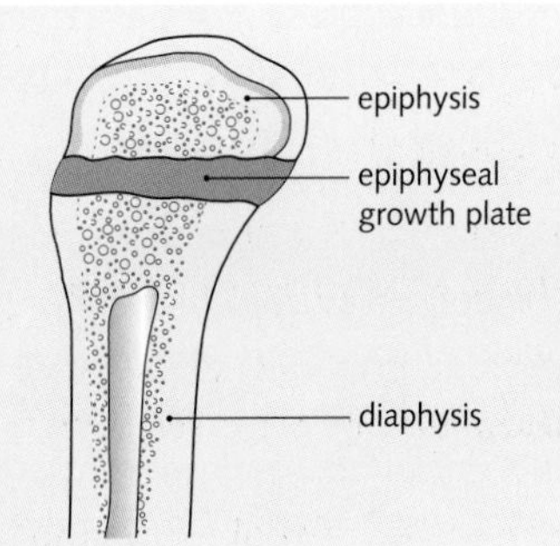

Fig. 9.2 The regions of a growing bone.

Other growth factors

Growth in specific tissues is also stimulated by a number of growth factors, many of which are small peptides that act in a paracrine (local) manner. Their relationship to GH is not known. The actions and secretion of several such peptides are described in Fig. 9.3.

INDIRECT CONTROL OF GROWTH

Many factors apart from GH control growth, including:

- Genetics—tall parents often have tall children.
- Adequate nutrition—however, excess nutrition does not increase height.
- Health—chronic disease affects height.
- Other hormones.

Other hormones

Growth problems can be caused by the abnormal secretion of a number of hormones, including:

- Insulin.
- Antidiuretic hormone (ADH).
- Parathyroid hormone and vitamin D.
- Cortisol.
- Sex steroids.

Fig. 9.3 The secretion of growth factors and their effects

Growth factor	Mode of delivery	Action on growth and development	Method and control of sectetion
Nerve growth factor (NGF)	Paracrine	Induces neuron growth and helps to guide growing sympathetic nerves to organs they will innervate (may also act on the brain and aid memory retention)	Secreted by cells in path of growing axon; regulation of secretion not yet understood
Epidermal growth factor (EGF)	Paracrine and endocrine	Promotes cell proliferation in the epidermis, maturation of lung epithelium and skin keratinization	Secreted by many cell types, i.e. not only epidermal cells (EGF is also found in breast milk); regulation of secretion not yet understood
Transforming growth factors (TGF-α, TGF-β)	Paracrine	Stimulate growth of fibroblast cells; TGF-α acts similarly to EGF; TGF-β especially affects chondrocytes, osteoblasts and osteoclasts	Secreted by most cell types but especially platelets and cells in placenta and bone; regulation of secretion not yet understood
Fibroblast growth factor (FGF)	Paracrine	Mitogenic effect in several cell types; may induce angiogenesis (formation of new blood vessels), which is essential for growth and wound healing	Secreted by most cell types; regulation of secretion not yet understood
Platelet-derived growth factor (PDGF)	Paracrine	Potent cell-growth promoter; chemotactic factor (involved in inflammatory response)	Secreted by activated blood platelets during blood-vessel injury
Erythropoietin	Endocrine	Stimulates the production of erythrocyte precursor cells	Secreted by the kidney in response to falling tissue oxygen concentration
Interleukins (IL) (33 known)	Autocrine and paracrine	IL-1 stimulates B-cell proliferation and helper T cells to produce IL-2; IL-2 autoactivates helper T cells and activates cytotoxic T cells	IL-1 is secreted by activated macrophages; IL-2 is secreted by activated helper T cells

Thyroid hormones

Thyroid hormones, described in Chapter 3, stimulate cell metabolism, promoting cell growth and division especially in the skeleton and developing central nervous system (CNS). Thyroid hormones also stimulate GH secretion from the pituitary.

Cortisol is described in Chapter 4; it inhibits pituitary GH secretion, so chronic ill health or stress can suppress growth.

Normal growth can only occur if both the hormonal milieu and the nutritional supply of proteins are suitable.

Fetal growth

In the fetus, a hormone called placental lactogen is secreted from the placenta. It stimulates fetal cartilage development and acts in a similar manner to prolactin on the maternal mammary glands.

Thyroid hormones are essential for the development of the skeleton and CNS. A deficiency in the fetus or neonate results in cretinism.

Puberty

Sexual maturation and the pubertal growth spurt are described in Chapter 11. The main hormones involved are:

- Gonadotrophins—luteinizing hormone (LH) and follicle-stimulating hormone (FSH).
- Sex steroids—oestrogen and testosterone, which stimulate increased IGF release, both directly and via increased GH.

DETERMINATION OF HEIGHT

A person's final height is determined simply by the rate and duration of growth.

During puberty, the epiphyseal growing plates at the end of the long bones begin to fuse. This fusion prevents further growth and, therefore, further height gain. Complete fusion occurs between 18 and 20 years of age in males, and earlier in females.

Fusion of the epiphyseal plates is stimulated primarily by GH and sex steroids; however, thyroid hormones also promote this effect. A simple increase in GH during puberty is not sufficient to increase final height since the bones simply mature faster and stop growing.

Only the bones that grow in this manner are prevented from responding to further GH. The jaw and skull can continue to grow past puberty; this effect is seen in GH excess. Ultimately, height is determined by multiple genetic factors.

Short stature, defined as a height less then the 5th centile, is associated with poor academic achievement and anxiety. Growth rates less than the 25th centile will result in a child dropping down centiles on a growth chart. Growth retardation can be primary, secondary or idiopathic. Primary disorders reflect an intrinsic bone defect and include achondroplasia and some causes of intrauterine growth retardation. Secondary disorders occur in the presence of other factors that limit bone growth. Malnutrition, chronic disease and endocrine disorders, such as Cushing's, can cause secondary growth retardation. Idiopathic short stature is the most common cause of short stature and is a variant of normal.

DISORDERS OF GROWTH

Excess of growth hormone

Excess GH prior to epiphyseal fusion causes gigantism, proportional abnormal growth. Since the epiphyses also fuse at an earlier age, the child may have an unremarkable height in adulthood. Diabetes is very common in this group because of the opposing actions of GH and insulin on blood glucose.

An excess of GH is slightly more common in adults where it manifests as acromegaly (prevalence 60 per million). The signs and symptoms are shown in Fig. 9.4 (see also Fig. 19.7). The long bones can no longer lengthen, so there is no increase in height. However, the soft tissues and other bones can still grow, causing the distinctive features of this condition. Acromegaly is a serious condition, associated with an increase in mortality from cardiovascular disease, respiratory disease and malignancy. A therapeutic reduction in plasma GH is effective in reducing this excess mortality.

GH-secreting pituitary adenomas are the most common cause of acromegaly. These adenomas can cause other symptoms by compressing surrounding structures (e.g. pituitary stalk compression). Assessment of acromegaly should therefore include demonstration of excess GH, localization of the tumour, global assessment of anterior pituitary function and assessment of metabolic and structural complications.

skull
- enlarged head circumference

face
- skin coarse and thickened resulting in prominent nasolabial folds and supraorbital ridge
- large lower jaw
- spaces between lower teeth due to jaw growth
- large nose
- large tongue

liver and kidneys
- enlarged organs

hands
- large, square and spade-like

blood
- 1 in 10 are hypercalcaemic
- 1 in 4 have glucose intolerance, some are diabetic

feet
- large and wide

brain
- mental disturbances
- insomnia

eyes
- loss of peripheral vision due to pituitary tumour compressing optic nerve

heart
- enlarged (predisposes to cardiomyopathy)

blood pressure
- 1 in 3 are hypertensive (predisposes to ischaemic heart disease)

bones
- predisposes to osteoarthritis owing to increased body size and altered bone structure

skin
- increased greasy sweating
- temperature intolerance

Fig. 9.4 The symptoms and signs of acromegaly.

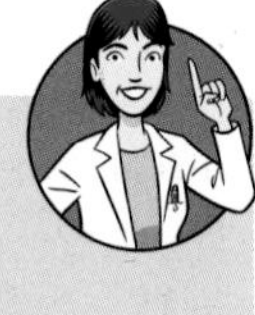

Tall stature is most often caused by tall parents; an excess of growth hormone is very rare.

Diagnosis and treatment

Excess GH can be diagnosed by high IGF-1 levels, but the best test is to measure GH levels following an oral glucose tolerance test. GH levels should fall with the rise in glucose. Computed tomography (CT) or magnetic resonance imaging (MRI) scans can be used to confirm the presence of a functional pituitary adenoma.

Somatotroph adenomas are removed surgically. Following the operation, the patient must be routinely monitored for GH levels and other pituitary hormones throughout life. If surgery is not appropriate then bromocriptine or octreotide (a GHIH analogue) can be used.

Deficiency of growth hormone

The deficiency of GH in children is called dwarfism. It is detected by short stature along with either:

- Dropping between growth chart centiles (i.e. not following the expected course).

- Being significantly shorter than mean parental height (MPH).

The most common cause of dwarfism is a deficiency of GHRH from the hypothalamus; craniopharyngiomas can also be responsible. See Chapter 2 for more details.

Diagnosis and treatment

GH deficiency is diagnosed using a stimulation test. GH levels are measured after exercise or a dose of clonidine, both of which should raise GH levels. Insulin-induced hypoglycaemia is no longer routinely used in children due to the potential risk of severe hypoglycaemia. GH deficiency is treated with subcutaneous injections of synthetic GH before bedtime every night.

Genetic short stature

Children can be short as a consequence of genetics without pathological correlates. These children have short parents and they start growing below the 5th centile at the normal rate with a normal age of pubertal onset. Mean parental height (MPH) is the average of the parents' height plus 7 cm in boys or minus 7 cm in girls. Final height is usually within 10 cm in either direction of the MPH. Constitutional delay in growth and maturation involves delayed puberty and a delayed pubertal growth spurt, but the normal adult height is attained.

10 Endocrine syndromes of neoplastic origin

Objectives

By the end of this chapter you should be able to:

- Describe the theories of MEN tumour formation.
- List the common tumours associated with each of the MEN syndromes.
- Describe the theories behind ectopic hormone secretion.
- List tumours that secrete hormones ectopically, along with the relevant hormone.

Endocrine organs can undergo neoplastic change and non-endocrine organs can acquire an endocrine phenotype as a result of neoplastic change. When several different endocrine tumour types affect a single individual they are usually part of a multiple endocrine neoplasia (MEN) syndrome. These syndromes result when several endocrine disorders share a common genetic basis. There are three patterns referred to as MEN-I, MEN-IIa, MEN-IIb. These syndromes are rare, but they can cause tumours in young adults. They are usually inherited and genetic testing can be used to determine the risk in family members.

Other endocrine syndromes are caused when tissues outside the endocrine system give rise to 'ectopic' hormone-secreting tumours. These tumours can present with symptoms pertinent to the hormone that is being secreted.

MULTIPLE ENDOCRINE NEOPLASIA SYNDROMES

MEN syndromes are clusters of endocrine tumours that often occur in the same patient. The tumours are rare, usually aggressive and arise in multiple tissues; they occur earlier than single sporadic tumours. The underlying cause is probably genetic, since these syndromes are usually inherited in an autosomal dominant fashion although some cases are sporadic.

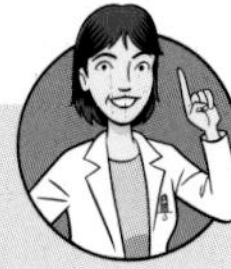

MEN syndromes are rare, but they may be life threatening.

The following patterns of MEN have been described:

MEN-I, MEN-IIa, MEN-IIb (Fig. 10.1) and FMTC.

MEN-I (Wermer's syndrome)

The most common tumours are:

- Parathyroid hyperplasia – most common.
- Pancreatic islet-cell tumours/duodenal tumours.
- Pituitary adenoma (secrete growth hormone, prolactin or ACTH).

The pancreatic islet-cell tumours may secrete ectopic hormones (e.g. glucagonoma or insulinoma) and the duodenal tumours may secrete gastrin causing Zollinger–Ellison syndrome (see Chapter 5, p. 73). Thirty per cent of the very rare Zollinger–Ellison tumours are caused by MEN-I.

Less commonly MEN-I is associated with:

- Parathyroid adenoma.
- Hyperplasia of thyroid parafollicular cells.
- Adrenal cortical hyperplasia.

MEN-IIa (Sipple's syndrome)

The main tumours of the MEN-II syndrome are:

- Phaeochromocytoma (often bilateral).
- Medullary cell carcinoma of the thyroid (MTC, often multi-focal, age of onset <30).

Occasionally, parathyroid hyperplasia can develop.

MEN-IIb

The very rare MEN-IIb is sometimes called MEN-III. MEN-IIb patients get both phaeochromocytomas and MTC, although the MTC is usually more aggressive and is present before 5 years of age. Patients also have

Fig. 10.1 The principal tumours and hormones associated with the three MEN syndromes

Syndrome	Associated tumours	Hormones secreted
MEN-I	Parathyroid hyperplasia, pancreatic islet-cell, pituitary adenomas	PTH, insulin, prolactin
MEN-IIa	Medullary carcinoma of the thyroid, phaeochromocytomas	Calcitonin, adrenaline
MEN-IIb	Medullary carcinoma of the thyroid, phaeochromocytomas, neuromas	Calcitonin, adrenaline

MEN, multiple endocrine neoplasia; PTH, parathyroid hormone.

a marfanoid appearance (long axial bones). Two other types of tumour develop in the skin and submucosa throughout the body:

- Neuromas (tumours of neurons).
- Ganglioneuromas (tumours of neuronal ganglia).

Familial medullary thyroid carcinoma (FMTC)

Medullary thyroid cancer can also occur in a hereditary pattern without the other endocrine abnormalities. 75% of MTC is not familial. Calcitonin is a good plasma marker for following the progression of MTC.

MEN-1 is caused by loss-of-function of a tumour suppressor gene, the *MEN-I* gene, which produces a protein that regulates cell proliferation. Patients typically have a germline mutation in one allele and acquire somatic mutations in the other allele. MEN-II syndromes are caused by gain-of-function mutations in the *RET* proto-oncogene. The precise genetic location of this mutation determines the exact phenotype. If family members test positive for these mutations, they can be treated with prophylactic surgery.

ECTOPIC HORMONE SYNDROMES

Ectopic hormones

'Ectopic' means out of place. The term 'ectopic hormone' is used when a tissue secretes a hormone that it does not normally secrete. The hormone is released in an uncontrolled manner by a tumour (benign or malignant). The tumour can be:

- Endocrine tissue secreting unusual hormones.
- Non-endocrine tissue secreting any hormone.

Symptoms are usually caused by the excess of the ectopic hormone while the tumour is still small. Examples of syndromes caused by ectopic hormone secretion are listed in Fig. 10.2.

Treatment

The tumours are treated in a similar manner to any symptomatic tumour, i.e.:

- Surgical removal.
- Irradiation.
- Chemotherapy.

Aetiology of ectopic hormones

The exact mechanism behind ectopic hormone release is not fully understood, and it may vary between tumours; there are two main theories:

- The tumour originates from cells that normally secrete small amounts of hormones, e.g. cells of the bronchial mucosa normally secrete adrenocorticotrophic hormone (ACTH) and anaplastic carcinoma of the lung secretes ectopic ACTH.
- Mutations associated with the transformation to neoplasia activate dormant genes resulting in ectopic hormone production.

Types of ectopic hormone

Ectopic hormones are almost always peptide hormones because their synthesis requires expression of

Fig. 10.2 Examples of syndromes caused by ectopic hormone secretion

Syndrome	Hormone secreted by tumour cells	Tumour
Hypercalcaemia	PTH or PTH-like peptide	Squamous cell carcinoma of the lung, breast carcinoma
Hyponatraemia	ADH	Oat cell carcinoma of the bronchus, some intestinal tumours
Hypokalaemia (symptoms of Cushing's syndrome caused by ACTH excess take longer to develop)	ACTH and ACTH-like peptides	Oat cell carcinoma of the bronchus, medullary carcinoma of the thyroid, thymic carcinoma, islet-cell tumours
Gynaecomastia	Human placental lactogen	Carcinoma of the bronchus, liver or kidney
Galactorrhoea	Prolactin	Carcinoma of the bronchus, hypernephroma
Polycythaemia	Erythropoietin	Hypernephroma, carcinoma of the uterus
Hypoglycaemia	Insulin (rare)	Hepatomas, large mesenchymal tumours
No syndrome	Calcitonin	Oat cell carcinoma of the lung

ACTH, adrenocorticotrophic hormone; ADH, antidiuretic hormone; PTH, parathyroid hormone.

only a single gene. Steroid-hormone synthesis requires the expression of a complicated series of enzymes.

The ectopic hormone is often not an exact version of a normal hormone, e.g. breast cancer cells secrete PTH-related peptide. This would fit the second theory of aetiology, since the normal processing enzymes may not be present.

Development of the reproductive system

11

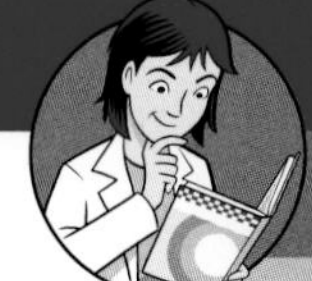

Objectives

By the end of this chapter you should be able to:

- Explain how gender is determined from a genetic and endocrine perspective.
- Describe the early development of the gonads along with the fate of the three types of cell.
- Describe the two ducts that form the male and female internal genital tracts.
- List the structures formed by these ducts in the male and female.
- Describe the development of the external genitalia.
- Describe the development of the breasts, especially the line along which they develop.
- Describe the endocrine changes that characterize puberty.
- List the changes that occur during male and female puberty.

The development of the reproductive system begins 4 weeks after conception and continues through to puberty. The majority of the structures are derived from the middle embryological layer, the mesoderm. However, the cells that will give rise to the gametes (sperm and oocytes) are derived from the endodermal yolk sac.

Sexual development can be thought of in three stages: genetic sex determination, gonadal sex determination and phenotypic sex determination. Between weeks 4 and 7, there are no morphological differences between male and female development, although the genetics are different. Differences begin to appear by the 7th week when the indifferent genitalia develop to form distinct reproductive systems for each sex.

Sexual development is arrested soon after birth until puberty. At puberty the gonads are reactivated by luteinizing hormone (LH) and follicle-stimulating hormone (FSH) secretion, and sex steroids (e.g. oestrogen and testosterone) are produced. These cause secondary sexual development and the attainment of sexual maturity.

Key words

Ectoderm: outer embryological layer that forms the skin and nervous system

Mesoderm: middle embryological layer that forms many organs and the cardiovascular system

Endoderm: inner embryological layer that forms the intestines and the germ cells

Mesenchyme: support tissue derived from the mesoderm

EMBRYOLOGICAL DEVELOPMENT OF SEX

Genetic determination of gender

The gender of a fetus is determined at conception by the sex chromosome in the sperm that fertilizes the oocyte (chromosome 23, which can be either X or Y). A single gene on the Y chromosome, called the sex-determining region of the Y chromosome (*Sry*), is responsible for the male (XY) phenotype. The protein transcribed by this is called testis-determining factor (TDF). The *Sry* gene is detected in cases of gender reversal including XX males. The absence of this gene and protein results in a female (XX) phenotype. The amount of gene product from the X chromosomes is the same in both sexes. In females one X chromosome is inactivated, forming a 'Barr body'. Certain genes that are present on both the X and Y chromosomes (the pseudoautosomal genes) remain active on both X chromosomes.

Early development

Gonads

The *Sry* gene is not activated until the 7th week of gestation. For the first 6 weeks, development is identical in both sexes. The bipotential gonads begin to form during the 5th week. Three types of cell form the gonads (Fig. 11.1):

- Mesenchymal cells, developing support tissue from the mesoderm.
- Mesothelial cells, coelomic epithelium that forms the lining of body cavities.
- Primordial germ cells, the developing gamete-producing cells.

The mesothelium and mesenchyme proliferate to form a bulge called the gonadal or genital ridge. This is found at the back of the developing abdominal cavity, associated with the developing mesonephros; these are ridges of tissue that act as primitive kidneys until the permanent kidneys develop.

The mesenchyme forms an inner medulla, while the mesothelium forms an outer cortex. The cortex has finger-like projections that reach into the medulla; these are called primary sex cords. The primordial germ cells that arose in the yolk sac migrate from the hindgut via the dorsal mesentery to enter the genital ridge and join the primary sex cords. The indifferent gonads are now complete (Fig. 11.2). Rarely primordial germ cells migrate to extragonadal sites and may give rise to teratomas.

Genital ducts

While the indifferent gonads are developing, two genital ducts are formed from the mesoderm (Fig. 11.3):

- Mesonephric (Wolffian) duct—this duct drains the urine from the mesonephros; it forms the male genital ducts, e.g. epididymis, vas deferens, seminal vesicles.
- Paramesonephric (Müllerian) duct—this funnel-ended duct lies laterally to the mesonephric duct; it forms the female genital ducts, e.g. uterine tubes, uterus, upper vagina.

External genitalia

The external genitalia also begin to develop around the 4th week. Initially, five mesenchymal swellings covered with ectoderm develop around the cloacal membrane; this membrane covers the blind end of the hindgut and urethra, both of which are endodermal structures. These five swellings are also shown in Fig. 11.4:

- One genital tubercle.
- Two urogenital folds.
- Two labioscrotal folds.

The genital tubercle enlarges to form the phallus—glans penis or the clitoris. The cloacal membrane divides into two and then ruptures to form:

- Urogenital orifice, though the vagina remains covered by the hymen.
- Anus.

A ligament, called the gubernaculum, forms between the indifferent gonad and the labioscrotal swellings through the inguinal canal. It guides the descent of the testes into the scrotum and forms the round ligaments of the uterus and ovaries. Failure of descent of the testis, cryptorchidism, carries a risk of testicular cancer and subfertility, and must be detected and treated early.

Fig. 11.1 The origins and fates of the cells that form the gonads

Cells	Origins	Structure at 6 weeks	Adult structure
Mesothelial cells	Mesodermal lining of the peritoneum	Cortex of the gonadal ridge and primary sex cords	Ovarian follicles or seminiferous tubules
Mesenchymal cells	Surrounding mesoderm	Medulla of the gonadal ridge	Leydig cells in the testes, and supporting stroma in the ovaries
Primordial germ cells	Migrate from the endodermal lining of the yolk sac	Primary sex cords	Gamete-producing male spermatogonia and female oocytes

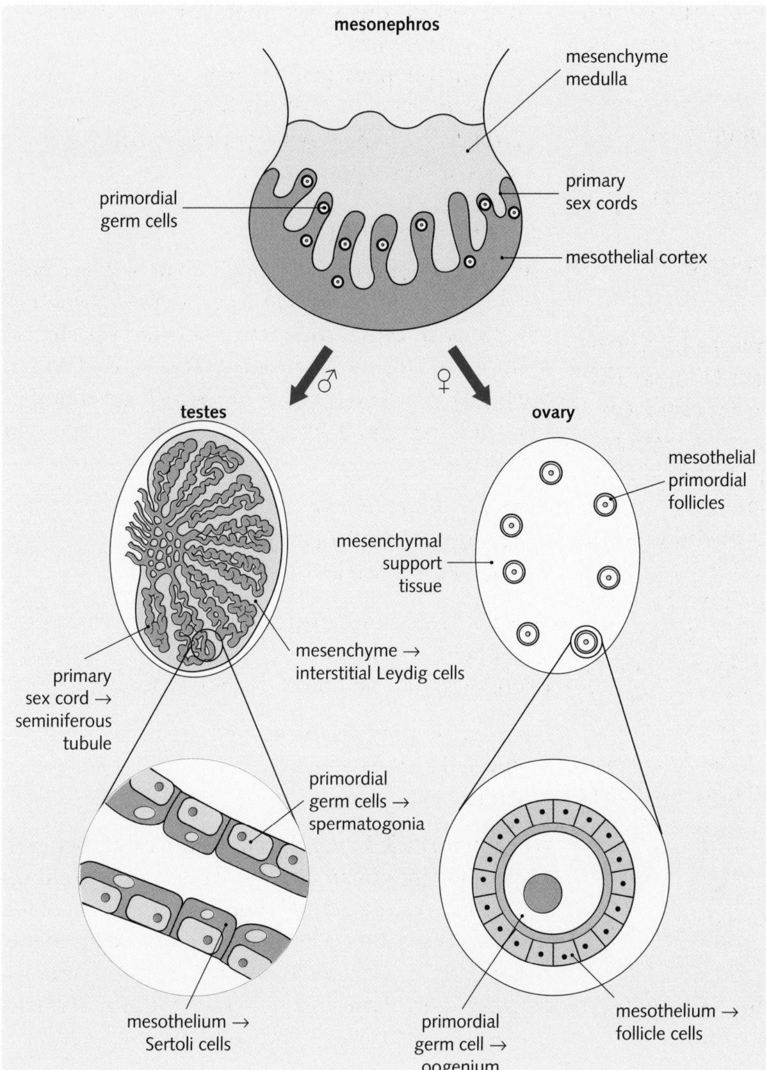

Fig. 11.2 The development of the male and female gonads.

As long as the Sry region is present and functional, the male phenotype is observed. Therefore people with aneuploid combinations, such as XXY (Klinefelter's syndrome) or XXXY are male. People with XX can be male as a result of translocation of the *Sry* gene to one of the X-chromosomes. People with the XY karyotype can be female due to inactivation of Sry region of the Y chromosome. The female phenotype is considered to be the default sex.

Male development

The testes

As the 6th week ends, the *Sry* gene is transcribed and testis-determining factor (TDF) is produced. This factor acts on the primary sex cords, which differentiate into the seminiferous cords. These separate from the surrounding mesenchyme to form the seminiferous tubules. The fate of the three cell types in the testes is shown in Fig. 11.2:

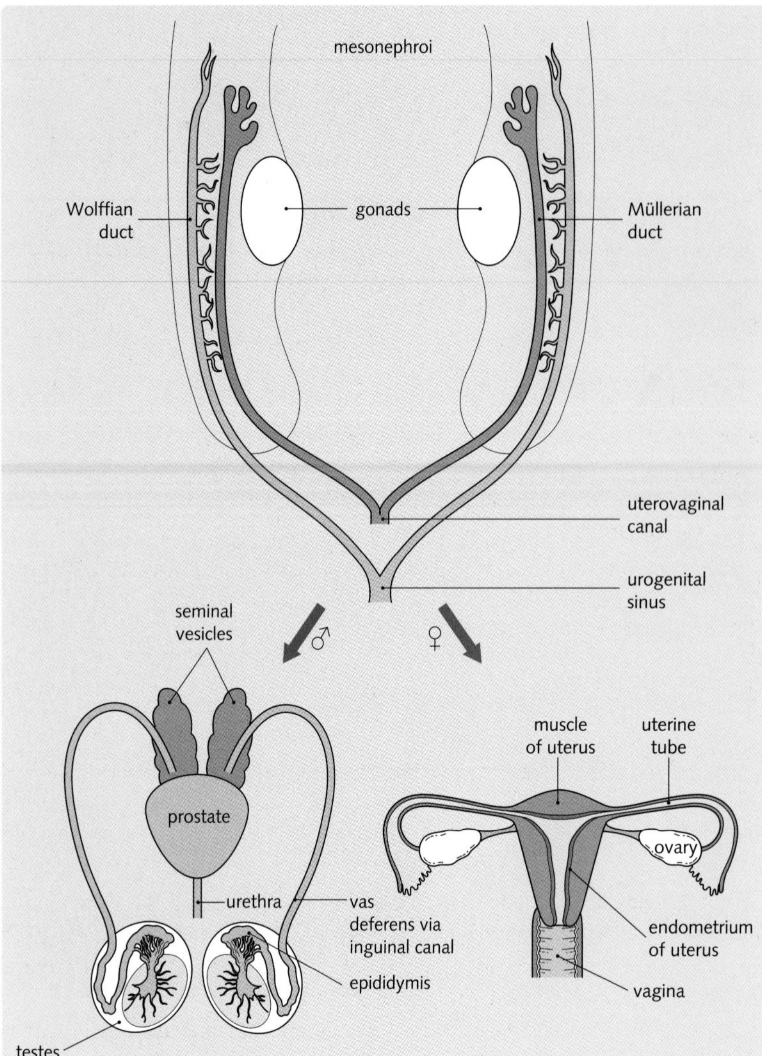

Fig. 11.3 The development of the male and female internal genitalia.

- Mesenchyme gives rise to interstitial (Leydig) cells.
- Mesothelium forms Sertoli cells.
- Primordial germ cells form spermatogonia.

The testes enlarge and separate from the mesonephros. They follow the path of the gubernaculum to reach the scrotum via the inguinal canal. The layers of the abdominal wall travel ahead of the testis into the inguinal canal, passing into the scrotum to form the layers of the scrotal wall and spermatic cord. A thin fold of peritoneum also descends; however, its connection with the abdomen (called the processus vaginalis) is lost. The small peritoneal sack remains in the scrotum as the tunica vaginalis. The testes finish their descent around the 7th month; they retain their abdominal blood vessels and lymphatic drainage. This migration and the formation of the scrotum is shown in Fig. 11.5.

Internal genitalia

The Leydig cells of the testes begin to secrete androgens (e.g. testosterone, androstenedione) from the 8th week. These androgens stimulate the further development of the mesonephric ducts, which differentiate into the:

- Epididymis.
- Ductus deferens.
- Seminal vesicles.
- Ejaculatory ducts.

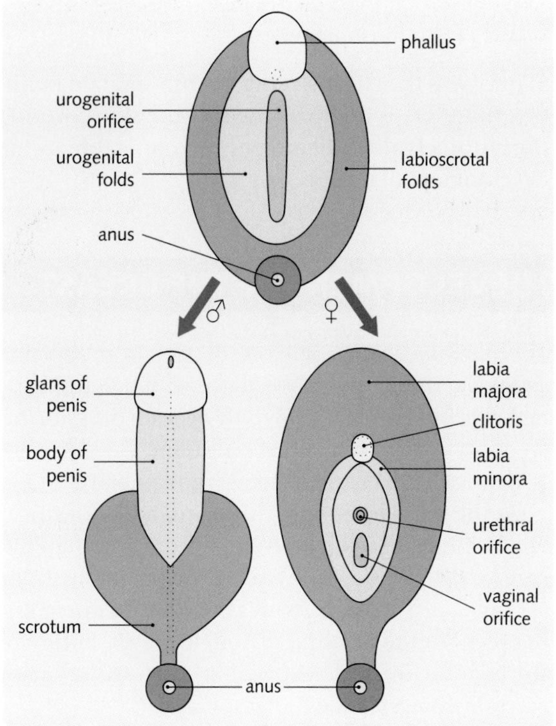

Fig. 11.4 The development of the male and female external genitalia.

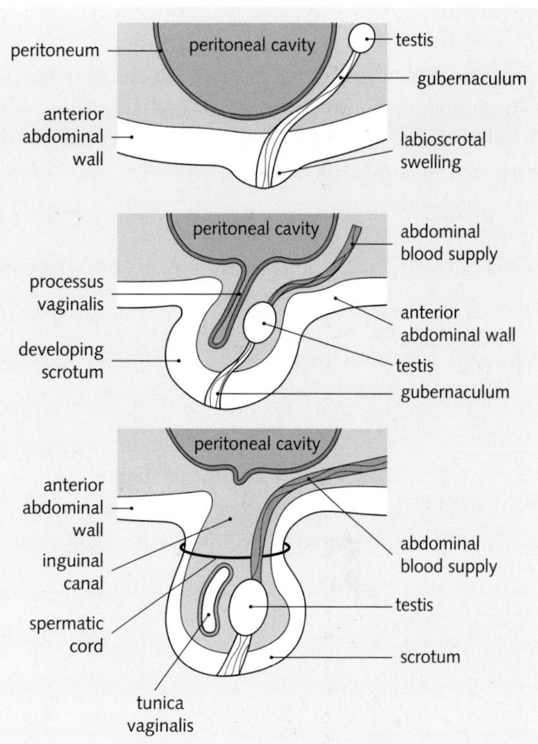

Fig. 11.5 The migration of the testes through the anterior abdominal wall.

The Sertoli cells also secrete Müllerian inhibiting substance (MIS)—a hormone that causes the paramesonephric ducts to regress (see Fig. 11.3).

The prostate develops from the urogenital sinus, the precursor of the urethra, as endodermal outgrowths surrounded by mesenchyme.

External genitalia

Dihydrotestosterone (DHT) is formed from testosterone secreted by the Leydig cells and is also responsible for the development of the male external genitalia shown in Fig. 11.4:

- Phallus enlarges to form the glans (distal end) of the penis.
- Urogenital folds fuse ventrally to form the body of the penis.
- Labioscrotal folds fuse to form the scrotum.

DHT is also responsible for the developing prostate.

All of these structures remain covered in ectoderm that forms the skin covering the penis. A clear ventral line called the scrotal and penile raphe remains from the fusion process. The ectoderm over the glans breaks down to form the foreskin (or prepuce), which remains attached to the glans, preventing retraction of the foreskin until late infancy.

The urethra is an endodermal structure that is enclosed by the urogenital fusion. Failure of this process results in hypospadias which is the most common malformation of the penis when the urethra opens onto the ventral surface of the penis (see Chapter 14).

Female development

The ovaries

Female sex is determined by a number of genes on the X chromosome. *Sry* overrides these genes (e.g. the XXY genotype in Klinefelter syndrome is phenotypically male). The genes of both X chromosomes are needed for normal female development; therefore, the XO genotype in Turner syndrome usually results in infertility and ovarian degeneration with the formation of a streak gonad. The signals involved in female development have not been determined.

The primary sex cords degenerate and secondary sex cords develop from the mesothelium. The primordial germ cells migrate into these new cords, which then break up to form primordial follicles. The mesenchymal medulla forms the connective tissue stroma that supports these follicles. The primordial germ cells develop into oogonia, which undergo mitotic division to increase the number of germ cells. They enter the first prophase of meiosis before birth, after which further mitosis is not possible; there is no stem-cell system equivalent to that found in males. The cells are called oocytes once the meiotic division has begun.

A primordial follicle is composed of:

- A single oocyte from the primordial germ cell.
- A single layer of follicular cells from the mesothelium, which surround the oocyte.

At birth about 750,000 primordial follicles are present; their meiotic division will only be completed many years later just before ovulation (see Fig. 11.2).

The ovaries separate from the mesonephros and become suspended in the pelvis by their mesentery.

Internal genitalia

The internal genitalia develop due to the absence of testosterone and MIS; the unstimulated mesonephric ducts regress, while the paramesonephric ducts develop. The funnel-shaped end nearest the ovary forms the:

- Uterine (fallopian) tubes.
- Uterine endometrium.

The other two layers (including the muscle) of the uterus are formed from surrounding mesenchyme (see Fig. 11.3).

The formation of the vagina is poorly understood; it develops in part from the paramesonephric duct (upper third) and the urogenital sinus (lower two-thirds). The vaginal epithelium is derived from the endodermal urethra, and the other layers develop from the surrounding mesenchyme. The hymen is formed from the thin tissue plate covering the urogenital sinus from which the vagina develops.

External genitalia

The external genitalia also develop due to the absence of testosterone (see Fig. 11.4):

- Phallus forms the clitoris.
- Urogenital folds do not fuse completely, and they form the labia minora.
- Labioscrotal folds do not fuse completely, and they form the labia majora.

Skin covers the clitoris, labia majora and labia minora, but there is no breakdown of the skin covering the clitoris (called the prepuce) comparable to the development of the foreskin.

DEVELOPMENT OF THE BREAST

The mammary glands (breasts) develop from apocrine sweat glands (i.e. those associated with hair follicles) in the mesenchymal layer directly beneath the skin; this accounts for their very superficial nature. Development is identical in males and females until puberty.

At the 4th week of development, a line of thickened ectoderm (skin) develops from the inguinal region to the axilla; this is called the mammary ridge (or milk line). In humans, this ridge normally regresses except in the pectoral region; however, failure of regression can cause extra nipples (polythelia) or accessory breast tissue (polymastia) to form.

In the 6th week, single mammary buds develop as downgrowths into the mammary ridge on either side. The buds then branch into structures which eventually become the lobules of the breast, Under the influence of placental hormones (e.g. human placental lactogen), lumina form inside the lobules and go on to form 15–20 lactiferous ducts. The surrounding mesenchyme develops into the fat and connective tissue of the breast. The functional glandular components of the lactiferous ducts in females are called alveoli; they develop under the influence of oestrogen at puberty. The supporting structures, including adipose tissue and the Coopers ligament, develop from the surrounding mesoderm.

The nipple is formed by depression of the skin before birth. Shortly after birth, the skin surrounding the nipple pit begins to grow, raising the nipple to form the usual shape.

POSTNATAL DEVELOPMENT

Soon after birth, the anterior pituitary gland begins to secrete gonadotrophins (LH and FSH) at roughly adult levels. Within 2 years, secretion declines rapidly to very low levels that are maintained until puberty. Sexual maturation is halted and the reproductive organs cease to develop.

Adrenarche

At about 8 years of age, the zona reticularis of the adrenal cortex reaches maturity. It begins to secrete adrenal androgens (see Chapter 4). This event is called adrenarche. These weak androgens contribute to the growth of pubic and axillary hair at puberty, especially in females. They do not cause puberty or the growth spurt.

PUBERTY

Puberty is when the sexually immature child becomes a sexually fertile adult. Prepuberty girls and boys develop pubic and axillary hair. This prepubertal phase is the result of the adrenache, i.e. the production of weak androgens from the adrenal gland. Puberty per se is the reactivation of gonadotrophin (LH and FSH) release after the dormancy of childhood. The age of pubertal onset varies widely between individuals (females 8–13 years; males 9–14 years). Puberty is characterized by a number of processes:

- Pubertal growth spurt.
- Development of secondary sexual characteristics.
- Achievement of fertility.
- Psychological and social development.

Gonadarche and the initiation of puberty

From an endocrine perspective, puberty is marked by the onset of pulsatile gonadotrophin release from the anterior pituitary gland during the night. Gonadotrophins stimulate the production of sex steroids (i.e. testosterone and oestrogen) from the gonads; the activation of the gonads is called gonadarche.

The onset of puberty is not fully understood; however, the CNS integrates a number of signals. According to the gonadostat hypothesis, a reduction in hypothalamic sensitivity to the negative feedback of the sex steroids causes the hypothalamus to secrete higher levels of gonadotrophin-releasing hormone (GnRH) in a pulsatile manner. Secretion of growth hormone (GH), thyroid-stimulating hormone (TSH) and adrenocorticotrophic hormone (ACTH) is also increased. Other evidence favours the central maturation of the CNS and its common final communication pathways between the hypothalamus GnRH neurons and the pituitary.

Body weight and puberty

Over the last few decades the onset of puberty has occurred at an increasingly young age. This change is often attributed to improved nutrition and rising body weight. In fact, achieving a body weight of 47 kg is a better predictor of the start of periods than age.

In recent years, a possible mechanism for this effect has been found. The hormone leptin is secreted by adipose tissue, and is a hormonal indicator of body fat: higher levels of leptin are present with increasing body fat. Leptin may be the trigger for GnRH activation. Puberty cannot begin without leptin, but evidence suggests that it is only one of a number of factors. The exact details of the causal relationship between a critical metabolic mass derived from lean body weight, body fat and total body water and the onset of puberty remains unclear.

The pubertal growth spurt

The earliest developmental event in puberty is an increase in growth velocity called the growth spurt. It occurs about 2 years earlier in females, giving a temporary height advantage. The initial rise in growth velocity is slight, so growth of the breasts or testes is usually noticed first.

The increase in growth rate is caused by increased GH and sex steroid secretion. Sex steroids also cause bone maturation. As the bones mature, the growing plates (epiphyses) fuse, preventing further growth. This fusion occurs 2 years earlier in females, giving males an extra 2 years of growth. This largely accounts for the increased height of adult males.

Puberty in the male

Puberty usually occurs between 9 and 14 years of age in boys; however, it is considered normal if it occurs between 9 and 16 years of age. Once the testes have developed, male pubertal changes are brought about by the secretion of androgens such as DHT and testosterone.

Testes development and early puberty

Growth of the testes from <2 mL to >4 mL is often the first sign of puberty noticed in boys around 12 years. The increase is mainly due to proliferation of the seminiferous tubules under the influence of FSH. LH stimulates the interstitial Leydig cells to secrete testosterone. The scrotum becomes larger, thicker and pigmented; pubic hair growth follows.

Spermatogenesis begins once the testes have enlarged and matured and is associated with a rise in serum inhibin B. Nocturnal emissions and daytime ejaculations are often around 13–14 years of age at Stage 3 of Tanner's male genital staging with fertile ejaculations around 15 years.

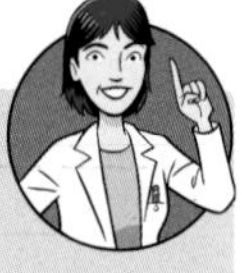

Clinically, male puberty has begun when the testes reach 4 mL. This is measured with an orchidometer.

Penile development and late puberty

The penis begins to enlarge after the testes about the same time the growth spurt is noticed. The penis doubles in size during puberty to reach an average size of 9.5 cm flaccid or 13.2 cm erect.

Klinefelter's syndrome (XXY) is associated with small testicles, abnormal spermatogenesis and infertility. The syndrome is also associated with delayed motor learning. Treatment is with testosterone. Women with Turner's syndrome lack part of the X chromosome (or a whole X chromosome) needed for normal ovarian development and the acquisition of normal secondary sexual characteristics. These women are often amenorrhoeic, infertile and have abnormal breast and pubic hair development. Treatment is with oestrogen to promote sexual development and growth hormone to encourage growth.

Facial and axillary hair growth usually starts at about 15 years of age. The sebaceous glands in the skin are also activated, often causing acne.

The breaking of the voice is also a late feature. The larynx, cricothyroid cartilage and laryngeal muscles enlarge to give an Adam's apple.

Tanner's stages are used to assess puberty milestones and compare individuals. The stages are based on testis, scrotum and penile growth and pubic hair in the male. Stage 1: height increases 5 cm per year, no pigmented pubic hair, testes <2 cm long, no penis growth; Stage 2: height increases 5 cm per year, some pubic hair, testes 2.5–3.2 cm long, increased penis dimensions; Stage 3: height increases 7.5 cm year, dark pubic hair, increase penis dimensions, voice breaks, increased muscle mass; Stage 4: height increases 10 cm per year, adult pubic hair quality, increase penis dimensions, axillary hair; Stage 5: No height increase from 17, adult pubic hair distribution, penis mature age 16.5, testes length >4.5 cm.

Puberty in the female

Puberty usually occurs between 8 and 13 years of age in girls, however, it is considered normal between 8 and 15 years of age. The changes caused by oestrogens and progesterone are shown in Fig. 11.6.

Breast development and early puberty

The development of breast buds is often the first sign of puberty noticed in girls. The breast then continues

Fig. 11.6 The changes caused by oestrogen and progesterone during female puberty

Oestrogen-mediated changes	Progesterone-mediated changes
Fat deposition and proliferation of the ductal system in the breasts, causing growth	Proliferation of the secretory lobules and acini in the breast
Growth of the vagina and maturation of the epithelium	Contribution to vaginal and uterine growth
Growth of the clitoris	Initiation of cyclical changes in endometrium and ovary

to grow under the influence of oestrogen while the ductal system develops, the number of lobules remains the same from infancy (see Fig. 11.6). Pubic hair begins to grow about 6 months later.

Menarche and late puberty

The uterus begins to enlarge after the development of pubic hair. The onset of menstruation (periods) is called menarche. The mean age of menarche is 13 years, making it a late feature of puberty. In the ovary, follicular development begins and the first ovulation occurs 10 months after menarche, on average, i.e. the early menstrual cycles are often anovulatory and infertile.

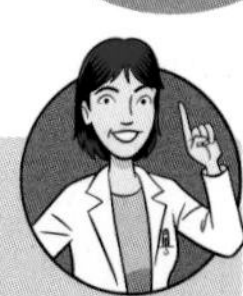

Tanner's stages and the female

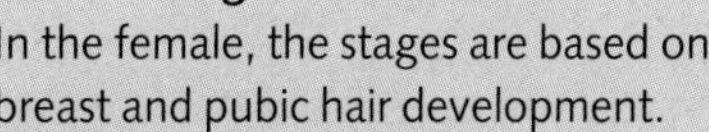

In the female, the stages are based on breast and pubic hair development.

Breast development

Stage 1: preadolescent, only papillae are elevated; Stage 2: breast bud develops with papillae and breasts elevated; Stage 3: juvenile smooth stage with further growth of breasts and areolae; Stage 4: areolae and papillae project above the breasts; Stage 5: adult pattern with areolae on the same level as the rest of the breasts.

Pubic hair development

Stage 1: preadolescent, no pubic hair; Stage 2: sparse hair on labia majora; Stage 3: darker, courser and curlier pubic hair, spreads over pubis; Stage 4: adult type pattern but covers smaller area; Stage 5: adult pattern. Hypogonadism can occur as a result of failure of the hypothalamic–pituitary–gonadal axis at any level. Hypergonadotropic hypogonadism occurs as a result of the gonad itself not producing enough sex steroid to inhibit the release of LH and FSH. Hypogonadotropic hypogonadism can be the result of a failure in GnRH release or a failure of the pituitary response to GnRH. Perinatal hypogonadism causes ambiguous genitalia, prepubertal hypogonadism prevents puberty and postpubertal hypogonadism causes infertility and sexual pathologies.

12 The female reproductive system

Objectives

By the end of this chapter you should be able to:

- Describe the structure and location of the ovaries.
- Describe the development of an ovarian follicle in the first half of the cycle.
- Describe the structure and location of the uterus and cervix.
- Describe the structure and location of the vagina and vulva.
- Describe the structure and location of the adult female breast.
- Describe the synthesis and regulation of the three types of ovarian sex steroid.
- List the major effects of oestrogens and progestogens.
- Describe the hormonal changes during the menstrual cycle.
- Describe the ovarian changes during the menstrual cycle.

The female reproductive system must perform five main functions:

- Oogenesis and ovulation—production and release of oocytes (female gametes).
- Fertilization—allowing the sperm and oocyte to meet and fuse.
- Pregnancy—providing a suitable environment for the fetus to grow.
- Parturition—expelling the fetus with minimal trauma to the mother and baby.
- Lactation—providing the baby with nutrition.

After menarche (the start of periods), the female body prepares for pregnancy every month until menopause. This process is regulated by four main hormones (Fig. 12.1):

- Follicle-stimulating hormone (FSH).
- Luteinizing hormone (LH).
- Oestrogen.
- Progesterone.

These hormones regulate all of the processes described above. In the absence of pregnancy, the hormone levels rise and fall in the same pattern every month. These fluctuations, and the changes they cause, are called the menstrual cycle. The menstrual cycles continue until the menopause (p.143).

ORGANIZATION

The female reproductive system consists of six main components:

- Ovaries—produce oocytes and female sex steroids (e.g. oestrogens).
- Uterine (fallopian) tubes—connect the ovaries to the uterus; they are the normal site of fertilization.
- Uterus—supports the implantation and development of the fetus.
- Vagina—normal site for the deposition of sperm.
- Vulva—the structures surrounding the introitus (external orifice of the vagina).
- Breasts—produce milk.

The ovaries lie inside the peritoneal cavity, while all the other components lie outside; the ovarian end of the uterine tubes open into this cavity. The peritoneum covers the uterus and uterine tubes to form a fold called the broad ligament. Each of these components is discussed individually in the following sections. Their anatomical locations are shown in Fig. 12.2, and their blood supply, lymphatics and innervation are shown in Fig.12.3.

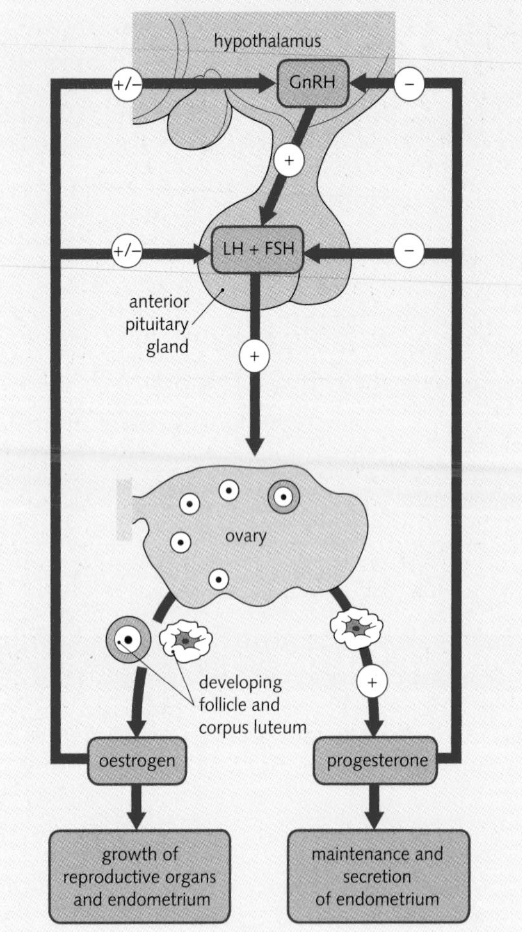

Fig. 12.1 Hormonal regulation of the female reproductive system. (FSH, follicle-stimulating hormone; GnRH, gonadotrophin-releasing hormone; LH, luteinizing hormone.)

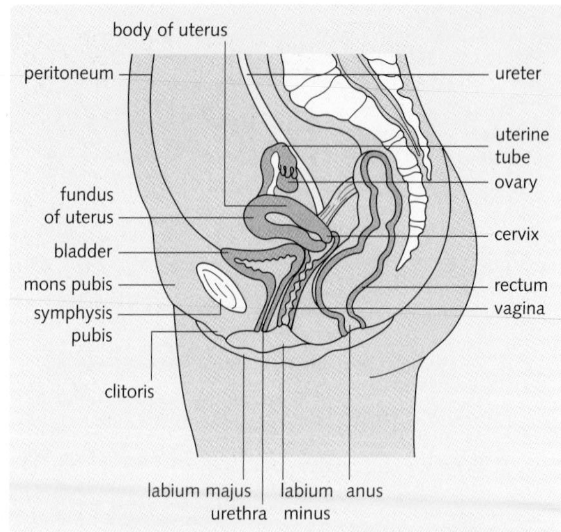

Fig. 12.2 Sagittal section of the female pelvis showing the locations of the reproductive organs.

Ovaries

The ovaries are two oval organs that produce oocytes (female gametes) and sex steroid hormones in response to pituitary gonadotrophins (LH and FSH). The position of the ovaries is variable, but they usually lie lateral to the uterus, fixed to the posterior of the broad ligament. The opening of each uterine tube (infundibulum) lies lateral to each ovary, allowing oocytes to enter the infundibulum at ovulation.

The ovaries are held on the surface of the broad ligament by a fold of peritoneum called the mesovarium, which is continuous with the germinal epithelium that forms their outer surface. Ovarian nerves, arteries and veins enter the hilum of the ovary from the mesovarium. The relationship of the ovaries to the uterus, uterine tubes and ligaments is shown in Fig. 12.4.

Two peritoneal ligaments attach to the ovary:

- Suspensory ligament of the ovary—from the mesovarium to the pelvic wall; it contains the blood vessels and nerves.
- Round ligament of the ovary—from the ovary to the fundus (top) of the uterus; it is a remnant of the upper section of the gubernaculum.

Microstructure

The ovary has three components (Fig. 12.5):

- Surface—simple cuboidal epithelium called the germinal epithelium, which has nothing to do with the origin of the germ cells despite its name.
- Cortex—composed of connective tissue stroma supporting thousands of follicles. Every month a group of preovulatory primary follicles begin to enlarge and synthesize steroid hormones. One of these follicles, the dominant follicle, will eventually ovulate and form a postovulatory corpus luteum whilst the others will regress (atresia). Therefore, the cortex supports preovulatory, postovulatory and degenerating follicles.
- Medulla—composed of supporting stroma, it contains a rich network of vessels and nerves that enter the ovary from the mesovarium.

The uterine (fallopian) tubes

The uterine tubes are two 'J' shaped tubes lying in the upper border of the broad ligament. The tubes extend

Fig. 12.3 Blood supply, lymphatics and innervation of the female reproductive organs

Organ	Arterial supply	Venous drainage	Innervation	Lymphatic drainage
Ovaries	The ovarian arteries from the aorta via the suspensory ligaments	Forms the pampiniform plexus that drains into the ovarian veins in the suspensory ligaments	Autonomic nerves via the suspensory ligaments	Para-aortic lymph nodes
Uterine tubes	Uterine and ovarian arteries	Uterine and ovarian veins	Uterovaginal plexus and suspensory ligaments	Iliac, sacral and aortic lymph nodes
Uterus	Uterine arteries, branches of the internal iliac arteries	Forms a plexus in the broad ligament that drains into the uterine veins	Uterovaginal plexus in the broad ligament	Iliac, sacral, aortic (and inguinal) lymph nodes
Vagina	Uterine arteries from the internal iliac arteries	Vaginal venous plexus that drains into the internal iliac veins	Uterovaginal plexus in the broad ligament	Iliac and superficial inguinal lymph nodes
External genitalia	Pudendal arteries	Pudendal veins	Pudendal and ilioinguinal nerves, S2–S4	Superficial inguinal lymph nodes
Breasts	Internal thoracic, lateral thoracic and intercostal arteries	Axillary and internal thoracic veins	Intercostal nerves, mainly T4	Axillary and parasternal lymph nodes and the contralateral breast

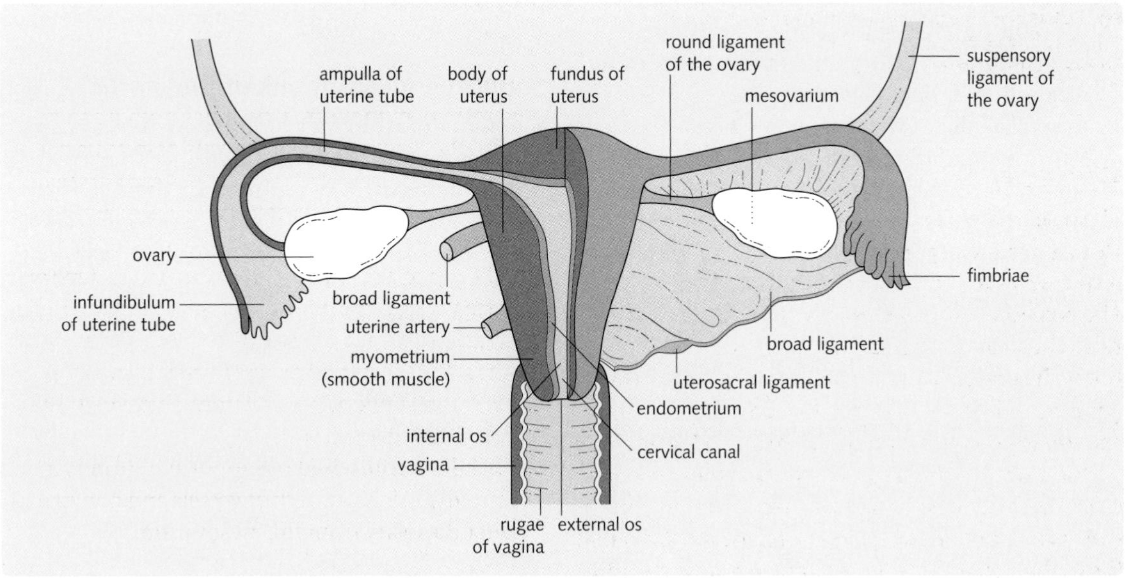

Fig. 12.4 Structure of the ovaries, uterine (fallopian) tubes and uterus.

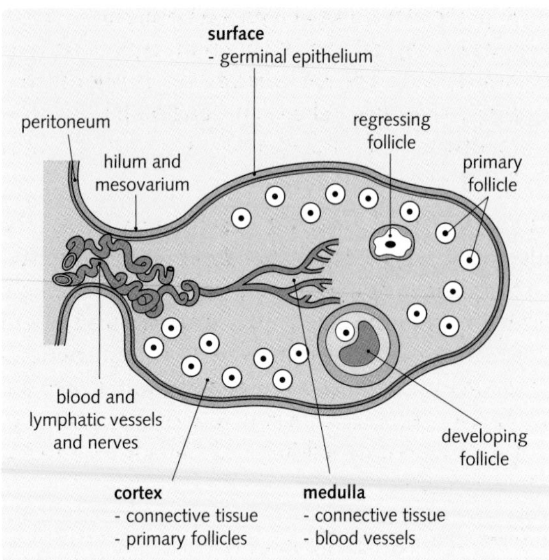

Fig. 12.5 Microstructure of an ovary.

from their opening into the peritoneal cavity near the ovaries to the fundus (top) of the uterus where they open into the uterine cavity. As a result, there is a connection between the peritoneal cavity and the external reproductive tract. Infection can travel up this route; however, the cervix acts as a barrier. The uterine tubes are described in four parts, from lateral to medial:

- Infundibulum—the funnel-shaped opening of the tube that is closely related to the ovary; it collects the oocytes from the surface of the ovary using ciliated, finger-like fimbriae.
- Ampulla—the widest section; is where fertilization normally occurs.
- Isthmus—connects the ampulla to the uterus.
- Uterine section—the section of the tube that penetrates the uterine muscle.

The uterine tubes are lined by ciliated and secretory cells that waft the oocyte towards the uterus and supply it with nutrients. Two layers of spiral muscle surround this lining and help move the oocyte and sperm by peristalsis. These muscles are sensitive to sex steroids (e.g. oestrogen) so that motility is most rapid when sex steroid levels are highest. The 'morning-after' pill uses oestrogen to increase this motility so that the oocyte is ejected before the uterus is ready for implantation, thus preventing pregnancy. If motility is slow there is a risk of ectopic pregnancy, in which implantation occurs in the uterine tube. The relationship of the uterine tubes to the uterus, ovaries and broad ligament is shown in Fig. 12.4.

Uterus and cervix

The uterus is a pear-shaped, muscular organ that can enlarge greatly to accommodate the growing fetus. It is lined by a specialized epithelium called the endometrium. The uterine tubes join superiorly, and the vagina is inferior. These relationships are shown in Fig. 12.4.

The uterus is described in three sections:

- Fundus—above the entry point of the uterine tubes.
- Body—this is the usual site of implantation.
- Cervix—the lower part ; links the uterus and vagina.

The cylindrical cervix is structurally and functionally distinct from the rest of the uterus. The junction of the cervix with body is called the internal os, and that with the vagina the external os. The passage between these two junctions is called the endocervical canal. The ureters pass 1 cm lateral to the internal os on either side; this relationship is important when considering cervical carcinoma as the ureter may become infiltrated by the carcinoma. The external os can be visualized in the conscious patient using a speculum, and the surrounding cells are sampled in a smear test.

The cervix and all structures superior are sterile areas. This sterility is maintained by the frequent shedding of the endometrium, thick cervical mucus and the narrow external os of the cervix.

Support and ligaments of the uterus

A number of structures hold the uterus in position and prevent prolapse into the vagina. The main support is derived from the tone of the pelvic floor formed by the levator ani and coccygeus muscles. The other supporting structures are called 'ligaments', though most of them are not actually ligaments. The functions, relations and locations of these structures are common exam questions:

- Broad ligament—a double layer of peritoneum that surrounds the uterus with the uterine tubes forming its superior border; it does not support the uterus.
- Round ligament—from the uterus body (anteroinferiorly to the insertion point of the uterine tubes) to the labia majora through the inguinal canal; it is the remnant of the lower sections of the gubernaculum. It holds the uterus

in an anteverted position and is a minor support. (The fundus lies superior and anterior to the cervix.)

- Uterosacral ligaments—from the cervix either side of the rectum to the piriformis muscle over the sacrum; these structures support the uterus.
- Transverse cervical (cardinal) ligaments—from the cervix and superior vagina to the lateral pelvic walls; these structures support the uterus.
- Pubocervical ligaments—from the cervix to the pubis bone; they do not support the uterus.

Microstructure of the uterus

The body and fundus are composed of three tissue layers (Fig. 12.6):

- Serosa—the peritoneal covering.
- Myometrium—the thick smooth muscle layer; it is sensitive to hormones, e.g. oxytocin.
- Endometrium—the inner lining of the uterus that varies through the menstrual cycle; it is sensitive to hormones, e.g. oestrogen and progestogen.

The endometrium is further divided into two layers:

- Deep basal layer—this changes little through the menstrual cycle and is not shed at menstruation.
- Superficial functional layer—a hormone-sensitive layer that proliferates in response to oestrogen and becomes secretory in response to progesterone; it is shed at the end of the menstrual cycle and regenerates from cells in the basal layer.

The arterioles of the superficial endometrial layer lie alongside the glands of the endometrium. They have a characteristic spiral appearance, unlike the straight arterioles of the basal layer. As progesterone levels fall at the end of the menstrual cycle, the spiral arterioles respond by intermittent vasoconstriction. The superficial layer becomes ischaemic and undergoes necrosis; this causes the shedding and haemorrhage that is menstruation.

Microstructure of the cervix

The cervix consists mainly of collagen and small amounts of smooth muscle. The columnar epithelium lining the endocervical canal secretes mucus that changes in consistency during the menstrual cycle. Oestrogen promotes a thin, watery mucus that is very stretchable (high *spinnbarkeit*) and allows sperm to pass. Progesterone causes the production of a thick, viscous mucus that is impenetrable to sperm; this is

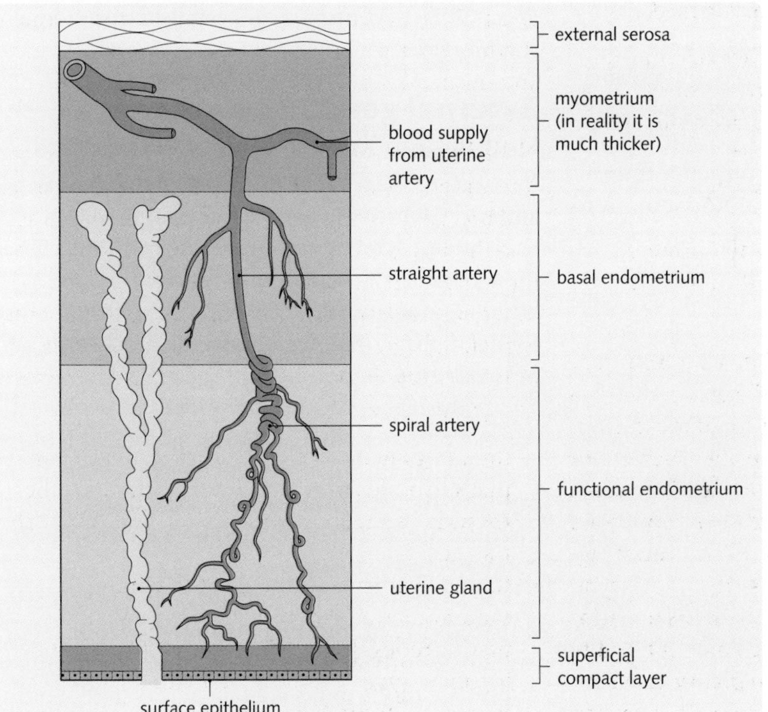

Fig. 12.6 Microstructure of the uterus.

the mode of action of progestogen-only oral contraception.

The cervix is divided into two sections:

- Endocervix—superior, related to the uterus body.
- Ectocervix—inferior, related to the vagina.

The anatomical definition of this division is different from the histological definition (Fig. 12.7). The anatomical division is generally located superiorly to the histological division.

During puberty and pregnancy, high oestrogen levels cause the simple columnar epithelium of the cervix to extend beyond the external os into the vagina; this is called cervical ectopy (ectropion). The acidic vaginal pH induces squamous metaplasia (changing to squamous epithelium) of the columnar epithelium. The cells that change are within an area called the transformation zone, and they are susceptible to dysplasia (precancerous changes). Cervical smears take samples of these cells to detect early signs of dysplasia allowing curative treatment (see pp. 144–45).

Vagina

The vagina is a 9-cm long muscular tube that runs upwards and backwards from the external genitalia (vulva) to the cervix. The urethra and bladder are anterior and the rectum posterior. In most women the cervix is inserted into the anterior wall of the vagina at an angle of 90°; this is called the anteverted position of the uterus.

The cervix projects into the vagina creating a small dome with the external os at the centre. The vaginal lumen around the cervix is divided into anterior, posterior and two lateral fornices. The posterior fornix is the deepest and it is covered by peritoneum on its internal surface. This is an important relationship since an object that penetrates this area (e.g. during a 'backstreet' abortion) will enter the peritoneal cavity, potentially causing peritonitis.

Fig. 12.7 Comparison of the endocervix and ectocervix

	Endocervix	Ectocervix
Anatomy	Above the internal os; covered by peritoneum anteriorly	Below the internal os; not covered by peritoneum anteriorly
Histology	Columnar endometrial epithelium; does not menstruate	Stratified squamous vaginal epithelium; does not menstruate

Microstructure

The structure of the vaginal wall allows expansion during intercourse and childbirth. The wall of the vagina is composed of four layers:

- Stratified squamous epithelial lining for protection.
- Elastic lamina propria.
- Fibromuscular layer (two layers of smooth muscle).
- Fibroelastic adventitia.

The wall contains few sensory fibres and no glands; the lining epithelium is lubricated by cervical mucus. During sexual arousal, the vagina is further lubricated by the secretions from the greater vestibular (Bartholin's) glands next to the introitus (external vaginal orifice) and the transudation of fluid across the vaginal epithelium.

Unlike the cervix, uterus and uterine tubes, the vagina is a non-sterile area; the main organism present is the commensal *Lactobacillus vaginalis*. During the menstrual cycle, oestrogen stimulates the cells of the vaginal epithelium to secrete glycogen. The lactobacilli digest this glycogen to release lactic acid and thus lower the pH of the vagina below 4.5; this prevents infection by other organisms. Other commensal organisms present include *Candida* and *Escherichia coli*. As in the gastrointestinal tract, antibiotics can disrupt the flora to cause overgrowth and infections such as candidiasis (thrush). Low oestrogen levels can also result in infection.

External genitalia (vulva)

The appearance of the vulva is shown in Fig. 12.8. The introitus or external vaginal orifice opens into the vestibule, which is the area between the labia. The short urethra opens anterior to the introitus within the vestibule. The labia minora are two hairless folds of skin that surround the vestibule; they fuse anterior to the urethral opening to form the prepuce (hood) of the clitoris. Beneath the prepuce lies the clitoris. The body of the clitoris is composed of two erectile corpora cavernosa that become engorged with blood upon sexual stimulation. The erectile tissue of the bulbs of the vestibule on each side of the vaginal opening are attached to the glans clitoris by thin bands of erectile tissue.

The labia minora lie within two larger, hair-bearing skin folds called the labia majora; the labia majora fuse posteriorly and extend anteriorly to the mons pubis. The mons pubis is a fat pad covered in pubic hair at the anterior of the vulva.

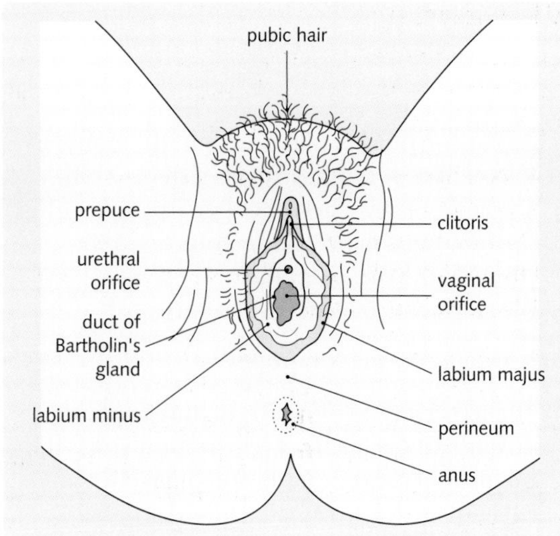

Fig. 12.8 Structure of the vulva.

Small glands located either side of the introitus are called the greater vestibular (Bartholin's) glands. During sexual arousal they secrete a lubricating mucus into the vestibule via small ducts that open into the vestibule.

Female breasts (mammary glands)

The breasts lie in the superficial fascia, two-thirds over the pectoral muscles on the anterior of the chest with one-third over serratus anterior. They are very superficial structures composed largely of fat; the size and shape varies between individuals. Their base, however, is constant and overlies the second to the sixth rib. They extend towards the axilla, and this axillary tail must be checked on examination. The pigmented skin around the nipple is called the areola. In white-skinned women, it permanently changes from pink to brown during pregnancy.

Microstructure

Embedded in the fatty tissue of the breast there are 15–20 glandular lobules with openings on the nipple. Each opening is a lactiferous duct that forms a lactiferous sinus beneath the areola. Within the breast, the lactiferous ducts branch extensively to end in secretory acini potentially capable of secreting milk. The ducts and lobules are surrounded by myoepithelial cells that contract in response to oxytocin and expel the milk on stimulation of the nipple. The internal structure of the breast is shown in Fig. 12.9.

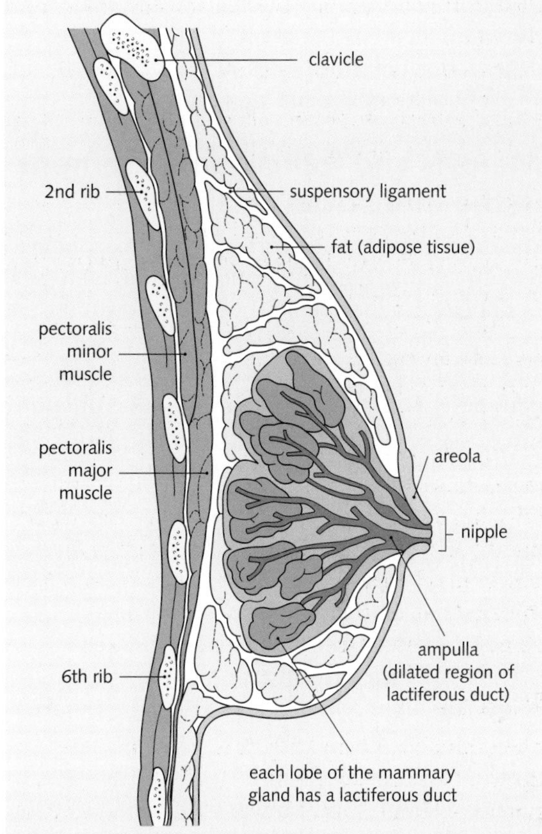

Fig. 12.9 Internal structure of the breast.

OOGENESIS

Meiosis in the female fetus

Oogenesis is the process by which haploid (23 chromosome) oocytes are formed from diploid (46 chromosome) stem cells called oogonia. This process requires a meiotic division that is begun before birth and ends when the oocyte is fertilized.

Oogonia are ovarian stem cells derived from the primordial germ cells in the yolk sac (see Chapter 11); initially they divide by mitosis to increase their numbers, peaking at around 7 million per ovary. In the second trimester of pregnancy all the oogonia develop into primary oocytes and enter the prophase (diplotene) of the first meiotic division. The meiotic division is arrested at this stage until menarche and the events of the menstrual cycle. Since no oogonia remain, further mitotic divisions to increase the number of oocytes are not possible. The entire reserve of oocytes is formed before birth. A single layer of flat granulosa cells surround each primary oocyte to form a primordial follicle. The follicles are located within the ovarian cortex. During fetal life there is atretric degeneration of the oocytes so that at birth around 1–2 million oocytes per ovary remain.

Meiosis and follicle development in the menstrual cycle

The primordial follicles containing primary oocytes remain unchanged until puberty and menarche. By puberty, around 400,000 oocytes per ovary are present. Once the menstrual cycle has become established, a few primordial follicles recommence growth on a daily basis. The stimulus for this growth is unknown but it occurs independently of gonadotrophins. FSH secretion then stimulates the development of a selection of these growing primordial follicles each month. The follicles pass through the following stages (see Fig. 12.10):

- Preantral (primary) follicle—the primary oocyte and a single layer of granulosa cells enlarge in size to form a multilaminar follicle—the granulosa cells divide to form layers and the zona pellucida (glycoprotein shell) forms around the primary oocyte. The surrounding ovarian cortex forms the secretory theca interna and theca externa. Towards the end of this phase, the most advanced late preantral follicles develop receptors for oestrogen and FSH on the granulosa cells and LH receptors on the theca cells so that they can respond to these gonadotrophins.
- Antral (secondary) follicle—a fluid-filled cavity called the antrum develops within the granulosa cell layer. The early antral follicles continue to develop FSH and LH receptors. The thecal cells of the mature antral follicles now bind LH and are stimulated to synthesize androgens, which are then aromatized to oestrogens by the FSH-stimulated granulosa cells (see below). The oestrogen output is mainly from the most advanced or dominant follicle, which ultimately will be released. Oestrogens in conjunction with FSH stimulate the appearance of LH receptors on the granulosa cells of the dominant follicle and the high levels of oestrogens provide positive feedback to the pituitary to induce the LH surge.
- Preovulatory (Graafian, mature) follicle—after the LH surge the primary oocyte of the dominant follicle completes the first meiotic division to form the secondary oocyte and first polar body. The secondary oocyte starts the second meiosis but goes into arrest at the second metaphase stage. There is a rapid expansion of follicular fluid and the granulosa cells now synthesize progesterone. The secondary oocyte becomes free floating within the expanded preovulatory follicle, which ruptures the surface of the ovary so releasing the secondary oocyte (ovulation).

The ovulated oocyte comprises:

- The secondary oocyte—the mature haploid oocyte that is capable of fertilization; it has the majority of the cytoplasm and organelles.
- First polar body—a small haploid cell that degenerates; it has virtually no cytoplasm.

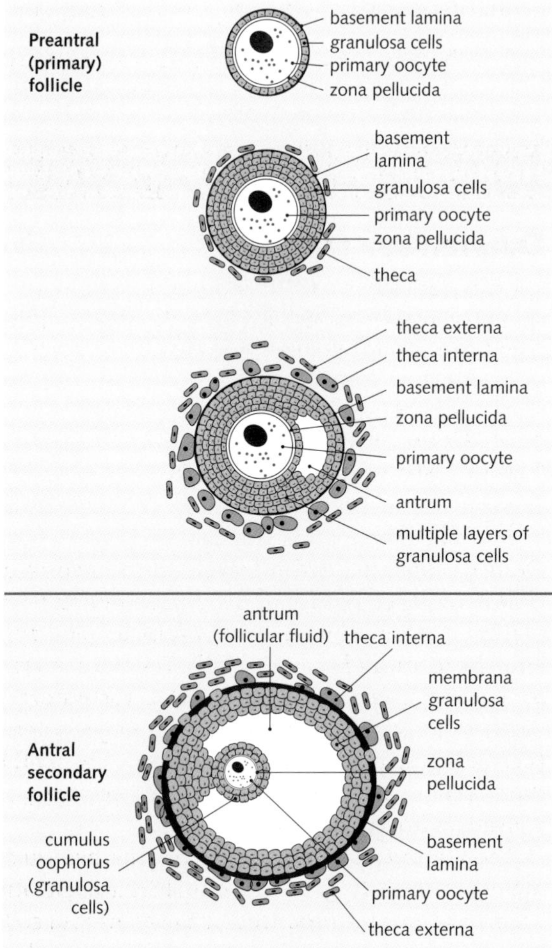

Fig. 12.10 Development of an ovarian follicle.

The ovulated secondary oocyte is surrounded by two layers:

- Zona pellucida—the glycoprotein layer (ZP3 glycoprotein is responsible for binding to sperm).
- Corona radiata (also called the cumulus oophorus)—a covering of granulosa cells from the follicle.

Meiosis at fertilization

With sperm entry, the second meiotic division of the secondary oocyte is completed. The calcium influx caused by the fusion of the sperm and secondary oocyte stimulates the completion of this division. Two haploid cells are produced:

- The mature ovum—the functional gamete; it has the majority of the cytoplasm and fuses with the male pronucleus (see Chapter 15).
- Second polar body—another small haploid cell that degenerates; it has virtually no cytoplasm.

With fertilization, the diploid one-cell zygote is formed.

HORMONES

Ovarian sex steroids

The ovaries produce a number of steroid hormones in response to gonadotrophins from the anterior pituitary. The main hormones produced are:

- Oestrogens, e.g. oestradiol.
- Progestogens, e.g. progesterone.
- Androgens, e.g. androstenedione.

Oestrogens

Oestrogens are secreted at the start of the menstrual cycle in response to LH and FSH. Their synthesis takes place in the developing ovarian follicle, requiring both the thecal and granulosa cells. The theca interna secretes androgens in response to LH. LH activates the enzyme that converts cholesterol to pregnenolone (i.e. the first step in steroid production), however the thecal cells lack the aromatase enzyme necessary to convert androgens to estrogens.

The majority of androgens cross the basement membrane into the granulosa cells. FSH activates the aromatase enzyme produced by the granulosa cells allowing the thecal androgens to be converted to oestrogens (mainly oestradiol-17β). The process of oestrogen synthesis is shown in Fig. 12.11. After ovulation, oestrogens are produced by the corpus luteum formed from the follicle.

Oestrogens are transported in the blood bound to sex-hormone-binding globulin (SHBG) and albumin. They act via intracellular receptors in the target cells. Oestrogens act on the anterior pituitary and hypothalamus to provide feedback which regulates the system. This feedback is usually negative, but high concentrations of oestrogens for prolonged periods result in a switch to the positive feedback required to induce the LH surge. The actions of oestrogens are shown in Fig. 12.12; the main actions are:

- Development of the reproductive organs and secondary sexual characteristics.
- Proliferation of the functional layer of uterus endometrium.
- Production of watery cervical mucus to allow sperm penetration.
- Production of glycogen by the vaginal epithelium.

Progestogens

Progestogens are secreted in the second half of the menstrual cycle by the corpus luteum. This structure is formed by the transformation of the granulosa and theca interna cells in the follicle after ovulation; LH maintains the secretory activity of these cells. The main progestogen is progesterone, which is synthesized from cholesterol in just two steps. During pregnancy, progesterone production is taken over by the placenta.

Progesterone is transported in the blood bound to corticosteroid-binding globulin (CBG) and albumin. It acts via intracellular receptors in the target cells. Progesterone acts on the anterior pituitary and the hypothalamus to provide negative feedback. The actions of progesterone are shown in Fig. 12.12; its main actions are:

- Maintenance of the uterine endometrium.
- Stimulation of uterine secretions.
- Production of viscid cervical mucus to form an impenetrable barrier.

Androgens

The androgens are precursors of oestrogens; however, small quantities are released systemically. They act with adrenal androgen to promote pubic and axillary hair growth during puberty.

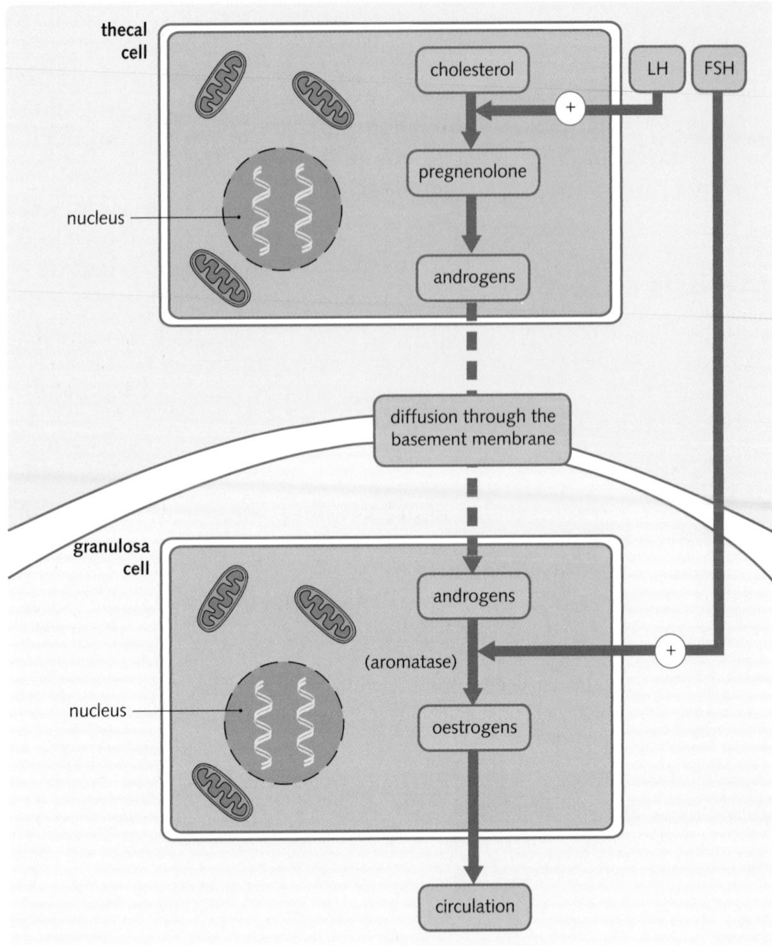

Fig. 12.11 Synthesis of oestrogens by the developing follicle. (FSH, follicle-stimulating hormone; LH, luteinizing hormone.)

Control of ovarian steroid production

Ovarian steroids are regulated in a similar manner to many other major hormones (as shown in Fig. 12.1). Gonadotrophin-releasing factor (GnRH) is synthesized by the hypothalamus and transported to the anterior pituitary gland in the portal veins. Here, it acts on gonadotroph cells to stimulate the release of gonadotrophins (i.e. LH and FSH). This process is described in more detail in Chapter 2.

Gonadotrophins reach the ovaries in the blood and stimulate the release of the ovarian sex steroids. Both LH and FSH stimulate enzymes involved in oestrogen synthesis. LH also allows the formation and maintenance of the corpus luteum that synthesizes progestogens amd oestrogens.

Oestrogens and progestogens feed back to the anterior hypothalamus to regulate their release. This feedback is usually inhibitory and it prevents excess secretion. Before ovulation, the oestrogen feedback becomes positive, triggering the surge in LH release that causes ovulation.

Other ovarian hormones

Inhibin and activin

Inhibin and activin are polypeptide hormones secreted by the granulosa cells of the ovarian follicles. Inhibin inhibits pituitary FSH secretion, while activin stimulates FSH secretion and inhibits androgen production but stimulates conversion to oestrogens. Together, they regulate FSH secretion and local sex steroid levels and the balance between oestrogens and androgens.

Relaxin

This is a polypeptide hormone secreted by the corpus luteum and placenta. It prepares the body for childbirth by causing cervical softening and relaxation of pelvic ligaments.

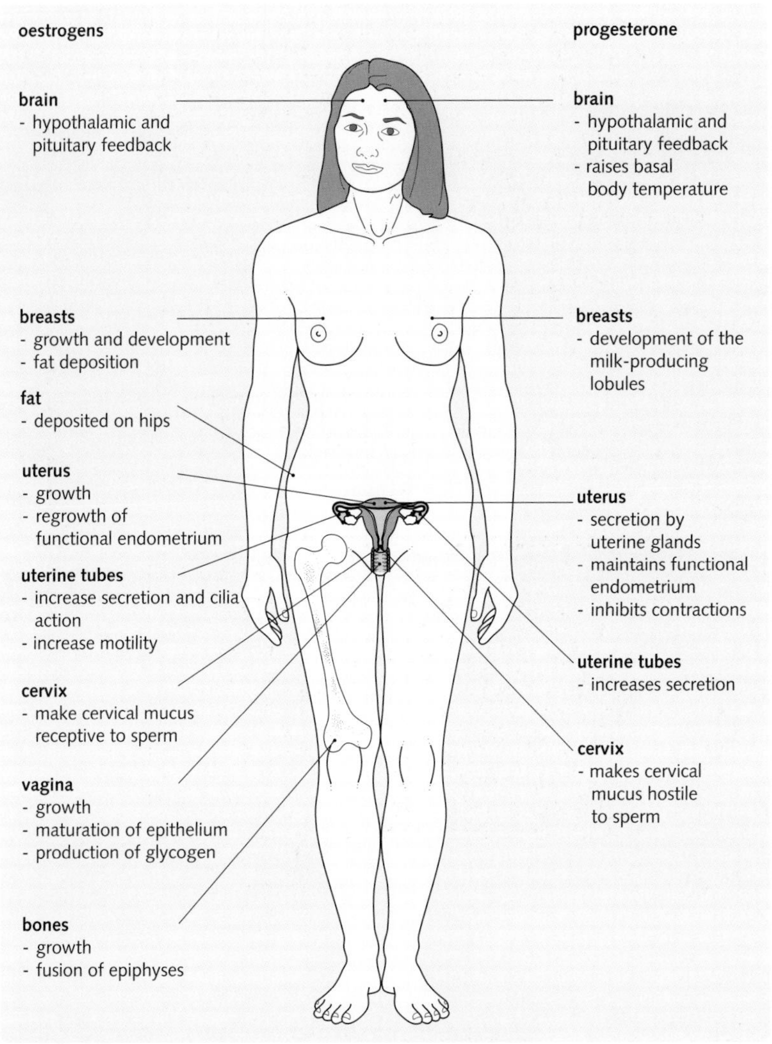

oestrogens

brain
- hypothalamic and pituitary feedback

breasts
- growth and development
- fat deposition

fat
- deposited on hips

uterus
- growth
- regrowth of functional endometrium

uterine tubes
- increase secretion and cilia action
- increase motility

cervix
- make cervical mucus receptive to sperm

vagina
- growth
- maturation of epithelium
- production of glycogen

bones
- growth
- fusion of epiphyses

progesterone

brain
- hypothalamic and pituitary feedback
- raises basal body temperature

breasts
- development of the milk-producing lobules

uterus
- secretion by uterine glands
- maintains functional endometrium
- inhibits contractions

uterine tubes
- increases secretion

cervix
- makes cervical mucus hostile to sperm

Fig. 12.12 Actions of oestrogens and progesterone.

THE MENSTRUAL CYCLE

The menstrual cycle is the process by which the female prepares for possible fertilization of the secondary oocyte. The system is driven by feedback loops between hypothalamic GnRH pulses, pituitary LH and FSH release and ovarian oestrogen, progesterone, inhibin and activin release. Unless interrupted by pregnancy or pathology, these feedback loops generate a cycle that lasts 28–32 days and begins on the first day of menstruation (also called a 'period'). A number of changes occur in the ovaries and endometrium; these are regulated by hormones. The hormonal, ovarian and endometrial changes are shown in Fig. 12.13.

The cycle is divided into two stages, each lasting about 14 days. Between these stages (about the 14th day) ovulation occurs.

Regulation of the cycle by the hypothalamic–pituitary axis

GnRH neurons in the hypothalamus intrinsically generate pulsatile GnRH release. FSH and LH act through endogenous opioids in the hypothalamus to modulate GnRH pulse frequency and amplitude. In turn, the amplitude and frequency of GnRH release dictates the pattern of LH and FSH transcription and release from the pituitary. LH then promotes androstenedione production in the theca cells and FSH stimulates oestrogen production in the granulosa cells and follicular growth.

The first half of the cycle

The first half of the cycle begins on the first day of menstruation and lasts until ovulation. The length of first half of the cycle is variable; if a woman has a long cycle it is the first stage that is prolonged.

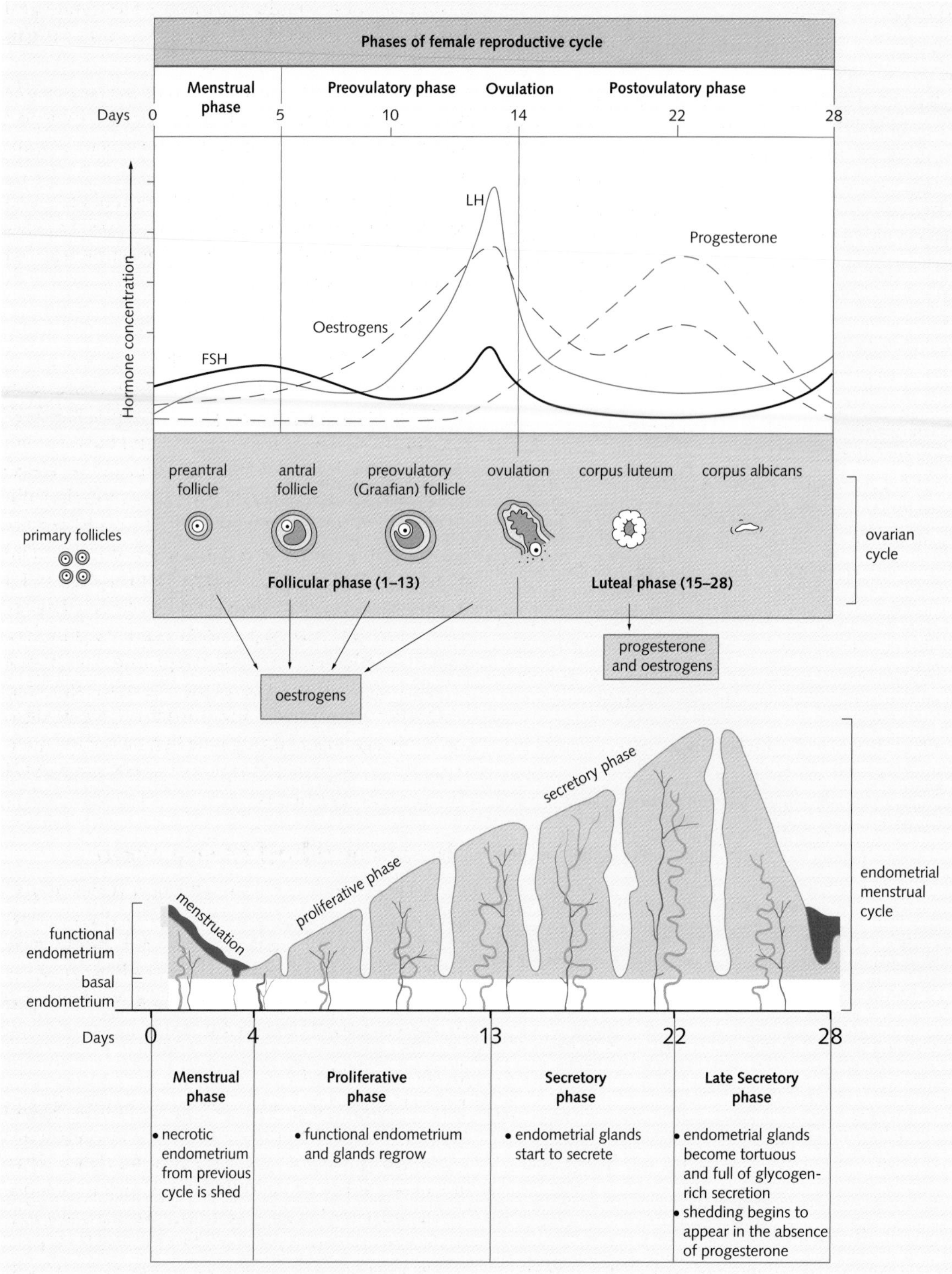

Fig. 12.13 The hormonal, ovarian and endometrial changes during the menstrual cycle. (FSH, follicle-stimulating hormone; LH, luteinizing hormone.)

Ovarian changes

This stage of the cycle is called the follicular stage in the ovary.

During menstruation, LH and FSH levels rise as oestrogen and progesterone production subside. As its name implies, FSH stimulates several antral (secondary) follicles to mature. Cell cooperation between the granulosa cells and the thecal cells allows oestrogen production to begin and for the next 12 days oestrogen levels rise exponentially. Most of the oestrogen output is from the dominant follicle.

The oestrogens stimulate synthesis of LH receptors in the granulosa cells and growth accelerates. With the LH surge, usually only one follicle will be released (the dominant follicle). The other follicles regress (a process called atresia).

Oral contraceptives: Administration of synthetic oestrogen and/or progestogen through the first half of the menstrual cycle prevents FSH secretion. This prevents follicular growth so that ovulation cannot occur.

The dominant follicle has a diameter of about 2.5 cm just before ovulation. The development of the follicle is shown in Fig. 12.10. It is composed of seven layers, from the inside out these are as follows:

- **Primary oocyte**—the female gamete, arrested in first meiotic prophase.
- **Zona pellucida**—a glycoprotein layer that surrounds the oocyte like an egg shell.
- **Granulosa cells**—cuboidal cells surrounding the oocyte; they secrete oestrogens.
- **Antrum**—fluid filled cavity within the granulosa cells.
- **Basement membrane/lamina**.
- **Theca interna**—a layer of stromal cells that secrete androgens.
- **Theca externa**—a non-secretory stromal cell layer.

Endometrial changes

The first half of the cycle is separated into two phases:

- Menstrual phase.
- Proliferative phase.

During the menstrual phase (days 1–4) the ischaemic and necrotic functional layer of the endometrium is lost. This sloughed tissue passes out of the vagina, along with blood from the degenerating spiral arteries.

The proliferative phase (days 4–13) is caused by the rising oestrogen levels. These stimulate cells in the basal layer of the endometrium to proliferate and form a new functional layer. Glands are formed in this layer but they are not yet active.

The rising oestrogen also stimulates secretion of a watery cervical mucus that facilitates sperm transport across the cervix. At other times, the mucus is scant and thick.

Oral contraceptives: Administration of progestogen through the first half of the cycle causes the cervical mucus to remain thick. This forms a barrier that prevents the passage of sperm.

Ovulation

At the end of the follicular stage, the dominant antral follicle secretes such large quantities of oestrogen that the feedback to the pituitary gland changes. The feedback turns from negative to positive and the very high oestrogen levels cause a dramatic surge in the release of LH and, to a lesser extent, FSH. LH causes the follicle to complete the first meiotic division and rupture through the germinal epithelium—a process called ovulation. The secondary oocyte and its first polar body are released into the peritoneal cavity; they are surrounded by the zona pellucida and a few granulosa cells. The released oocyte is swept into the uterine tubes by the wafting action of the cilia of the fimbriae.

Oral contraceptives: Administration of oestrogen and/or progestogen through the first half of the menstrual cycle can prevent the preovulatory surge of LH that stimulates ovulation.

The second half of the cycle

The second half of the cycle is the time between ovulation and menstruation; the average length is 14 days and this remains constant despite changes in cycle length. The length is determined by the lifespan of the corpus luteum (about 10 days). This stage of the cycle is called the luteal stage in the ovary.

Ovarian changes

The LH surge continues to act on the granulosa and theca cells in the empty follicle once ovulation has occurred. The cells change and become yellow. They are now called lutein cells (lutein means yellow, hence the name 'luteinizing' hormone) and the rump of the ruptured follicle is called the corpus luteum.

Over the next 10 days, these cells secrete high levels of progesterone and oestrogens, but they then spontaneously involute (shrink) and lose their secretory ability unless they are rescued by the signal of human chorionic gonadotrophin (hCG) produced by the implanting conceptus.

The progesterone and oestrogen secreted by the corpus luteum inhibit LH and FSH release from the pituitary gland. The falling LH levels fail to maintain the corpus luteum, so it undergoes involution. As a result, progesterone and oestrogen levels fall dramatically so their negative feedback to the pituitary gland is lost. FSH and LH secretion rise, causing ovarian follicles to grow, thus starting the next cycle.

Oral contraceptives: The use of oestrogen and/or progestogen in oral contraceptives aims to mimic the early stages of the second half of the menstrual cycle.

Endometrial changes

After ovulation, the progesterone secretion by the corpus luteum activates the endometrium by stimulating differentiation. A number of changes occur:

- Nutrients are stored in the cells.
- Glands become tortuous (irregularly shaped) in preparation for secretion.

About 5 days after ovulation, the glands begin to secrete a glycogen-rich 'milk' in preparation for a potential embryo; as a result the changes to the endometrium during the second half of the menstrual cycle are called the secretory phase.

As progesterone and oestrogen levels fall, the spiral arteries supplying the functional endometrium begin to coil and constrict causing ischaemia and necrosis. Blood leaks from the damaged vessels into the endometrium before the whole functional endometrium is shed. Menstruation occurs, and this marks the first day of the next cycle.

If pregnancy occurs then the implanting conceptus produces hCG, which binds to LH receptors on the luteal cells exerting a luteotrophic signal for the corpus luteum to maintain itself.

The role of peptides in the menstrual cycle

FSH controls the production of inhibin and activin in the granulosa cells. Inhibin A suppresses FSH release during the early follicular phase and inhibin B suppresses FSH during the late phase. Activin facilitates the release of FSH and enhances its actions.

13 Disorders of the female reproductive system

Objectives

At the end of this chapter, you should be able to:

- Describe the endometrial changes during the menstrual cycle.
- Discuss the presentation, diagnosis and treatment of pelvic inflammatory disease.
- Describe the hormonal changes and symptoms of polycystic ovarian syndrome.
- List the common types of ovarian cysts and tumours along with a brief description of each.
- Describe the presentation, diagnosis and treatment of endometriosis, and explain how it differs from adenomyosis.
- List the conditions that can be caused by excess oestrogen.
- Describe the presentation, diagnosis and treatment of fibroids and endometrial carcinoma.
- List the common causes of amenorrhoea, menorrhagia and dysmenorrhoea.
- Describe the diagnosis, treatment and natural progression of cervical intraepithelial neoplasia.
- Discuss common infections of the vagina and vulva.

DISORDERS OF THE OVARIES AND UTERINE TUBES

Pelvic inflammatory disease

Inflammation of the ovaries, uterine tubes or uterus is called pelvic inflammatory disease (PID), whereas inflammation specific to the uterine tubes is called salpingitis. PID can run an acute or chronic course and it is usually caused by the following organisms:

- Sexually transmitted diseases ascending from the vagina, e.g. *Chlamydia trachomatis* (60% of all PID) and *Neisseria gonorrhoeae* (30%).
- Direct infection following childbirth, surgery or the insertion of a coil.
- Infection from adjacent organs, e.g. from appendicitis.
- Blood-borne infection, e.g. tuberculosis.

These last three infections are usually caused by staphylococci, streptococci, *E. coli* or anaerobes; together they account for only 10% of PID.

Acute pelvic inflammatory disease

In acute PID the lining of the internal genital tract becomes inflamed and swollen; excess mucus is secreted along with a fibrinous exudate (pus). Acute PID can be asymptomatic, but moderate infection causes the following symptoms:

- Severely painful and tender lower abdomen.
- Fever, often with rigors.
- Vaginal discharge.
- Painful intercourse (dyspareunia).

On examination there is often abdominal guarding and vaginal examination will cause extreme pain. Acute PID must be treated with antibiotics since failure of treatment causes damage to the uterine tubes in 10% of cases. Recurrent asymptomatic infection with *Chlamydia trachomatis* can also cause damage and potentially infertility.

Chronic pelvic inflammatory disease

A failure to treat acute PID can also result in chronic PID. The uterine tubes can become sealed by the pus resulting in the following complications:

- Hydrosalpinx—severe swelling due to outflow obstruction.
- Pyosalpinx—an abscess develops in the uterine tube and adhesions form to surrounding structures, especially the ovaries.
- Infertility.

The patient may complain of menorrhagia and intermittent pelvic pain, often worse before menstruation. On vaginal examination, a tender swelling may be felt and further investigation by laparoscopy may be needed. It is usually treated by surgical removal of the affected organs, especially the uterine tubes.

Polycystic ovarian syndrome

Polycystic ovarian syndrome (PCOS) is a common but very complicated syndrome of ovarian dysfunction characterized by hormone dysfunction and multiple cysts in the ovaries. The 'cysts' are actually multiple immature follicles that develop in the ovaries and are visible on ultrasound examination. Twenty per cent of women have polycystic ovaries (PCO), although only a fraction develop symptoms. The symptoms are caused by the endocrine abnormalities, of which the most important are:

- Excess of LH and deficiency of FSH secretion from the anterior pituitary.
- High insulin levels and insulin resistance.
- Excess testosterone.

These endocrine abnormalities cause the following symptoms:

- Amenorrhoea or oligomenorrhoea (no or infrequent periods) with infertility.
- Hirsutism (male pattern hair growth).
- Acne.
- Weight gain.
- Cardiometabolic complications as a consequence of insulin resistance and elevated lipoproteins.
- Risk of endometrial cancer due to unopposed oestrogens.

PCOS is diagnosed from the history, ultrasound examination and raised LH:FSH ratio of >3:1. Treatment is aimed at treating the symptoms:

- Infertility is treated by raising pituitary FSH secretion, often by using the antioestrogen clomiphene.
- Insulin resistance can be treated by the diabetic medication, metformin, and this may also help infertility.
- Antiandrogen drugs are given with a combined oral contraceptive pill to improve the hirsutism though cosmetic treatment is often better.
- In severe cases, destruction of the follicles by laparoscopic ovarian 'drilling' will relieve symptoms for about a year.

Benign ovarian tumours and cysts

Benign ovarian masses are common during the reproductive years; however, it is often impossible to distinguish them from malignant ovarian masses from the history and examination alone. In this account, benign ovarian masses will be considered according the cell type of origin; follicle, epithelium, germ cells, stroma.

Cysts (fluid-filled masses) develop in the ovary during the normal menstrual cycle (i.e. the follicle and corpus luteum). These cysts reach 2–2.5 cm diameter, at which stage they are visible on transvaginal ultrasound examination but usually impalpable on pelvic examination; they should regress within 1 month. Persistent, large or abnormal cysts and solid masses merit further investigation as both can become malignant (Fig. 13.1).

Benign masses derived from the follicles

The most common cause of ovarian masses during the reproductive years result from abnormal development of ovarian follicles. Perturbed follicular development leads to the formation of functional (hormone secreting) ovarian cysts which are not neoplastic. They are larger than normal follicles and typically shrink without treatment. There are two variants of functional cyst:

- **Follicular cyst**—an unruptured and persistent follicle that forms in the absence of an LH surge. These cysts secretes oestrogen often causing menorrhagia (heavy periods).
- **Luteal cyst**—a persistent corpus luteum secreting progesterone, causing irregular bleeding and severe premenstrual syndrome (PMS). Can rupture and cause sharp pain. Risk increased by treatment with superovulatory fertility treatment (clomiphene)

Benign masses derived from the epithelium (ovarian adenomas)

Cystadenomas

These are benign tumours of the ovarian epithelium (cf malignant counterpart, p.136) that secrete fluid to form a cyst; they can grow to massive sizes. They account for 50% of benign ovarian tumours. There are two types:

- Serous—secretes a thin, watery substance.
- Mucinous—secretes protein-rich fluid called mucin.

Fig. 13.1 Common types of ovarian neoplasia

Tumour origin	Name	Frequency	Description
Epithelial cell	Serous cystadenoma	30%	Benign, clear-fluid filled cyst
	Serous cystadenocarcinoma	5%	Malignant, clear-fluid filled cyst
	Mucinous cystadenoma	10%	Benign, mucin-filled cyst
	Mucinous cystadenocarcinoma	0.5%	Malignant, mucin-filled cyst
	Endometrioid	8%	Benign, solid and brown
Germ cell	Benign teratomas	20%	Benign cyst with several tissue types
	Immature teratomas	0.1%	Malignant cyst with several tissue types

Endometriotic cysts

Endometriosis (see p. 137) can result in functional endometrial tissue being deposited on the ovaries. This tissue is stimulated by the hormonal changes of the menstrual cycle, which results in periodic bleeding. With time the blood becomes dark brown and thick; these cysts are, therefore, called chocolate cysts.

Brenner tumours

These are very rare, benign and solid tumours that resemble the transitional epithelium of the urinary tract. They are a type of fibroma.

Benign masses derived from the germ cells

Benign cystic teratomas

These tumours (also called dermoid cysts) are a common type of ovarian tumour. The tumour is composed of cells from all three germ layers (i.e. ectoderm, mesoderm and endoderm). Other recognizable structures and tissues may be present (e.g. teeth, bone, muscle and neural tissue). Complete organization is thought to be missing, as these tumours are parthenogenic (i.e. derived from either male or female cell). This is a common cause of ovarian mass in childhood.

Struma ovarii

These are very rare types of benign cystic teratoma composed mainly of thyroid tissue; they may present with hyperthyroidism.

Benign masses derived from the stroma

Malignant tumours in the ovarian stroma are exceedingly rare; however, the stromal mesenchyme of the ovarian cortex and medulla can become neoplastic. These rare benign tumours are often associated with hormone production:

- Thecomas—develop from the thecal cells; they often secrete oestrogens, causing endometrial hyperplasia and a higher risk of endometrial carcinoma.
- Granulosa cell tumours—develop from the granulosa cells; like thecomas they often secrete oestrogens, with similar effects.
- Androblastoma—the tumour resembles testicular cells (e.g. Sertoli and Leydig cells); they secrete androgens.
- Fibromas—solid, white tumour comprising fibrous tissue (also associated ascite and pleural effusion in the context of Meig's syndrome).

Malignant ovarian disease

Ovarian carcinoma is the most common gynaecological malignancy in the UK and the 5-year survival is poor because of late detection. It is a more common cause of death than cervical and uterine cancer combined. More than half the deaths occur in women over 55. Older women are at highest risk and postmenopausal women are predominantly affected. Risk is increased by the *BRCA1* gene and low parity (i.e. few children); the contraceptive pill has a protective effect. All large, abnormal or persistent ovarian masses should be considered malignant until proven otherwise.

As with benign ovarian masses there are many types, they are described according to their tissue of origin (see Fig. 13.1).

Malignant masses derived from the epithelium (ovarian carcinomas)

Cystadenocarcinomas

Benign cystadenomas may undergo malignant change to form malignant cystadenocarcinomas. The two types are:

- Serous—the most common type of ovarian malignancy (about 50%).
- Mucinous—accounts for 10% of ovarian malignancy.

Endometrioid tumours

These are primary tumours that resemble adenocarcinoma of the endometrium. They usually arise spontaneously, though rarely they develop from endometrioid cysts. Uterine adenocarcinoma is sometimes present.

Clear cell tumours

These are a less common type of endometrioid tumour with pale, glycogen-rich cytoplasm that resembles the secretory phase endometrium.

Malignant masses derived from the germ cells

Dysgerminomas

These are the most common malignant germ cell tumour; the cells resemble seminomas found in the male testes. They occur mainly in adolescents and young women; they are highly malignant.

Yolk-sac tumours

Derived from the endoderm of the yolk sac, these are highly malignant tumours that secrete α-fetoprotein (AFP), which can be detected in the blood. They occur mainly in adolescents and young women.

Solid teratoma

Teratomas that contain embryonal tissues are highly malignant. They occur mainly in adolescents.

Choriocarcinoma

These are highly malignant tumours that secrete human chorionic gonadotrophin (hCG); they are derived from trophoblastic tissue found in teratomas. Around 50% of patients have had a preceding molar pregnancy. They are rare in the UK and USA but more common in Asia. Formerly fatal, this tumour responds to chemotherapy.

Metastatic ovarian tumours

Tumours may metastasize to the ovaries, especially from:

- Endometrium.
- Breast.
- Stomach (Krukenberg tumour).
- Colon.

Diagnosis and treatment of ovarian masses

Symptoms

Ovarian masses are frequently asymptomatic. Pelvic or abdominal pain may occur; large masses can cause noticeable increases in abdominal girth. Advanced malignancy may cause appetite and weight loss, tiredness and general malaise. Ovarian masses are most commonly detected through pelvic examination or ultrasound scans.

Investigations

The definitive diagnosis of an ovarian mass can only be made from a biopsy taken during laparotomy. Initial investigations aim to determine which masses require surgical exploration. These investigations include:

- Pregnancy test—to eliminate the risk of ectopic pregnancy.
- CA-125—a blood-borne tumour marker.
- Ultrasound scan—determines the location, size and nature of the mass.

If a malignancy is suspected, further investigations to assess staging will determine treatment.

Unsuspicious (benign) ovarian masses can be followed-up using repeated pelvic examinations and ultrasound scans. They usually do not require treatment.

Staging

The staging of ovarian carcinoma is shown in Fig. 13.2.

Treatment

Ovarian carcinoma is usually treated at the initial investigative laparotomy. Suspicious masses are removed along with both ovaries, the uterus and the omentum. These tissues are sent for histological analysis and diagnosis. The surgeon will also explore the abdomen and pelvis for signs of metastases. Metastasis may occur via the intraperitoneal (pseudomyxoma peritoneii), haematogenous or

Fig. 13.2 Staging and prognosis of ovarian carcinoma

Stage	Description	Five-year survival (%)
I	Limited to one or both ovaries	80–100
II	Other pelvic sites involved	80–100
III	Sites involved above the pelvic brim within the peritoneal cavity	15–20
IV	Distant metastases	5

lymphatic routes. Surgery is followed by chemotherapy unless the carcinoma is stage I.

BRCA I or *BRCA II* tumour suppressor genes are involved in the hereditary breast and ovarian cancer syndrome. Mutations in the DNA mismatch repair gene *HNPCC* also cause a predisposition to ovarian cancer. Peutz–Jeghers syndrome, which results from a mutation in the *STK11* tumour suppressor gene, also causes a predisposition to ovarian and breast cancer.

Tumours of the uterine tubes

Tumours of the uterine tubes are extremely rare. Benign adenomatoid tumours can form in the superior border of the broad ligament (mesosalpinx). Primary adenocarcinoma of the epithelium rarely occurs in postmenopausal women, and it has an extremely poor prognosis due to late presentation.

DISORDERS OF THE ENDOMETRIUM AND MYOMETRIUM

Inflammation of the endometrium (endometritis)

Inflammation of the endometrium is called endometritis; it can follow an acute or chronic course. Acute endometritis is a bacterial infection, often following trauma (e.g. childbirth, surgical termination, cervical surgery or insertion of the coil). The endometrium usually avoids infection by frequent shedding (menstruation) and the thick cervical mucus. The main causative organisms are staphylococci, streptococci, clostridia and anaerobes.

Endometritis presents in a similar manner to PID, with lower abdominal pain, tenderness and fever. In severe cases, cervical obstruction can occur so the uterus fills with pus (pyometra). This is treated with antibiotics following cervical swabs to determine the organism and its antibiotic sensitivity.

Untreated acute endometritis or PID can cause chronic endometritis. Women develop menstrual irregularities, particularly heavy periods, and the infection may spread to affect other reproductive organs.

Adenomyosis

Adenomyosis is when the basal endometrium penetrates the myometrium (muscular layer of the uterus). Cells from the basal layer of the endometrium form small deposits within the smooth muscle that grow and stimulate proliferation of the muscle. The uterus develops a tumour-like mass or enlarges diffusely often causing menstrual pain and heavy periods. Symptomatic adenomyosis is usually treated by hysterectomy, since the basal cell layer is insensitive to hormones.

Endometriosis

Endometriosis is the presence of functioning endometrial tissue outside the uterus. It is a very common gynaecological disorder occurring in about 5% of women; however, many are undetected. The main locations of the ectopic endometrial cells are shown in Fig. 13.3. The two most common sites are the:

- Ovaries.
- Ligaments of the uterus.

The ectopic tissue still responds to oestrogenic stimuli, so cyclic proliferation and bleeding occurs. The bleeding often forms a cyst that enlarges every month. The size of the cyst is limited by rupture; this may cause adhesions.

The exact cause of endometriosis is still under debate however, there are three theories:

- Retrograde menstruation—menstrual debris enters the peritoneal cavity via the uterine tube in most women. A lack of immune activity could cause implantation and disease.
- Metaplasia of peritoneal epithelium—an unknown stimulus causes the epithelium to transform into endometrial tissue.

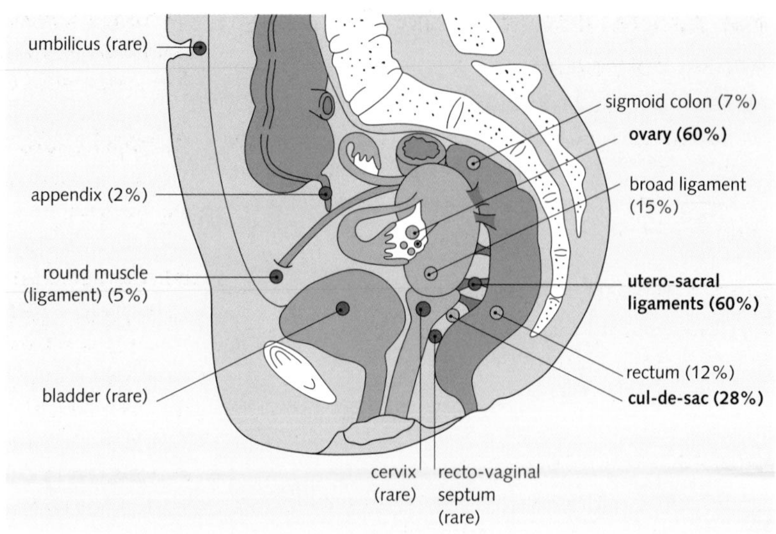

Fig. 13.3 Locations of endometriosis with the relative frequencies (multiple sites are common).

- Metastatic spread—emboli of endometrial tissue may travel via blood and lymph vessels to reach ectopic sites.

In 25% of women, endometriosis is asymptomatic. Women who do have symptoms may have:

- Lower abdominal pain during menstruation (75%).
- Constant pain if adhesions are present.
- Menstrual irregularities (60%).
- Deep dyspareunia (pain on intercourse; 30%).
- Infertility (30%).

Endometriosis is diagnosed from the history and by laparoscopy, which shows red spots. Since endometriosis is common, it is important to know if it is causing the presenting symptoms. This can be achieved by a short course (up to 6 months) of continuous GnRH analogues that stop cyclical sex steroid changes and endometrial symptoms (they downregulate the GnRH receptors). This investigation also acts as a treatment that persists after the GnRH analogue is discontinued.

Endometriosis can be further treated by:

- Continuous use of combined oral contraceptives.
- Medroxyprogesterone acetate (a progestogen).
- Laparoscopic ablation of the endometrial deposits and adhesions, often used if fertility is desired.
- Danazol—an antioestrogen and antiprogesterone with androgenic activity (up to 6 months).

Severe endometriosis may require hysterectomy and bilateral salpingo-oophorectomy (removal of the uterus, uterine tubes and both ovaries).

Endometrial hyperplasia

Endometrial hyperplasia is caused by an excess of oestrogens or unopposed oestrogen action (e.g. oestrogen replacement, oestrogen-secreting tumours or polycystic ovarian syndrome). Obesity is thought to increase the risk through the conversion of androstenedione, causing irregular and heavy menstruation. Endometrial hyperplasia is important because it causes irregular, heavy bleeding and it carries a higher risk of developing into endometrial carcinoma. A spectrum of malignant change is seen:

- Simple hyperplasia—diffuse enlargement, dilated glands; low risk of carcinoma.
- Complex hyperplasia—architecture of tissue change, but internal cell structure unaltered.
- Complex hyperplasia with atypia—like complex hyperplasia, but cells show atypical malignant changes; there is a high risk of carcinoma.

Endometrial hyperplasia is investigated by biopsy of the endometrium. If there is simple hyperplasia in patients who wish to remain fertile, conservative treatment with cyclical progesterone may be sufficient. In severe and atypical cases hysterectomy is recommended.

Functional endometrial disorders

Anovulatory cycles

At the extremes of reproductive age (i.e. around menarche and menopause) menstruation is frequently irregular. This is due to a failure of ovulation followed by excessive oestrogen secretion. The endometrial glands proliferate as a result.

Inadequate luteal phase

A failure in progesterone secretion from the corpus luteum causes inadequate endometrial differentiation resulting in infertility.

Oral contraceptives

Starting or changing the 'Pill' can cause break-through bleeding (bleeding in the middle of the cycle). It usually settles down within a few months, and it can be reduced by taking the pill at the same time every day. Higher doses of oestrogen may be needed if it does not settle. Prolonged use of oral contraceptives reduces the thickness of the endometrium and inactivates the glands, which reduces the amount of menstrual discharge. There is also a 50% lower risk of endometrial and ovarian cancer.

Menopausal changes

At menopause, ovulation and menstruation become irregular followed by complete cessation of the cycles and menstruation within a few months or years. The endometrium reverts to the prepubertal state and the columnar epithelium may undergo metaplasia to form squamous epithelium; cysts can also develop.

Neoplastic disorders

The most common types of uterine neoplasia are shown in Fig. 13.4.

Benign endometrial polyps

Endometrial polyps are very common around the menopause. They are benign tumours caused by the overproliferation of endometrial glands in response to oestrogen. The polyps are usually 1–3 cm in size, and they form smooth, firm nodules within the endometrium. They cause menstrual pain (dysmenorrhea) and irregularities and can be removed using forceps and a speculum.

Benign leiomyomas (fibroids)

Fibroids are benign tumours of the myometrium (muscle layer of the uterus); they are the most common tumours in the genital tract and affect 20% of menopausal women. The tumours are well-defined, monoclonal growths of the smooth muscle cells that often occur in several locations at the same time (Fig. 13.5). Fibroids are oestrogen dependent so they enlarge during pregnancy and with the use of oral contraceptive, but regress after the menopause.

The majority of fibroids are asymptomatic. In the remainder, symptoms are caused by the presence of a

Fig. 13.4 Types of uterine neoplasia

Uterine layer	Name	Frequency	Description
Endometrium	Endometrial hyperplasia	Common	Benign overgrowth of endometrium
	Oestrogen-sensitive endometrial carcinoma	Less common	Malignant tumour derived from endometrial hyperplasia
	Oestrogen-insensitive endometrial carcinoma	Less common	Malignant tumour that originates spontaneously
	Endometrial polyps	Common	Benign enlargement of endometrial glands
Myometrium	Leiomyoma	Very common	Benign smooth muscle tumour
	Leiomyosarcoma	Very rare	Malignant smooth muscle tumour

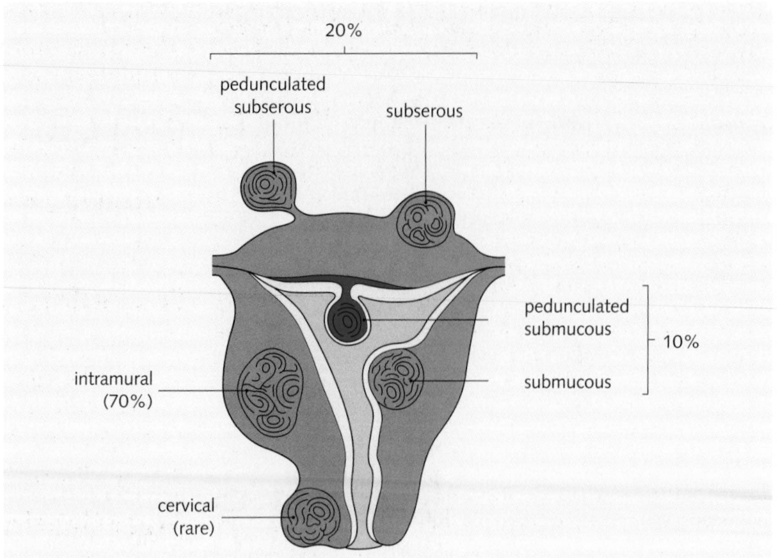

Fig. 13.5 Locations of fibroids with relative frequencies.

uterine mass and the extra endometrium required to cover it. Symptoms include:

- Menorrhagia—periods are heavy and prolonged.
- Pelvic pain—torsion of the fibroid can cause ischaemia and pain.
- Pelvic mass—large fibroids can be felt in the abdomen and compress surrounding structures.
- Infertility—interference with embryo implantation or causing recurrent spontaneous abortion.

Treatment is only needed if the fibroids are symptomatic and troublesome. Continuous GnRH agonists may cause the fibroid to regress, however women who have completed their families often choose hysterectomy. The fibroids can be removed, sparing the unaffected uterus (myomectomy), but adhesions are a common complication.

Endometrial carcinoma

Endometrial carcinoma is the commonest malignancy of the female genital tract. It is usually found during or after the menopause; two patterns are seen:

- Following endometrial hyperplasia—this affects menopausal women; the tumour is an oestrogen-dependent adenocarcinoma with a good prognosis.
- Independent of oestrogen—this affects post-menopausal women; it can follow endometrial squamous metaplasia and has a poor prognosis.

Endometrial carcinoma spreads mainly by local invasion. Initially, this affects the myometrium but the bladder and rectum may become involved with time. It presents with postmenopausal bleeding that becomes progressively more severe. This symptom must be investigated by hysteroscopy (viewing the endometrium through an endoscope inserted through the cervix) and endometrial biopsy (pipelle biopsy).

The staging of endometrial carcinoma is shown in Fig. 13.6. Early-stage carcinoma can be cured by hysterectomy and bilateral salpingo-oophorectomy (removal of the uterus, uterine tubes and both ovaries) followed by radiotherapy. Patients with inoperable carcinoma may benefit from high doses of progestogens and/or radiotherapy.

Other uterine carcinomas

Rarely, malignancy may develop from the stroma of the endometrium, usually with a poor prognosis. They present in a similar manner to endometrial carcinoma but an epithelial component is often present. There are three main types:

- Endometrial stromal sarcoma—consisting of stromal spindle cells.
- Adenosarcoma—malignant stromal and benign epithelial components.
- Carcinosarcoma—malignant stromal and epithelial components, may contain non-uterine tissues.

Fig. 13.6 Staging and prognosis of endometrial carcinoma

Stage	Description	Five-year survival (%)
I	Limited to the endometrium and myometrium, but not serosa	75–100
II	Limited to the uterus and cervix, but not serosa	60
III	Involvement of serosa and/or metastases to other pelvic organs	50
IV	Distant metastases	20

Leiomyosarcomas are extremely rare, malignant tumours of the myometrium that tend to occur after the menopause. They often metastasize by vascular spread to the lungs.

MENSTRUAL DISORDERS

Abnormal frequency, duration and volume of menstruation are common presentations of many gynaecological diseases. Normal menstruation:

- Occurs once every 22–35 days.
- Lasts less than 7 days.
- Less than 80 mL of fluid is discharged.

Amenorrhoea

If menstruation has not occurred within 42 days of the start of the last cycle, it is called oligomenorrhoea. An absence of menstruation for 6 months or more is called amenorrhoea; this is normal before puberty, during pregnancy, and after the menopause. Pathological amenorrhoea is divided into primary and secondary causes.

Primary amenorrhoea

This is when a girl fails to menstruate by 16 years of age.

Secondary amenorrhoea

This is when a woman who has begun to menstruate fails to have a period for 6 months or more. It is a relatively common disorder that affects about 1% of women of reproductive age. The most common causes of secondary amenorrhoea are shown in Fig. 13.7.

Investigation and treatment

Amenorrhoea is investigated with hormone tests (prolactin, FSH, LH and thyroid function tests) and an ultrasound scan of the pelvis. Treatment depends on the cause of the amenorrhoea.

Menorrhagia

Menorrhagia is excessive (>80 mL) menstrual bleeding; it may also be prolonged. Severe menorrhagia may result in iron-deficiency anaemia. The main causes are:

- Dysfunctional uterine bleeding (80%).
- Endometrial tumours and polyps that distort the endometrium.
- Adenomyosis.
- Chronic pelvic inflammatory disease.
- Hypothyroidism.

Fig. 13.7 Common causes of secondary amenorrhoea

Cause	Aetiology	Frequency (%)
Weight loss	Deficiency of leptin from fat prevents GnRH release	35
Polycystic ovaries	FSH deficiency and multiple endocrine abnormalities prevent follicle development	25
Pituitary insensitivity	Following the 'Pill', stress or illness	15
Hyperprolactinaemia	Microadenoma of the pituitary gland (see Ch. 2)	15
Primary ovarian failure	Premature menopause, possibly with autoimmune involvement	5

FSH, follicle-stimulating hormone.

Menorrhagia should be investigated if the woman is over 40 years of age, has intermenstrual bleeding or postcoital bleeding. Hysteroscopy, endometrial biopsy, transvaginal ultrasound, thyroid function tests and clotting studies are used to exclude pathology. In the majority of patients with menorrhagia no underlying pathology is found and the disease is termed dysfunctional uterine bleeding; this condition can also cause irregular bleeding. This is more common at the extremes of reproductive age and is due to an excess of endometrial prostaglandin synthesis that may cause excessive uterine contractions and abnormal blood clotting.

If an underlying cause is found it should be treated; otherwise dysfunctional uterine bleeding can be assumed. Menorrhagia can be treated with:

- Oral contraceptives.
- Mirena® (progestogen-releasing intrauterine system).
- Mefenamic acid (a non-steroidal anti-inflammatory drug).
- Tranexamic acid (fibrinolysis inhibitor).
- Endometrial ablation or hysterectomy if the bleeding is severe.

Dysmenorrhoea

Dysmenorrhoea means painful menstrual periods; it has either primary or secondary causes:

Primary dysmenorrhoea

This is caused by an imbalance in prostaglandin synthesis that results in ischaemia and hyperexcitability of the myometrium. Uterine spasms result, causing cramping pains before and at the start of menstruation. This disorder is very common soon after menarche when it affects about 75% of girls. It decreases with age, but NSAIDs or oral contraceptives usually help.

Secondary dysmenorrhoea

This affects older women, and is usually due to endometriosis or PID. Cramping pains are felt before menstruation; however, they persist and worsen through the period. The underlying pathology should be treated.

Premenstrual syndrome

Premenstrual syndrome (PMS) describes a negative mood and several physical symptoms that can occur in the luteal phase (days 14–28) of the menstrual cycle. Mild PMS is very common, but 5–15% of women suffer from life-disrupting symptoms regularly. The symptoms are shown in Fig. 13.8.

The cause remains unknown; however, fluctuating oestrogen levels may be responsible, possibly mediated via decreased levels of serotonin (5-hydroxytryptamine; 5-HT) in the CNS. Diagnosis is made from the history, and can be confirmed by keeping a diary of symptoms; these must correspond to the menstrual cycle. Treatment can be symptomatic (e.g. analgesia) or aimed at preventing oestrogen fluctuations (e.g. oral contraceptives or oestrogen patches).

> Menorrhagia refers specifically to heavy bleeding. A common cause is dysfunctional uterine bleeding but more serious disease (endometrial cancer) can be the cause and the symptoms can be distressing. Other distinguishable symptoms include; excessive bleeding frequency (polymenorrhoea), irregular bleeding (metrorrhagia), or a combination of excessive and frequent bleeding (menometrorrhagia). It is important to establish when bleeding occurs as post-coital bleeding can reflect underlying cervical ectropion, atrophic vaginitis, cervical dysplasia, sexually transmitted infection or cervical polyps.

Fig. 13.8 Symptoms of premenstrual syndrome

Psychological	Behavioural	Physical
Anxiety Depression Increased appetite Irritability Loss of libido Sleep disturbance Tension	Anger Impulsiveness and accident-prone behaviour Poor concentration Poor tolerance to stress	Acne Weight gain Breast tenderness and swelling Abdominal bloating Change in bowel habit Headache Pelvic pain

MENOPAUSE

The menopause is the cessation of menstruation (6-12 months after the last menses) and ovulation that usually occurs between the ages of 45 and 55 years (average 51). The term 'climacteric' includes the time before and after the menopause during which 'menopausal' symptoms are noticed.

The ovaries gradually become less sensitive to FSH and LH from about the age of 40 years because of the loss of follicles and receptors. This causes anovulatory cycles and a progressive decrease in oestrogen production. As oestrogen levels fall, FSH and LH secretion increases because of the lack of negative feedback. The ovaries resist this increase and the woman enters a period of oligomenorrhoea followed by amenorrhoea. After 6 months of amenorrhoea, the woman is said to have reached menopause. With time, the FSH and LH levels begin to decline along with oestrogen levels.

Other tissues are capable of secreting oestrogens independently, e.g. adipose tissue and the adrenal cortex. The oestrogens produced do not equal the premenopausal levels, so women become oestrogen deficient. The lack of oestrogen predisposes women to three main complications (Fig. 13.9):

- Osteoporosis.
- Heart disease.
- Collagen breakdown.

The climacteric period is symptomatic in 75% of women and severe in 40%. The climacteric symptoms are listed below (those caused by low oestrogen levels are in bold):

- **Hot flushes**; usually at night, often with sweating.
- **Dry, burning vagina** with dyspareunia (pain on intercourse).
- Painful joints.
- Headaches.
- Depression, anxiety, irritability and dizziness.
- Palpitations.
- Urinary incontinence and infection.

The menopause sometimes reduces libido.

Hormone replacement therapy (HRT) is the replacement of oestrogens via a tablet, implant or skin patch. It is often used to treat climacteric symptoms and prevent the long-term complications of oestrogen deficiency. There are three types of HRT:

- Cyclical combined HRT—continuous oestrogens, 12/28 days of progestogens; they cause regular withdrawal bleeds.
- Continuous combined HRT—continuous oestrogens and progestogens; they can only be used 12 months after the last menstrual period.
- Oestrogen only—continuous oestrogens; they can only be used if the woman has had a hysterectomy.

Progestogens must be included if the woman has not had a hysterectomy to prevent endometrial hyperplasia and carcinoma. Cyclical progestogens cause withdrawal bleeding (similar to using the Pill); after 1 year, the woman may use a continuous combined preparation in which progestogens are taken constantly to prevent withdrawal bleeds.

Fig. 13.9 Long-term complications of oestrogen deficiency following the menopause

Symptom/disease	Cause	Consequence
Osteoporosis	Accelerated bone loss	Increased risk of bone fractures, especially the femoral neck at the hip and crush fractures of the vertebrae
Cardiovascular disease	Oestrogens have a beneficial effect on the type of lipid in the blood and in doing so protect against cardiovascular disease	Increased risk of coronary artery disease, myocardial infarction and strokes
Loss of collagen	Weakening in the pelvic ligaments, joints, and muscles, and loss of elasticity in the skin	Predisposes to uterovaginal prolapse, immobility, muscle weakness and causes skin wrinkling

Long-term use of HRT may decrease osteoporosis but may increase the risk of breast cancer, deep vein thrombosis and cardiovasular disease.

The contraindications of HRT include:

- Oestrogen-dependent cancer (including breast cancer).
- Thromboembolic disorders.
- Liver disease with abnormal liver function tests (LFTs).
- Undiagnosed vaginal bleeding.
- Pregnancy or breastfeeding.

There is no male equivalent of the menopause. Men continue to produce testosterone and spermatozoa well into their 80s, but the amount and quality decline with age.

DISORDERS OF THE CERVIX

Cervical ectropion (ectopy)

Cervical ectropion is a normal physiological finding that has been called cervical erosion in the past. It describes the extension of the columnar epithelium of the endocervix beyond the external os under the influence of oestrogen. Any process that raises oestrogen levels can temporarily result in a cervical ectropion, including puberty, pregnancy and the first months of using the 'Pill'. In cervical ectropion, the columnar epithelium appears as a red ring around the external os compared with the pink squamous epithelium. With time, metaplasia occurs and the columnar epithelium converts to stratified squamous epithelium. The presence of cervical ectropion may account for small amounts of postcoital or intermenstrual bleeding; it may raise susceptibility to sexually transmitted infection.

Inflammation of the cervix

Cervicitis

Cervicitis is inflammation and infection of the cervix. It is usually asymptomatic, although vaginal discharge, postcoital bleeding, dyspareunia and pelvic pain may be present; on examination it may be inflamed and tender. The infection is often caused by:

- *Chlamydia trachomatis* (very common, see below).
- *Neisseria gonorrhoeae* (common, see below).
- *Trichomonas vaginalis* (see p. 147).
- Herpes simplex (see p. 148).

The infection is diagnosed using an array of swabs (cervical, *Chlamydia* cervical, and high vaginal) along with a wet mounted cervical smear for *Trichomonas*. Asymptomatic infection should be treated aggressively because of the risk of PID and infertility. The partner often requires treatment to prevent reinfection.

Chlamydia trachomatis This intracellular bacterium is sexually transmitted. It is thought to cause asymptomatic infection in about 5% of young, sexually active women. Although infection is usually asymptomatic, *Chlamydia* can cause urethritis (infection of the urethra), cervicitis and pelvic inflammatory disease (PID, see p. 133). It is usually diagnosed by direct fluorescent antibody tests (DFA) that require a special culture medium; it is treated using the antibiotics doxycycline or erythromycin.

Neisseria gonorrhoeae This Gram-negative diplococcus is an intracellular bacterium that is often called gonococcus; it is a sexually transmitted infection. Like *Chlamydia*, it usually causes asymptomatic urethritis, cervicitis and pelvic inflammatory disease. It is diagnosed by Gram stain and culture of the swab sample; it is treated with the antibiotics cefixime and ceftriaxone. *Chlamydia* is also present in 50% of gonococcus infections, so doxycycline is often given as well.

Neoplasia of the cervix

During puberty, the vagina becomes more acidic due to the presence of glycogen in the vaginal walls and the action of lactobacilli that colonize the vagina. The columnar epithelium of the endocervix reacts to the acid environment by transforming into stratified squamous epithelium—a process called metaplasia. This results in a transformation zone between the ectocervix and endocervix, which is susceptible to dysplasia (precancerous changes). The 'smear test' is used to identify and treat these dysplastic changes before they progress to cervical carcinoma.

Cervical intraepithelial neoplasia

The dysplastic changes leading to cervical carcinoma are called cervical intraepithelial neoplasia (CIN); they are graded from I to III according to the severity and depth of the changes. The risk and rate of progression to cervical carcinoma increases with each grade; however, all stages are treatable. All stages are asymptomatic and undetectable by simply looking at the cervix.

Risk factors

CIN is strongly associated with certain strains of human papilloma virus (HPV). Any factor associated with exposure to HPV increases the risk of CIN, including multiple sexual partners and early age of first intercourse. Cigarette smoking is also a risk factor.

The smear test

In the UK, women between the ages of 20 and 64 years are offered free Pap smears (smear tests) every 3 years until the age of 49 and every 5 years from 50 to 64 by their doctor. From 65, only those women with recent abnormal smears are offered tests. The test involves scraping cells from the cervix using a speculum to open the vagina and wooden spatula to take the sample. Between 2 and 5% of smears are reported as abnormal.

Since the sample is taken from the surface layer, the depth of epithelial involvement cannot be measured directly. The number and severity of dysplastic cells are used to estimate the grade of CIN (Fig. 13.10). This estimate is not entirely accurate. Classification of borderline smears can be improved by testing for the presence of oncogenic HPV strains.

Management of positive smears

Receiving a diagnosis of a positive (abnormal) smear test is commonly misinterpreted as a diagnosis of cervical cancer; the patient will often be afraid and anxious. It is important to explain that it is not a diagnosis of cancer but that follow-up smears/treatment is very important. The management is shown in Fig. 13.10.

Colposcopy

Abnormal smears are often followed up using colposcopy; this is usually performed at a hospital outpatient clinic. A colposcope looks like a pair of binoculars; it magnifies the cervix by 5–20 times. Acetic acid is applied to the cervix so that abnormal areas of cervical epithelium turn white. These areas are inspected and biopsied so that the depth of involvement can be assessed to accurately diagnose the grade of CIN. It is often treated immediately.

Treatment

Moderate to severe (II and III) CIN is treated by removal or destruction of the abnormal epithelium; this is usually performed in colposcopy using local anaesthetic. There are a number of methods of treatment:

- Large loop excision of the transformation zone (LLETZ).
- Laser therapy.
- Cone biopsy (grade III, may raise miscarriage risk).

Vaginal bleeding and discharge is common for about 2 weeks after treatment; sexual intercourse and the use of tampons should be avoided for 4 weeks after treatment. The treatment is followed up with a Pap smear test 6 months later and yearly smear tests for 5 years. Ninety per cent of women are cured; 10% require repeated treatment.

Cervical carcinoma

Cervical carcinoma is usually a squamous cell carcinoma arising in the transformation zone between the ectocervix and endocervix. There is a clear progression from CIN to carcinoma and both diseases have the same risk factors, including HPV infection.

Cervical carcinoma usually affects women after the menopause, but the incidence in younger

Fig. 13.10 Classification, natural history and treatment of cervical intraepithelial neoplasia

Grade	CIN I	CIN II	CIN III
Pap smear classification	Mild dysplasia	Moderate dysplasia	Severe dysplasia / carcinoma in situ
Extent of epithelium involved on biopsy	Third nearest the basement membrane	Two-thirds nearest the basement membrane	Full thickness
Percentage who progress to carcinoma if untreated	1%	8%	20%
Treatment	Follow-up in 6 months or refer to colposcopy	Refer to colposcopy	Refer to colposcopy

women is high enough to warrant population screening from the age of 20 years. The early stages are frequently asymptomatic; by the time of presentation advanced disease with poor 5-year survival is often present. Symptoms include abnormal vaginal bleeding (classically postcoital), vaginal discharge or renal failure in advanced stages; it can be detected through abnormal smear tests. The staging and 5-year survival figures are shown in Fig. 13.11. Invasion of the ureters (which pass 1 cm lateral to the internal os) in stage IIb is a poor prognostic feature.

Suspected cervical carcinoma is investigated by colposcopy with biopsy; if advanced disease is suspected then imaging techniques are used to identify the extent of invasion and metastases:

- Stage Ia—cone biopsy or simple hysterectomy.
- Stage Ib/IIa—radical hysterectomy (includes parametrium and pelvic lymph nodes) or pelvic radiotherapy.
- Stage IIb—combination of radical surgery, chemotherapy and radiotherapy.

Cervical polyps and benign cervical tumours

Cervical polyps are small, round, benign growths of the cervix that often protrude through the external os. They are very common, affecting about 5% of women; they may cause irregular vaginal bleeding or vaginal discharge. They are treated by surgical excision that is often performed in outpatients.

Other benign tumours of the cervix are uncommon though leiomyomas (smooth muscle tumours) can occur.

A new era for cancer management

Vaccines against HPV-16 (found in 50% of cervical cancer) can prevent women from getting both HPV-16 infection and cervical cancer. This may usher in a new paradigm for cancer prevention.

DISORDERS OF THE VAGINA AND VULVA

Infections

The female genital tract is susceptible to many infections, including a number that are sexually transmitted. A summary of the most common female sexually transmitted infections is shown in Fig. 13.12.

Infections of the vagina

Vaginal discharge is a common symptom that can be caused by infections of the cervix (e.g. *Chlamydia*, discussed on p. 144) and vagina (e.g. thrush). The most common causes of vaginal discharge are not sexually transmitted, instead they are caused by overgrowth of normal vaginal flora. This is caused by a rise in vaginal pH (as occurs in pregnancy and diabetes) or loss of the lactobacilli (as occurs when taking antibiotics). These diseases are:

- Bacterial vaginosis.
- Candidiasis (thrush).

Nonetheless, women presenting with vaginal discharge are investigated for a number of sexually transmitted diseases (STDs) due to the high prevalence of

Fig. 13.11 Staging and prognosis of cervical carcinoma

Stage	Description	Five-year survival (%)
Ia	Carcinoma only in cervix, <5 mm	95
Ib	Carcinoma only in cervix, >5 mm	85
IIa	Invasion outside the cervix but not the parametrium (surrounding tissue, including ureters)	75
IIb	Invasion outside the cervix including the parametrium (± ureters)	55
III	Invasion of ureters, lower third of the vagina, or pelvic walls	30
IV	Invasion of bladder, rectum or outside the pelvis	10

Fig. 13.12 Common sexually transmitted infections in women

Infection	Site of infection	Organism	Symptoms	Treatment
Pelvic inflammatory disease	Upper genital tract	*Chlamydia trachomatis* (atypical bacteria) or *Neisseria gonorrhoeae*	Abdominal pain and tenderness, dyspareunia, pus discharge	Doxycycline or ceftriaxone
Gonorrhoea	Cervix	*Neisseria gonorrhoeae*	Urinary frequency, dysuria, pus discharge	Penicillin or ceftriaxone
Trichomoniasis	Vagina	*Trichomonas vaginalis* (parasite)	Itching, discharge	Metronidazole
Thrush	Vagina	*Candida albicans* (fungus)	Itching, white discharge	Clotrimazole (vaginal pessary)
Herpes	Vulva	Herpes simplex virus	Burning red blisters that may recur	Aciclovir if recurrent
Warts	Vulva	Human papilloma virus	Growths on the vulval skin	Podophyllotoxin cream
HIV and AIDS	Systemic	Human immunodeficiency virus	Chronic, progressive immunodeficiency	Combination antiretroviral therapy
Hepatitis	Systemic (liver)	Hepatitis virus B, C and E	Chronic liver disease	(Interferon-α)
Syphilis	Systemic (vulval lesion)	*Treponema pallidum*	Ulcerated nodules, but may become systemic	Penicillin

sexually transmitted infection. The main vaginal infections are described below.

Bacterial vaginosis

This disease is usually caused by the overgrowth of the anaerobic bacteria *Gardnerella vaginalis*, although other anaerobes may be responsible. It is classically associated with a smooth, white vaginal discharge with a distinctive 'fishy' smell. It is diagnosed if the discharge has:

- pH >5.5.
- Ammonia smell when mixed with potassium hydroxide.
- Clue cells on microscopic examination.

It is treated using the antibiotic metronidazole.

Candidiasis

Overgrowth of the yeast (a type of fungi) *Candida albicans* is responsible for thrush. Infection causes the following symptoms:

- Vulval itching and soreness.
- Redness of the vulva and vagina.
- Thick, white vaginal discharge.

It is diagnosed by microscopy of the vaginal discharge that reveals dark purple yeast spores or filaments when stained with potassium hydroxide. A vaginal tablet (pessary) of clotrimazole is used to treat the infection; the partner(s) may also need to be treated to prevent recurrence.

Trichomoniasis

This is an infection with the sexually transmitted flagellated parasite *Trichomonas vaginalis*. It is often asymptomatic, but an accompanying rise in vaginal pH may cause symptoms including:

- Thin, watery (may be green or foamy) vaginal discharge.
- Some itching and redness.

It is diagnosed by viewing the vaginal discharge mounted on saline under a microscope; the organism can be identified by the movement seen. Oral metronidazole cures 90% but a second vaginal swab should be performed 2 months later. The partner(s) should also be treated.

Infections of the vulva

The vulva is susceptible to sexually transmitted viral infections similar to those that affect skin on other areas of the body:

Herpes simplex

This is caused by the herpes simplex virus (usually HSV type II though HSV type I can also cause vulval disease). About 25% of patients experience acute symptoms including:

- Localized itching and burning.
- Multiple painful red vesicles.
- Ulceration of vesicles causing more pain.
- Dysuria if the area round the urethra is involved.
- Fever and malaise.

Vesicles appear ~3 days after infection and take up to 2 weeks to heal, during which time the virus is shed and can be transmitted. The virus cannot be transmitted if vesicles are not present, but some vesicles may be hidden. The virus enters the dorsal root ganglion of sensory nerves supplying the infected area. It usually lies dormant, but it may cause recurrent attacks in 5% of patients.

Herpes simplex can be diagnosed from viral culture of fluid in the vesicles and antibody screening. It is treated symptomatically (e.g. anaesthetic cream), although the antiviral agent aciclovir can reduce the frequency and duration of recurrent attacks. The virus can be transmitted to other body parts via the hands; the eyes are particularly susceptible. The presence of herpes vesicles in late pregnancy is an indication for caesarean section.

Genital warts

These are benign growths of the epithelium caused by human papilloma viruses (HPV), of which there are many types. Some HPV strains infect the vulval skin, causing small cauliflower-shaped warts that may cause itching and burning. The infection can spread to the vagina and cervix, and it is readily passed onto sexual contacts. Certain strains of HPV can predispose to dysplastic changes in the cervix, vulva and anus that may lead to carcinoma; these strains rarely cause obvious growths.

Vulval warts are treated with podophyllotoxin cream, cryotherapy or minor surgery if they cause the patient distress. Smear tests should be repeated annually.

Bartholin's cyst

This disease is caused by bacterial infection of the greater vestibular (Bartholin's) gland and duct found either side of the introitus (vaginal orifice); it is a common vulval disorder. If the duct becomes obstructed, a cyst can form that presents as a vulval swelling. The main causative bacteria are staphylococci, *E. coli* and gonococci.

Cysts require surgical treatment and antibiotics to prevent abscess formation.

Systemic sexually transmitted infections

Other sexually transmitted diseases cause systemic illness and often have a chronic course. They are briefly described in Fig. 13.12; recent infection with syphilis can result in a genital lesion at the site of infection.

Neoplasia of the vagina

Tumours very rarely develop in the vagina, though they may spread to the vagina from the cervix and endometrium. The majority of tumours that do develop are squamous cell carcinomas found in the upper third of the vagina in elderly women. Adenocarcinoma, melanoma and sarcoma are even rarer, but tend to affect younger women.

Vaginal carcinoma presents with abnormal vaginal bleeding, pelvic pain and the detection of a lump. It is investigated by smear test and ultrasound scan to determine the origins of the carcinoma. The treatment of cervical and endometrial carcinoma are described on p. 146 and p. 140, respectively. Squamous cell carcinoma is mainly treated with radiotherapy, though surgery and chemotherapy may also be required.

Vulval dystrophies

The vulval dystrophies are non-neoplastic, chronic disorders of the vulval skin; they mainly affect menopausal or postmenopausal women, but they may affect prepubescents. They are distinct from the physiological vulval atrophy caused by oestrogen deficiency following the menopause. There are two patterns of vulvar dystrophy:

- Lichen sclerosus.
- Squamous cell hyperplasia (also called hypertrophic dysplasia or leucoplakia).

These diseases are compared in Fig. 13.13. Both conditions present with vulval itching and pain on contact leading to superficial dyspareunia; they can undergo malignant change. They are investigated using a colposcope (p. 145) and biopsy of suspicious areas under local anaesthetic. Treatment is shown in Fig. 13.13.

Neoplasia of the vulva

Malignant tumours

Vulval intraepithelial neoplasia (VIN)

Precancerous changes can be detected in the vulva (VIN) in a similar manner to the cervix (CIN; see

Fig. 13.13 Comparison of lichen sclerosus and squamous cell hyperplasia

Feature	Lichen sclerosus	Squamous cell hyperplasia
Epidermis	Thin	Thick
Dermis	Hyalinized (degeneration and replacement with collagen) and oedematous	Oedematous
Inflammatory cells present	Lymphocytes	Plasma cells
Appearance	Shiny, white and crinkly plaques	Thick, white/grey areas with deep skin-folds
Treatment	Vaseline or topical steroids	Topical steroids

p. 144). These changes are associated with HPV (wart virus) infection, smoking and the vulval dystrophies described above. The affected vulva may feel itchy and sore, and there may be a lump or ulcer. It is investigated using a colposcope and biopsy to determine the extent of cellular dysplasia; it is graded in a similar manner to CIN to determine treatment (Fig. 13.14). Appropriate treatment ensures a 5-year survival of 100%; untreated VIN may progress to vulval cancer. The risk is significantly higher for VIN III.

Vulval carcinoma

Vulval carcinoma is an uncommon malignancy that mainly affects elderly women. It is usually a squamous cell carcinoma predisposed by HPV infection and smoking; 30% occur as a progression from VIN. They present with similar symptoms to VIN and are investigated with colposcope examination and biopsy. The staging system and 5-year survival are shown in Fig. 13.15. Vulval carcinoma is treated surgically (radical vulvectomy and lymph node dissection to various extents) and with radiotherapy in stages III and IV.

Other malignancies

Since the vulva is covered with skin, it can develop similar malignant tumours to other areas of skin. The melanocytes can give rise to malignant melanoma, and the vulval ducts can develop cancerous Paget's disease.

Benign tumours

The vulva is prone to the same benign tumours as other areas of skin. One of the most frequent tumours is papillary hidradenoma. This is a benign growth of the sweat (eccrine) glands.

DISORDERS OF THE FEMALE BREAST

The most common presenting complaint involving the breast is a lump. Fig. 13.16 shows the most common causes and their associated features.

Congenital abnormalities

Supernumerary nipples

Failure of the fetal mammary ridge to regress can cause extra nipples (polythelia) to develop. The extra nipple is usually just below a normal breast, however they can be found anywhere along the line of the

Fig. 13.14 Classification and treatment of vulval intraepithelial neoplasia

Grade	VIN I	VIN II	VIN III
Classification	Mild dysplasia	Moderate dysplasia	Severe dysplasia/ carcinoma in situ
Treatment	Topical steroids and regular follow up	Topical steroids and regular follow up	Surgical excision or destruction

Fig. 13.15 Staging and prognosis of vulval carcinoma

Stage	Description	Five-year survival (%)
I	Tumour confined to vulva and perineum, <2 cm	>90
II	Tumour confined to vulva and perineum, >2 cm	80–90
III	Tumour involves lower urethra/vagina/anus and/or unilateral lymph nodes	50–80
IV	Distant metastases, involvement of upper urethra/bladder/rectum/pubic bone and/or bilateral metastases	5–30

Fig. 13.16 Types of breast lump and associated features

Disease	Most common age group	Frequency	Features of lump
Fat necrosis	Any	Rare	Single, hard and irregular
Mammary duct ectasia	Older women before the menopause	Common	Tender; near the areola
Nodular fibrocystic change	Older women before the menopause	Very common	Single or multiple firm nodules
Cystic fibrocystic change	Just before the menopause	Very common	Rapidly growing smooth, rounded cysts
Fibroadenoma	Younger women (25–35 years)	Common	Single firm, highly mobile, non-tender lump
Phyllodes tumour	Older women	Less common	Single, large, rubbery lump
Duct papilloma	Middle-aged women	Common	Lump near the nipple with bloody discharge
Carcinoma	Middle-aged to elderly women	Common	Single hard lump with stromal interference

mammary ridge (axilla to inguinal rings) and very rarely in other locations. It is a common disorder affecting about 1% of people, though the extra nipple is often mistaken for a mole.

Accessory breast tissue

In females, accessory breast tissue (polymastia) can also develop, although it is usually not noticed until puberty. The extra tissue is usually in the axilla, but it can form in the same locations as extra nipples. The accessory breast tissue may be associated with a nipple to form an extra breast.

Congenital nipple inversion

The nipple is usually inverted at birth; development of the areola should cause it to rise. If this process fails the nipple may be permanently inverted, causing difficulty in breastfeeding. It is important to differentiate between congenital inversion and a recent inversion that may suggest a malignancy.

Inflammatory disorders and infections

Acute mastitis and breast abscess

When the woman is lactating, the breast is prone to bacterial infection through cracks in the nipple and areola. The usual organisms responsible are *Staphylococcus* and *Streptococcus*.

The initial infection causes an acute inflammation of the breast called mastitis, in which the breast becomes tender and enlarged. It should be treated with antibiotics to prevent breast abscesses that must be drained surgically. Chronic mastitis can also develop, but it is very rare.

Mammary duct ectasia

Mammary duct ectasia is a chronic inflammatory condition of unknown origin that causes the lactiferous ducts near the nipple to dilate. It is most common just before the menopause in women who have had children. The dilated duct fills with a creamy, protein-rich fluid that causes a green discharge from the nipple and tender lumps near the areola. The possibility of carcinoma must be excluded by biopsy or surgical excision. The dilated ducts are prone to infection, which requires antibiotic treatment to prevent abscess formation.

Fat necrosis

Relatively minor trauma to the breast can result in necrosis of the adipose tissue (fat cells). This necrosis prompts an inflammatory reaction that can cause fibrous scarring, producing a hard, irregular lump in the breast. These lesions can mimic carcinomas, including characteristic interference with the normal breast connective tissue such as skin dimpling. This condition is relatively rare, and it can only be differentiated from a malignancy by excision biopsy.

Fibrocystic change/fibroadenosis

Fibrocystic change is caused by benign growth of the breast tissue resulting in tender lumps. It is a very common disease that affects 50% of women, though only 10% are symptomatic. It is most common in older women before menopause.

The overgrowth occurs in two tissues:

- Epithelial lining of the ducts and lobules.
- Fibrous stroma.

A variation in hormonal response results in a growth imbalance between the fibrous and epithelial tissues causing solid nodules and fluid-filled cysts to develop. The nature of this imbalance can vary, resulting in three patterns of change (described below); these may coexist.

Simple fibrocystic change

Overgrowth of both tissues is seen in simple fibrocystic change producing a mixture of fibrous nodules and epithelial cysts. The imbalance in tissue overgrowth is a local effect, and many microscopic areas display these changes. Larger growth imbalances can cause symptomatic fibrocystic change.

Single or multiple fibrous nodules can develop, and these frequently become tender towards the end of the menstrual cycle (i.e. premenstrually). It is difficult to differentiate the single lumps from a carcinoma except by biopsy or excision.

Palpable epithelial cysts are most frequent close to the start of the menopause. They can be distinguished from lumps by palpation (smooth, rounded and flocculent) and their appearance on X-ray mammograms and ultrasound scans. Cysts contain a watery fluid that can be aspirated and examined for evidence of malignancy; this aspiration also treats the cyst. Simple fibrocystic change is entirely benign.

Epithelial hyperplasia

If the epithelial overgrowth predominates, the condition is called epithelial hyperplasia. It is a benign change, but it has an increased risk of breast carcinoma (two times normal risk). The risk of carcinoma is higher if the epithelial cells show signs of dysplasia, called atypical hyperplasia (five times normal risk).

Sclerosing adenosis

If the fibrous overgrowth predominates, the condition is called sclerosing adenosis. This rare variation is entirely benign. It can compress the surrounding glands and cause a histological appearance of solid cords that can be confused with invasive carcinoma on histological and X-ray (mammogram) examination.

Benign neoplasia

Fibroadenoma

Fibroadenomas are common, solitary, benign lumps that occur mostly in young women (below 35 years of age). Lumps develop from the mammary ducts and stroma in response to hormonal stimuli. They contain glandular epithelial components from the duct and fibrous components from the stroma, so they may be caused by a type of fibrocystic change instead of being true benign tumours. The lumps are usually firm, rubbery, and non-tender; they are highly mobile and can slip away during palpation (hence the name 'breast mice').

Phyllodes tumour

Phyllodes tumours resemble fibroadenomas, but they are often much larger. They can occur at any age after puberty, but usually affect older women. These lesions are usually benign, but a spectrum of dysplasia is seen: 10% are malignant.

Duct papilloma

Duct papillomas are benign growths of the mammary duct epithelia. These solitary tumours usually develop in the lactiferous duct just below the nipple in middle-aged women. In younger women, they usually develop in the smaller ducts. They cause a lump and bloody nipple discharge. The tumour is surgically excised and the breast is examined by mammography to reveal any underlying carcinoma.

Multiple duct papillomas are rare and have an increased risk of breast carcinoma.

Malignant neoplasia

Breast carcinoma is the most common cancer in women, affecting about 1 in 12 at some point in their life. The risk of breast cancer increases with age, being very rare before 25 years but moderately common by 40 years of age. There are a number of risk factors for breast cancer:

- Family history—including the recently discovered autosomal dominant *BRAC 1* and *BRAC 2* mutations.
- Geographical—there is a higher risk in developed countries.
- Excess oestrogen exposure—this can be caused by many factors (e.g. early menarche, late menopause, HRT, no pregnancies) but probably not the 'Pill'.
- Epithelial hyperplasia—see the section on fibrocystic change.

Classification of breast carcinoma

The vast majority of breast cancers are adenocarcinomas. These can develop in three patterns according to their location in the breast:

- Invasive ductal carcinoma (50%).
- Invasive lobular carcinoma (30%).
- Mixed ductal and lobular carcinoma (10%).

The other 10% are rarer forms of breast cancer (see below).

All three patterns of adenocarcinoma can be preceded by non-invasive carcinoma in situ. With time, roughly 25% of these will develop into invasive carcinoma, but early mastectomy usually prevents this. Two forms are seen, identified by location:

- Intraductal carcinoma.
- Intralobular carcinoma.

Three other types of carcinoma occur more rarely. They have a better prognosis than invasive adenocarcinoma. They are:

- Tubular carcinoma.
- Mucoid carcinoma.
- Medullary carcinoma.

Presentation

The majority of breast cancers present as lumps or from mammogram screening. All lumps should be investigated as if they were malignant. This includes:

- Ultrasound or attempted aspiration to differentiate cysts and lumps.
- Fine-needle aspiration or excision biopsy of lumps.

Excision biopsy is only carried out on lumps or cysts with a history or appearance suggestive of malignancy. There are a number of signs of carcinoma that suggest excision biopsy is needed or that prompt investigation in the absence of a lump. These are mostly caused by interference with the breast stroma or lymphatic drainage:

- Skin dimpling.
- Recent nipple inversion.
- Bloody nipple discharge.
- Peau d'orange (skin with the appearance of orange peel).
- Surface erythema or ulceration.
- Paget's disease of the nipple.

Paget's disease is an eczema-like rash around the nipple caused by local spread of invasive ductal carcinoma.

The features of a lump or cyst that suggest malignancy are:

- Large, hard or growing masses.
- Fixing of mass to underlying structures.
- Enlargement of the affected breast.
- Blood-stained cystic fluid.
- Recurrence.
- Enlarged axillary lymph nodes.

Spread, prognosis and staging

Invasive breast carcinoma can spread by three routes:

- Local spread—within the breast or into surrounding structures, e.g. skin, nipple, pectoral muscles and the chest wall.
- Lymphatic spread—to the axillary, internal thoracic lymph nodes and the other breast.
- Vascular spread—especially to the bone (especially vertebral bodies), lungs, pleura and ovaries (called a Krukenberg tumour).

Metastasis involves the invasion of cells through a basement membrane and dissemination to a distant site. Breast cancer commonly metastasizes to the local lymph nodes, bone, lung, liver and brain. Symptoms can occur as a consequence of local disruption at the site of metastasis, for example visual field defects in the case of brain metastases. However, biochemical abnormalities can also occur giving rise to systemic symptoms. Bony metastasis can cause hypercalcaemia with resultant bone pain, fatigue, constipation, nausea and fits. Be wary of hypercalcaemic symptoms in a woman.

The prognosis of breast cancer is predicted by the stage of the tumour. This is determined from the TNM system, which assigns scores according to three measures (Fig. 13.17):

Tumour size, **N**odal involvement and **M**etastases.

In general, low scores have a better prognosis, e.g. 80% 5-year survival if no nodes are involved. The presence of metastases is a particularly poor prognostic sign, reducing the 5-year survival to 10%.

Treatment

The options for treating breast cancer are the same three for most cancers, namely:

- Surgery.
- Radiotherapy.
- Chemotherapy.

Surgical removal of the tumour is necessary if a cure is to be achieved. There are two options depending on the size of the tumour:

- Simple mastectomy (removal of the affected breast).
- Lumpectomy (removal of the lump) along with a large area of surrounding tissue.

Radiotherapy is used to prevent local and lymphatic spread. The breast, chest wall and surrounding lymph nodes are often irradiated.

Chemotherapy is aimed at preventing metastatic spread. The standard cytotoxic drugs are used along with tamoxifen, which is an oestrogen receptor blocker. This drug causes symptoms of an early menopause in younger women.

As breast cancer carries such a high mortality rate, it is often the first paradigm for new approaches to cancer care. Emerging technologies include the use of microarray global gene expression data to identify genes which are prognostic of outcome and predictive of cancer occurrence in order to better tailor therapy. 'Pharmacogenomics' is the process of identifying genes which predict a patient's response to therapy. 'Systems biology' is an attempt to understand cellular behaviour as complex genetic networks. Systems biology approaches are needed in breast cancer where several genetic perturbations are involved. They will hopefully identify better combinatorial therapies.

Fig. 13.17 TNM staging system of breast cancer

Stage	0	1	2	3
Tumour (T)	None	<2 cm	2–5 cm	>5 cm
Nodes (N)	None	Nodes involved but mobile	Nodes involved but immobile	
Metastases (M)	None	Metastases		

The male reproductive system

14

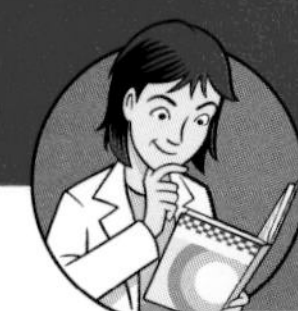

Objectives

By the end of this chapter you should be able to:

- Describe the structure and function of the testes.
- Describe the structure of the penis and the mechanism of erection.
- Describe the course and layers of the spermatic cord, and explain how these relate to the abdomen and scrotum.
- Describe the structure and location of the prostate.
- Name three hormones involved in the male reproductive system, along with their origins and actions.
- Describe the process of spermatogenesis. Explain the roles of the Sertoli and Leydig cells.
- Describe how continuous fertility is achieved in the male.
- Name and briefly describe three congenital abnormalities of the testes.
- Compare testicular torsion and epididymo-orchitis.
- Describe the differential diagnosis of a scrotal lump.
- Name three types of testicular carcinoma, the cells they are derived from and the age groups they affect.
- Describe the aetiology, presentation and treatment of benign prostatic hyperplasia.
- Describe the location, presentation and treatment of prostatic carcinoma.
- Discuss four sexually transmitted diseases, including their presentation and treatment.
- Recognize gynaecomastia and male breast carcinoma.

The male reproductive system encompasses the testes, the prostate, the seminal vesicles and the penis. Its principal functions are:

- Sperm production (spermatogenesis) and release.
- Production of hormones involved in male reproduction and libido.

After puberty, the testes begin to produce sperm and they continue to do so until death. This process is regulated by four main hormones (Fig. 14.1):

- Follicle-stimulating hormone (FSH).
- Luteinizing hormone (LH).
- Testosterone,
- Inhibin B.

The ejaculation of sperm is controlled by neural stimuli from the autonomic nervous system. The sperm are ejected with seminal fluid that protects them and provides nutrients.

ORGANIZATION

The male reproductive system consists of five main components:

- Testes—produce the sperm.
- Epididymis—stores and matures the sperm.
- Vas (ductus) deferens—transports sperm from the epididymis to the penis.
- Prostate and seminal vesicles—secrete seminal fluid to support ejaculated sperm.
- Penis—deposits sperm in the vagina.

All of these components lie outside the peritoneal cavity. Each of these components is discussed individually in the following sections. Their locations are shown in Fig. 14.2 and their blood supply, lymphatics and innervation are shown in Fig. 14.3.

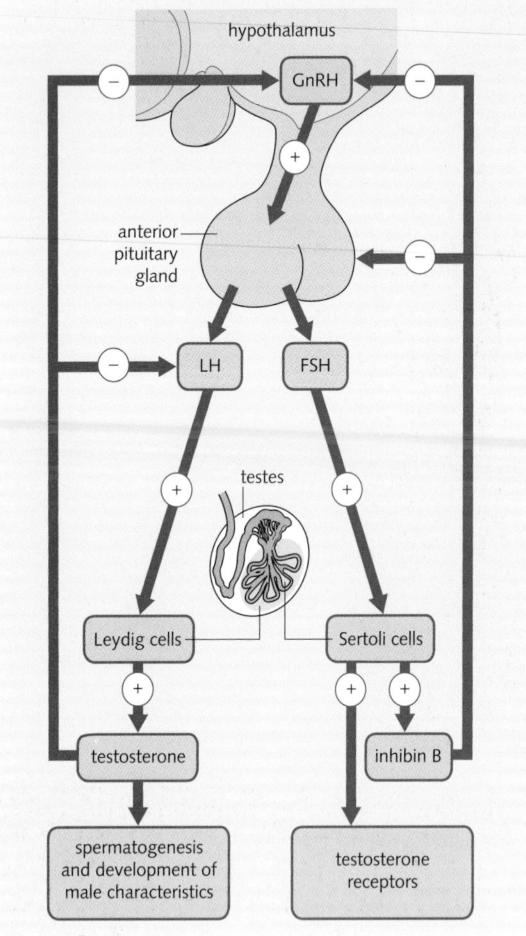

Fig. 14.1 Hormonal regulation of the male reproductive system. (FSH, follicle-stimulating hormone; GnRH, gonadotrophin-releasing hormone; LH, luteinizing hormone.)

Testes

The testes are two oval-shaped organs that produce sperm (the male gametes) in response to gonadotrophins (LH+FSH) from the pituitary gland and testosterone from the Leydig cells of the testes. They are suspended in the sac-like scrotum by the spermatic cord; this keeps their temperature 2–3°C lower than body temperature. If their temperature rises then sperm production ceases. Each testis is surrounded by a capsule of three layers (starting nearest the testis):

- Tunica vasculosa—loose connective tissue with blood vessels.
- Tunica albuginea—fibrous connective tissue.
- Tunica vaginalis—derived from peritoneum, it also surrounds the epididymis.

Microstructure

Fibrous septa divide each testis into about 300 lobules, each containing 1–4 seminiferous tubules that produce sperm. The seminiferous tubules are closed loops lined with a specialized epithelium that contains two types of cells:

- Spermatogonia that undergo meiosis to give rise to haploid spermatozoa.
- Sertoli cells that support the developing sperm and secrete testicular fluid into the tubules.

In between the seminiferous tubules there are vessels and clusters of testosterone-secreting interstitial (Leydig) cells. The microstructure of the seminiferous tubules is shown in Fig. 14.4.

Inside the testis, the loops of the seminiferous tubules drain into the rete testis. These are convoluted networks of ducts, lined by simple cuboidal epithelial cells with microvilli, most cells bearing a single long flagellum. All the vessels that support the testis enter the testis capsule at the rete testis. The sperm pass from the rete testis to the epididymis via about 15 efferent ductules lined by ciliated epithelium.

Epididymis

The epididymis is a firm, comma-shaped structure attached posteriorly to the top of the testis within the scrotum. Normally it can be distinguished from testis by palpation. It is described in three sections:

- Head—superior section where the efferent ductules enter.
- Body—in between the head and tail.
- Tail—inferior section, continuous with the vas deferens.

The epididymis contains a single, tightly coiled tube formed by the fusion of the efferent ductules from the rete testes. Testicular fluid is partially reabsorbed by the tall columnar epithelium with long microvilli (stereocilia). The sperm pass slowly through this tube to reach the vas deferens at the tail of the epididymis. The epididymis is surrounded by a fibrous capsule that is separated from the testis by the tunica vasculosa and tunica albuginea, except at the head where the testis and epididymis join. The tunica vaginalis surrounds the testis and the fibrous capsule of the epididymis.

Scrotum

The scrotum contains both testes, epididymides and the start of vasa deferentia. The skin is usually pigmented and wrinkled with a line down the midline called the scrotal raphe.

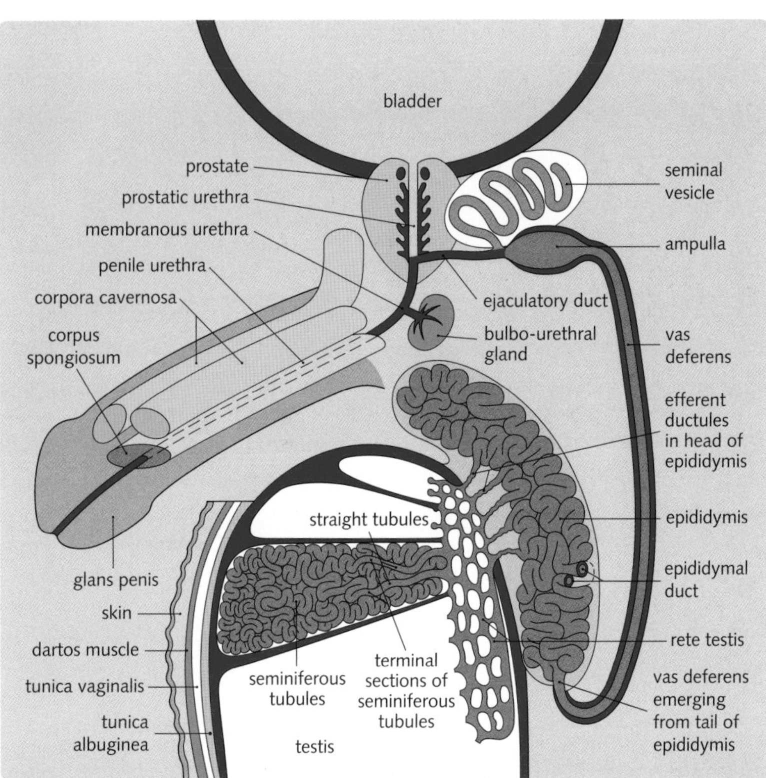

Fig. 14.2 Arrangement of the male reproductive system. This diagram is not to scale.

Fig. 14.3 Blood supply, lymphatics and innervation of the male reproductive organs

Organ	Arterial supply	Venous drainage	Innervation	Lymphatic drainage
Testis	Testicular arteries from the aorta via the spermatic cord	Pampiniform plexus, which forms the testicular veins. Left drains into the left renal vein, right into the inferior vena cava	Sympathetic innervation via the splanchnic nerves	Para-aortic lymph nodes
Scrotum	Pudendal arteries	Scrotal veins	Branches of the genitofemoral, ilioinguinal and pudendal nerves	Superficial inguinal lymph nodes
Prostate	Vesicular and rectal branches of the internal iliac artery	Prostatic venous plexus drains into the internal iliac veins	Parasympathetic via splanchnic nerves; sympathetic from inferior hypogastric plexus	Internal iliac and sacral lymph nodes
Penis	Internal pudendal arteries	Venous plexus, which joins the prostatic venous plexus	Branches of the pudendal nerve	Superficial inguinal lymph nodes

Microstructure

The wall of the scrotum is formed by five layers; three of these continue as the covering of the spermatic cord. All five are continuous with the abdominal wall from which they are derived. They are described in Fig. 14.5 and their development is shown in Fig. 11.5. Two muscles are found in the scrotum:

- Dartos muscle—contracts the scrotal skin in response to cold.
- Cremasteric muscle—retracts the testis towards the abdomen prior to ejaculation. Sumo wrestlers can train themselves to retract the testes for their protection. Clinically, the cremesteric reflex is more active in children.

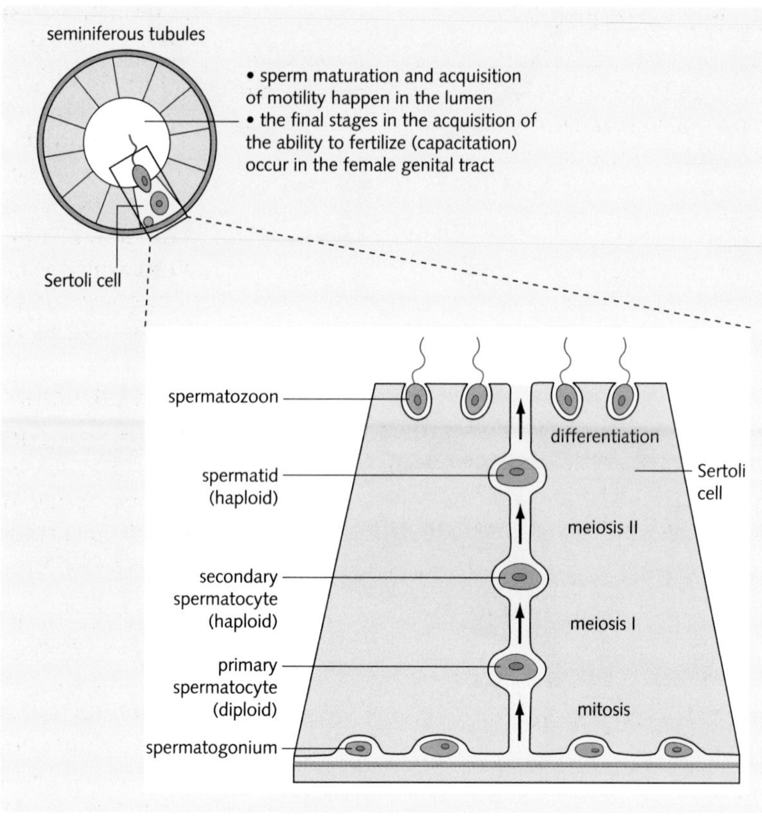

Fig. 14.4 Microstructure of the seminiferous tubule.

Fig. 14.5 Layers of the abdominal wall, spermatic cord and scrotum

Abdominal layer	Spermatic cord layer	Scrotal layer
Skin	None	Skin
Superficial fascia	None	Dartos muscle
External oblique aponeurosis	External spermatic fascia	External spermatic fascia
Internal oblique muscle and fascia	Cremasteric muscle and fascia	Cremasteric muscle and fascia
Transversalis fascia (not the muscle)	Internal spermatic fascia	Internal spermatic fascia

Vas (ductus) deferens

The vas deferens is the continuation of the epididymis on each side of the scrotum. It transports sperm from the epididymis to the ejaculatory ducts during the emission phase of an ejaculation (see p.159). It has three muscular layers to propel the spermatozoa along its 40 cm length and a lining epithelium similar to that found in the epididymis. The vas deferens is palpable in the scrotum; this allows male sterilization (vasectomy) with only minimal incisions.

Once the vas deferens enters the abdomen in the spermatic cord, it passes along the lateral wall of the pelvis, external to the peritoneum. It crosses the ureter and descends to the base of the bladder. The duct widens into the ampulla before the junction with the duct of the seminal vesicle.

Spermatic cord

The spermatic cord is formed at the deep inguinal ring of the abdominal wall and passes along the inguinal canal and then inferiorly in the scrotum to the testis. It contains nine structures:

- Vas deferens.
- Testicular artery.
- Artery to the vas.
- Cremesteric artery.
- Pampiniform plexus of veins.
- Genital branch of the genitofemoral nerve.
- Autonomic nerves (including the sensory nerves that transmit pain from the testis).
- Lymph vessels.
- Remnants of the processus vaginalis.

These structures are surrounded by three fascial layers from the anterior abdominal wall (see Fig. 14.5).

Seminal vesicles and ejaculatory ducts

The seminal vesicles are two 6-cm long, pear-shaped structures found above the prostate between the bladder and rectum. They secrete a fructose-rich, alkaline fluid that forms 70% of ejaculated semen. The fibrinogen component is responsible for semen forming a coagulum when the male ejaculates. The duct of the seminal vesicles joins the vas deferens at the ampulla behind the prostate. Together they form the 1-cm long ejaculatory ducts that pass forward into the prostate gland. The ejaculatory ducts open into the prostatic urethra just before it leaves the prostate (see Fig. 14.2).

Microstructure

Each seminal vesicle is formed from a slightly coiled tube that is 15 cm long. It is covered by two layers of smooth muscle and an external fibroelastic layer. The tube is lined by tall, secretory columnar epithelium.

The ejaculatory ducts have no muscular coverings. They are lined by tall, columnar cells and smaller, rounded cells.

Prostate

The prostate is a chestnut-sized gland that surrounds the prostatic urethra at the base of the bladder. The posterior surface is palpable by rectal examination; it should feel regular and firm with a midline groove. The prostate secretes seminal fluid into the urethra during ejaculation. This fluid is rich in bicarbonate buffers (to neutralize vaginal acidity), nutrient citric acid and fibrinolytic enzyme to liquefy semen.

Inferior to the prostate, the two small bulbourethral (Cowper's) glands secrete sugar-rich mucus into the membranous urethra. This fluid may lubricate the urethra and contribute to pre-ejaculatory emissions from the penis.

Microstructure

The prostate gland is composed of three concentric rings of glands surrounded by smooth muscle and a fibrous capsule. The smooth muscle contracts during ejaculation to squeeze the prostatic secretions into the urethra. The three types of gland are:

- Inner periurethral (mucosal) glands—these secrete directly into the urethra, which they surround.
- Outer periurethral (submucosal) glands—these secrete into the urethra via short ducts. The outer and inner periurethral glands comprise the central zone, and can undergo benign prostatic hypertrophy
- Peripheral zone glands—this ring of glands is incomplete anteriorly; they secrete via long ducts and can give rise to prostatic cancer.

The glands are lined by tall columnar epithelium with a few flat basal cells. Their secretory activity is dependent on testosterone.

Penis

The penis is the outlet for urine and semen. The internal structure of the penis is shown in Fig. 14.6. It is described in three sections:

- Root—fixed attachment to the perineum and pubic arch.
- Body—the free pendulous portion;.
- Glans—the sensitive, distal end that includes the external opening of the urethra.

The edge of the glans that joins the body of the penis is called the corona. The penis is composed of three cylinders of erectile tissue, each surrounded by a fibrous capsule called the tunica albuginea. Surrounding these structures is a layer of thin, pigmented skin; over the glans this skin is called the

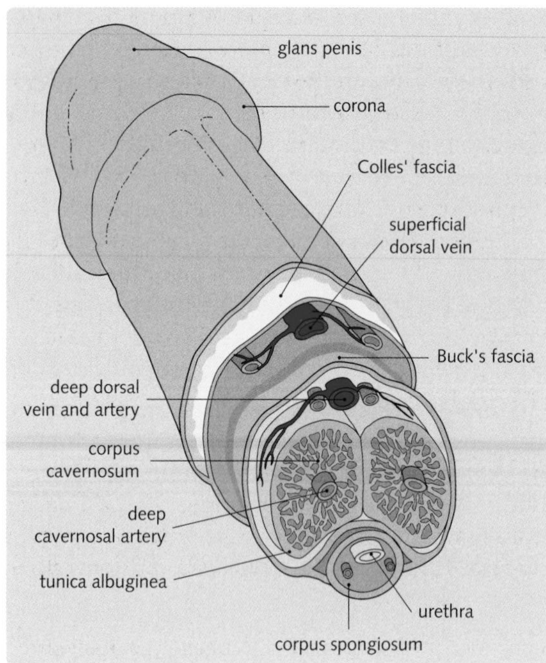

Fig. 14.6 Internal structure of the penis.

foreskin or prepuce. The three cylinders of erectile tissue are:

- Two corpora cavernosa—these large cylinders form the dorsum (upper surface) and sides of the free body of the penis; they are extensions of the crura in the root of penis.
- One corpus spongiosum—this smaller ventral (lower surface) cylinder surrounds the spongy urethra; it forms the whole of the glans and is the extension of the bulb of penis at the root.

The majority of vessels and nerves supplying the penis are found on the dorsal (upper surface) side. The arteries within the corpora cavernosa are called the deep arteries (branch of the internal pudendal artery).

Microstructure and mechanism of erection

Erection is the result of relaxation of the helicine arteries which supply the corpus cavernosa and relaxation of the smooth muscle within the cavernosa. Mounting pressure obstructs venous drainage and blood pools in vascular spaces causing penile rigidity. Erection is mediated by adrenergic, noradrenergic and nonadrenergic, noncholinergic (NANC) systems. Parasympathetic stimulation causes relaxation of corporal smooth muscle and erection. Ejaculation requires sympathetic stimulation, which inhibits the parasympathetic system causing a loss of erection.

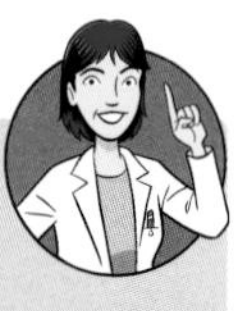

Remember 'point and shoot' to recall the function of the parasympathetic and sympathetic innervation of the penis.

SPERMATOGENESIS

Early spermatogenesis

Spermatogenesis is the process by which haploid (23 chromosome) spermatozoa are formed from diploid (46 chromosome) stem cells called spermatogonia. Spermatogonia are found close to the basement membrane of the seminiferous tubules in the basal compartment of the tubule. There are three types:

- Dark A cells (Ad)—these are the true self-regenerating stem cells; they divide by mitosis to produce more spermatogonial stem cells and, at intervals, pale A cells (Ap).
- Pale A cells (Ap)—these represent the first step towards differentiation into spermatocytes; they divide by mitosis to produce more Ap cells and, after the fifth, mitosis, form type B cells.
- B cells—these divide by mitosis to produce primary spermatocytes.

The mitotic cell divisions of spermatogonia are incomplete, so that the daughter cells remain connected by thin cytoplasmic bridges. These bridges remain throughout the development of the spermatocytes and spermatids until the spermatozoa are released into the lumen of the seminiferous tubule.

Meiosis

The primary spermatocytes undergo meiosis, which is the special form of cell division that produces haploid gametes. The first division forms two haploid secondary spermatocytes. The second meiotic division occurs soon afterwards to form four haploid spermatids. Meiosis takes place only within the adluminal intratubular compartment of the seminiferous tubules formed by the tight junctions of the Sertoli cells.

As meiosis progresses, the germinal cells migrate from the basal compartment to the adluminal compartment of the Sertoli cells and are closely associated with the Sertoli cell microenvironment. The Sertoli cells perform a number of functions that are essential for spermatogenesis:

- They provide nutrients and remove waste.
- They phagocytose excess cytoplasm or poorly developing spermatids.
- Tight junctions between cells prevent antibodies reaching the haploid cells; they form a blood–testes barrier.
- They produce androgen-binding protein to raise the local androgen concentration, which is necessary for meiosis to take place.

Spermiogenesis

Having completed the meiotic division, the haploid spermatids are small, spherical cells that must still develop the structure of a mature spermatozoon. This process is called spermiogenesis and takes place within the microenvironment of Sertoli cells in four stages:

- Golgi phase—the Golgi apparatus begins to form an acrosomal vesicle over the nucleus while the centrioles migrate to the other end of the cell. One of the centrioles begins to form the tail.
- Cap phase—the acrosomal vesicle surrounds the front of the nucleus while the nucleus condenses.
- Acrosome phase—the nucleus becomes smaller and lengthens squeezing the acrosome and cell membrane together. Mitochondria migrate towards the tail to form the 'middle piece' while microtubules condense behind the nucleus to form the neck or 'manchette'.
- Maturation phase—excess cytoplasm is 'pinched off' and phagocytosed by the Sertoli cell. The completed spermatozoon is then released into the lumen of the seminiferous tubule by breaking off the cytoplasmic bridges,termed spermiation.

Final maturation

The maturation from spermatogonia to released spermatozoa in the seminiferous tubule lumen takes about 64 days, and its rate is not affected by external factors such as temperature. Further maturation occurs as they pass through the epididymis to make the spermatozoa motile and capable of fertilization. The spermatozoa are pushed through the rete testis and efferent ductules by the movement of testicular fluid, caused by the action of the cilia, to reach the epididymis.

The epithelium of the epididymis secretes glycoproteins that bind to the surface of the spermatozoa, causing the phospholipid membrane to be remodelled. The epididymis is also capable of removing degenerate or poorly formed spermatozoa by phagocytosis. Spermatozoa pass through the epididymis by the movement of testicular fluid and peristalsis.

The fully mature spermatozoa are stored in the epididymis until they are ejaculated or broken down. The epididymis contracts during orgasm to transport the spermatozoa into the vas deferens. The vas deferens has a thick muscular layer that propels the sperm along the duct at ejaculation.

Continuous fertility

After puberty males are always fertile, though their fertility may decline with age. Continuous fertility is achieved because there is a population of stem cells in the testes (cf. ovaries):

- Successive cycles of spermatogenesis start every 16 days (the spermatogenic cycle) at each point in the tubule.
- Sertoli cells are arranged in bands in which cycles of spermatogenesis begin randomly at different times.
- Cycles are at different stages in different segments of the seminiferous tubules and are phase advanced or retarded.

Mature spermatozoon

Mature spermatozoa have a distinct head and tail (Fig. 14.7). The head is composed largely of condensed chromatin in the pointed nucleus; the front is surrounded by a giant lysosome called the acrosome that allows the spermatozoa to penetrate the oocyte.

The tail is a long and specialized flagellum derived from one of the centrioles. It has the usual pattern of microtubules with nine outer pairs around a central pair; this structure is called the axoneme. There are four sections of the tail:

- Neck—this narrowing contains the centrioles connected to the axoneme.
- Middle piece—the axoneme is surrounded by elongated spiral mitochondria. These release energy to drive the axoneme by the anaerobic respiration of fructose.
- Principal piece—this forms the majority of the tail. It contains fibres, which are not present in the smaller end piece.
- End piece.

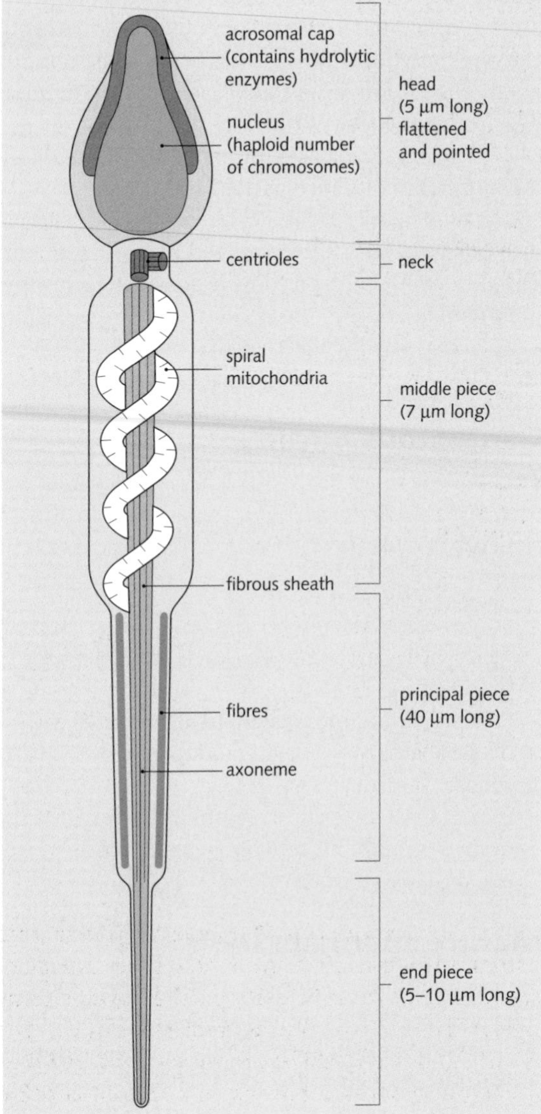

Fig. 14.7 Microstructure of a mature spermatozoon. This diagram is not to scale.

Normal ranges for semen

Semen analysis is clinically important means of identifying male infertility. WHO guidelines give the following normal ranges for semen analysis: volume >2 mL; sperm concentration >20 M/mL; total sperm count >40 M/ejaculate; motility >50% forward; normal morphology >30% (WHO 1992) or 15% (WHO 1999). A sperm count of <10 M/mL is bordering on subfertility

HORMONES

Testicular sex steroids

The testes secrete 95% of the male sex steroids called androgens; the adrenal cortex is responsible for the remaining 5%. The main androgen is testosterone.

Testicular androgens are secreted by the interstitial Leydig cells found between the seminiferous tubules. They convert cholesterol into the steroid testosterone by a series of reactions. The Leydig cells also secrete small quantities of oestrogens and progestogens as by-products of testosterone synthesis.

Testosterone is a strong androgen. However, some target tissues can convert it to the more potent form called dihydrotestosterone (DHT). The conversion requires the 5-reductase enzyme and occurs in the:

- Sertoli cells.
- Prostate gland.
- Skin.

Testosterone is transported in the plasma by sex-hormone binding globulin (SHBG) or albumin. It acts via intracellular receptors to regulate protein synthesis producing the actions shown in Fig. 14.8. The main actions are:

- Growth and development of male reproductive tract.
- Development of male secondary sexual characteristics (e.g. male hair pattern, muscle growth).
- Stimulation of spermatogenesis.
- Stimulation of growth and the fusion of the growth plates of the long bones (see Chapter 9).

Control of testicular steroid production

Testosterone synthesis and release is controlled by the same hormones in the male as oestrogen synthesis in the female. Gonadotrophin-releasing hormone (GnRH) from the hypothalamus is transported to the anterior pituitary gland by the portal veins. It stimulates the gonadotroph cells to secrete gonadotrophins (LH and FSH). This process is described in more detail in Chapter 2.

LH acts on the Leydig cells to stimulate the first step in testosterone production. Testosterone feeds back to the hypothalamus and pituitary gland to inhibit LH release, but it has little effect on FSH.

FSH acts on the Sertoli cells; it increases the number of testosterone receptors to stimulate spermatogenesis.

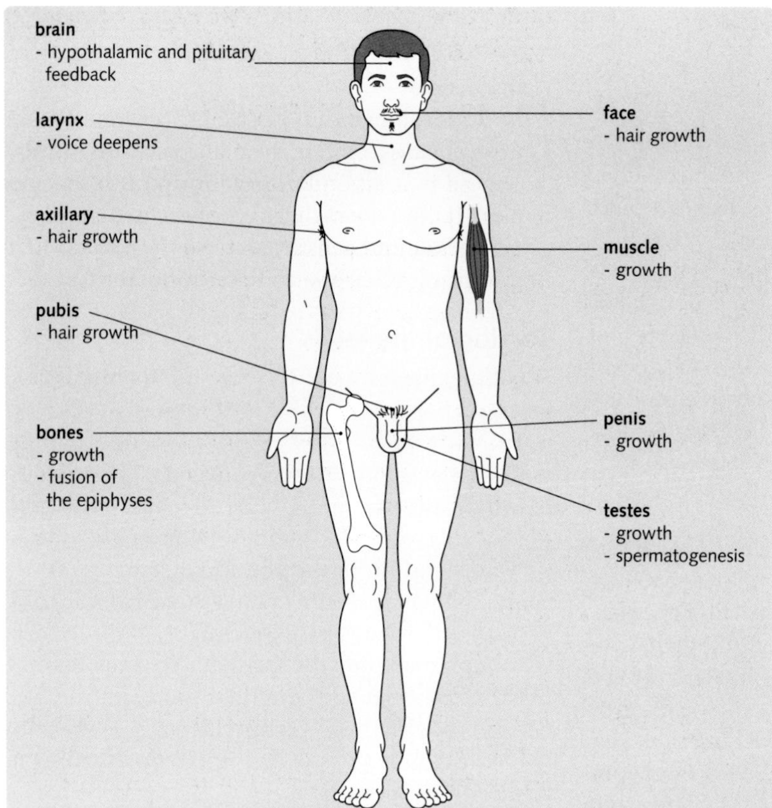

Fig. 14.8 Actions of testosterone.

It also causes inhibin B release from the Sertoli cells, which feeds back to the hypothalamus and pituitary gland to inhibit further FSH release. Inhibin has little effect on LH and therefore regulates sperm production without inhibiting testosterone levels.

Other testicular hormones

The fetal Sertoli cells produce the Müllerian inhibiting substance (MIS; described in Chapter 11). This hormone prevents development of the female internal genitalia by causing the Müllerian ducts to regress.

DISORDERS OF THE TESTES AND EPIDIDYMIS

Congenital abnormalities and regression

Cryptorchidism

Cryptorchidism is the medical term for testes that have failed to descend into the scrotum. It is a common finding in newborns (3–4%), especially premature babies, and it can affect one or both testes. An undescended testis must be distinguished from a testis retracted due to cold (by the cremasteric muscle). It is only undescended if it cannot be massaged into the scrotum or cannot be felt at all. An impalpable testis usually lies in the inguinal canal or at its abdominal entrance (deep inguinal ring). The descent of the testis and formation of the scrotum are described in Chapter 11.

In the majority of babies, this condition resolves with no treatment. However, if the testes still have not descended after a year, their development can be affected. Failure to treat the condition at this stage causes a high risk of infertility because the spermatogonia (stem cells) need cooler temperatures to survive. Testosterone production is not affected because the Leydig cells are not as sensitive. Cryptorchidism also carries a higher risk of germ-cell testicular cancer in later life. It is corrected by surgically fixing the testes in the scrotum—an operation called orchidopexy.

Abnormalities of the tunica vaginalis

Congenital hernia

The processus vaginalis is a tube of peritoneum that connects the tunica vaginalis to the abdominal cavity through the inguinal canal in the fetus. This structure is shown in Fig. 11.5; a persistent processus vaginalis is shown in Fig. 14.9. If it fails to close then intestines may pass into the scrotum causing an indirect inguinal hernia (through the inguinal canal). This condition is more common in the presence of undescended testes. It must be corrected surgically to prevent the risk of bowel obstruction and ischaemia due to the narrow inguinal ring. Femoral and direct inguinal hernias are very rare in neonates.

Congenital hydrocoele

If the processus vaginalis persists but is too small for a hernia to form, then peritoneal fluid may enter the tunica vaginalis causing a hydrocoele. This presents as a transluminable swelling within the scrotum that cannot be distinguished from the testis. It often regresses without treatment, but if not it should be drained. Recurring or large hydrocoeles require surgical correction. Throughout life hydrocoeles are the most common cause of intra-scrotal swelling; the fluid may be a sign of inflammation or neoplasia of the testis.

Trauma and vascular disturbances

Testicular haemorrhage

Haematoma

Trauma to the groin can cause bleeding within the testes. If the bleeding remains within the intact tunica albuginea it is called a testicular haematoma. It is extremely painful.

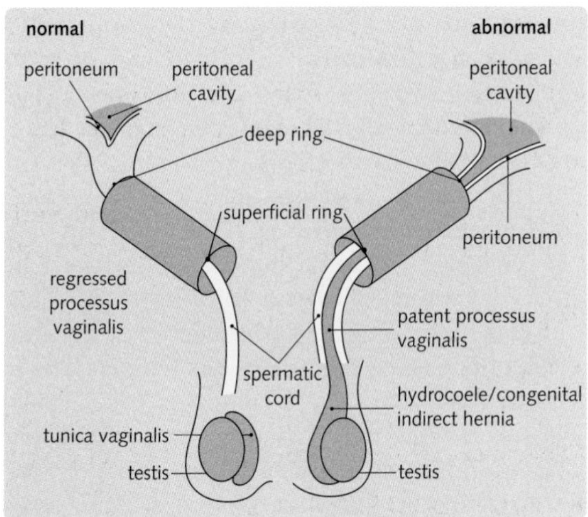

Fig. 14.9 Diagram of a normal testis and one with a persistent processus vaginalis causing a hydrocoele or indirect hernia.

Hematocoele

If the tunica albuginea splits, blood can collect in the tunica vaginalis forming a hematocoele. This can also be caused by a testicular tumour in the absence of trauma. If the haemorrhage is not drained the blood can coagulate and constrict around the testis, potentially causing ischaemia and necrosis of the testis.

Torsion of the testis

Torsion of the testis occurs when the spermatic cord becomes twisted, blocking the blood vessels from a testis. It can only occur if the testes are free to rotate within the scrotum due to a congenital abnormality. Normally the tunica vaginalis attaches to the spermatic cord close to its origin from the epididymis to prevent rotation. In the abnormal state the tunica vaginalis attaches further along the spermatic cord. If the testis rotates excessively, the pampiniform venous plexus within the spermatic cord can become twisted and occluded. Arterial blood continues to enter the affected testis but cannot leave, so the testis swells and undergoes venous infarction leading to haemorrhagic necrosis.

Testicular torsion is most common in children and adolescents following mild trauma, especially sporting injuries. It presents with the sudden onset of pain and tenderness in one testicle. On palpation the affected testis is high in the scrotum and the spermatic cord may be thickened. With time, the pain becomes severe with vomiting and dull abdominal pain as the affected testicle swells.

It can be difficult to distinguish the later stages of torsion from acute orchitis. Since testicular torsion is an acute surgical emergency an unclear diagnosis needs surgical exploration. Without treatment the testis will undergo necrosis and need to be removed. Early surgery (before about 6 hours) can untwist and save the testicle; both testes should be secured to the scrotum to prevent recurrence.

Varicocoele

When the pampiniform plexus in the spermatic cord becomes varicose (dilated and tortuous) it is called a varicocoele. It is found in about 10% of young men and in 90% of these the spermatic cord on the left is affected. This may be due to the higher pressure in the renal vein compared with the inferior vena cava (see Fig. 14.3). The underlying cause is not known, although rapidly developing varicocoeles may very rarely be caused by carcinoma of the left kidney obstructing the left testicular vein.

The testes should be examined with the patient standing up because the blood often drains out of the plexus when they lie down. This response is inhibited if there is an underlying obstruction (e.g. renal carcinoma). The full varicocoele feels like a 'bag of worms' above the testes.

Occasionally varicocoeles present with discomfort, but the vast majority are asymptomatic. The excess blood can warm the testes reducing the fertility of the patient. Varicocoeles are seen in around 35% of men with primary infertility and in 80% of men with secondary infertility and is a commom cause of male infertility. Varicocoeles can be treated surgically, but this is only considered if discomfort or infertility are present.

Inflammation and infection

Acute orchitis and epididymitis

Inflammation of the testis is called orchitis, while inflammation of the epididymis is called epididymitis. These two conditions often occur together and they are managed in a similar manner. The following acute bacterial infections are the most common causes of epididymo-orchitis:

- *Escherichia coli* and other coliforms (from a urinary tract infection; UTI).
- *Chlamydia trachomatis* (sexually transmitted disease; STD).
- *Neisseria gonorrheae* (STD).

Patients complain of either one or two painful, tender and enlarged testes, which may be accompanied by a secondary hydrocoele, general malaise, fever or headache. It is diagnosed from the history and examination of the urine, but surgical exploration is often performed to exclude testicular torsion. Antibiotics are used to treat the infection otherwise scarring and infertility can develop.

Other infections

Mumps

The mumps virus often causes viral orchitis if it infects post-pubertal males. It tends to cause a single tender and enlarged testis. Rarely it can cause infertility if the disease is bilateral.

Tuberculosis

Tuberculosis (TB) can infect the epididymis and testis from the blood or urinary tract. It causes chronic granuloma with caseous necrosis that can persist long after infections at other sites have been successfully treated.

Syphilis

The rare tertiary stage of *Treponema pallidum* infection (i.e. syphilis) can produce the characteristic chronic syphilitic granuloma (called gumma) in the testes.

Autoimmune granulomatous orchitis

Granulomatous orchitis is a rare autoimmune disease that causes chronic inflammation of the testis and destruction of the seminiferous tubules. The tight junctions between the Sertoli cells normally prevent an immune reaction against the developing haploid sperm, but this barrier appears to break down.

It presents in a similar manner to a testicular tumour; the affected testis becomes firm and enlarged, sometimes with a secondary hydrocoele.

Epididymal cysts

Epididymal cysts often develop in adult life and are found in the head of the epididymis. The cysts contain either a watery fluid or a milky fluid containing sperm (this can be called a spermatocoele). They usually present as painless swellings that can be distinguished from the testis and transluminated. If they cause symptoms they can be removed surgically.

Neoplastic disorders

Tumours of the testes are important because they are the most common type of cancer in young adult males. They are often highly malignant but frequently curable with early detection. If undetected they can spread to the para-aortic lymph nodes or, by blood, to the lungs and liver. Patients often present with:

- A painless, enlarged, hard testis or testicular lump.
- Secondary hydrocoele.
- Gynaecomastia [due to human chorionic gonadotrophin (hCG) or oestrogen secretio].
- Metastases to the lungs or liver.

Testicular ultrasound is used to distinguish cystic swellings from testicular tumours. Two tumour markers can be detected in the blood; these are used in diagnosis and monitoring treatment:

- α-Fetoprotein (AFP).
- hCG.

Other tests are aimed at detecting any tumour spread:

- Chest X-ray to check the lungs.
- Abdominal computed tomography (CT) for liver and lymph nodes.

Testicular carcinoma is treated by orchidectomy (removal of testis) using an inguinal incision. The spermatic cord should be clamped before the testis is removed to help prevent venous spread. If the testis appears normal and on-the-spot biopsy analysis does not reveal malignancy, then the testis can be returned to the scrotum. Confirmed carcinoma is followed up with radiotherapy or chemotherapy depending on the type of testicular tumour. The prognosis also depends on the type of tumour, but it is generally very good. If the lymph nodes are not involved there is almost a 100% 5-year survival rate.

There are two groups of testicular tumour:

- Germ-cell tumours (97%).
- Sex-cord stromal tumours (3%).

The different types within these groups are shown in Fig. 14.10.

Germ-cell tumours

Germ-cell tumours develop from the gamete-producing spermatogonia in the seminiferous tubules. They are predisposed by undescended testes. There are three types of germ-cell tumours, described below.

Seminoma

This tumour accounts for 50% of germ-cell tumours, and it is most common in 40- to 50-year-olds. It presents as a painless enlargement of one testis and histology reveals a creamy-white tumour. Ten per cent of tumours secrete hCG as an ectopic hormone. They usually spread via the lymphatics. They are very sensitive to radiotherapy, so the prognosis is good.

Teratoma

These tumours are most common in 20- to 30-year-olds. Teratomas are composed of a number of tissue types derived from endoderm, mesoderm and ectoderm. Well-differentiated tumours are usually benign; more commonly, the tissues are undifferentiated and immature causing a highly malignant tumour (cf. ovarian teratomas). There are a number of categories of teratoma according to their histological appearance. They often secrete α-fetoprotein and hCG because they develop from yolk sac and trophoblast tissues. They metastasize early to the lungs and have a poorer prognosis than seminomas, but they are very sensitive to chemotherapy.

Mixed tumours

Some tumours contain different types of teratomas or a combination of seminoma and teratoma tissues. Their behaviour and prognosis depends largely on the types of teratoma involved.

Sex-cord stromal tumours

Tumours that develop from the other tissues in the testes are called sex-cord stromal tumours. They account for only 3% of testicular tumours. There are three types, described below.

Leydig-cell tumours

These are also called interstitial or stromal-cell tumours. They can occur at any age and are usually benign. They frequently secrete testosterone or oestrogens which can affect the reproductive system.

Sertoli-cell tumours

These are also called androblastomas or sex-cord tumours. They can occur at any age, but they are most common between 40 and 50 years of age. They are often benign, but they may secrete ectopic oestrogens.

Fig. 14.10 Frequency of types of testicular tumour and the age group they commonly affect

Tumour type	Tumour	Main age group (years)	Testicular malignancy (%)
Germ-cell tumours	Seminoma	40–50	50
	Teratoma	20–30	35
	Mixed tumour	20–40	12
Sex-cord stromal tumours	Leydig-cell tumour	Any	<1
	Sertoli-cell tumour	40–50	<1
	Primary lymphoma	65+	2

Primary lymphoma

In the elderly, lymphomas can develop in the testes; aggressively malignant non-Hodgkin's lymphomas are the most common type of testicular tumour in those aged 65 years or over.

DISORDERS OF THE PROSTATE

Inflammation and infection

Bacterial prostatitis

The prostate can become inflamed due to bacterial infection; this can follow an acute or chronic course.

Acute

Bacteria reach the prostate from the urethra so the common causative organisms are those which cause urinary tract infections or are sexually transmitted, namely:

- *E. coli* and other coliforms (UTI).
- *Neisseria gonorrhoeae* (also called gonococcus; an STD).
- *Chlamydia trachomatis* (STD).

Patients present with increased urinary frequency, penile and testicular pain and systemic illness (e.g. fever). The prostate gland becomes enlarged and acutely tender on rectal examination. Severe inflammation can obstruct the urethra, causing urinary retention and abscesses may develop leading to a urethral discharge of pus.

It is diagnosed from urine culture and treated with appropriate antibiotics (e.g. trimethoprim or erythromycin).

Chronic

Failure to cure acute prostatitis can lead to chronic prostatitis. It can also be caused by tuberculosis infection, often from the kidney or epididymis. The symptoms are similar to acute prostatitis but ill-defined and less severe. It is managed in the same manner as an acute infection or with treatment for TB.

Abacterial prostatitis

Chronic prostatitis can also be caused by non-infective disease in which anti-inflammatory drugs may ease symptoms. The exact aetiology is unknown but theories include:

- Allergy, since it is associated with asthma.
- Autoimmune disease.
- Urine reflux.

PSA screening

Serum levels of prostate-specific antigen (PSA) are used to screen for prostate cancer and to monitor recurrence after treatment. After prostatectomy, an early rise in PSA levels indicates a metastatic recurrence and a late rise indicates a local recurrence of disease. Unfortunately, the specificity of this screen is low such that PSA levels also rise as a consequence of prostatitis, benign prostatic hyperplasia, urologic operations and some drugs. Alternative markers are now being investigated using proteomic analysis of serum.

Benign prostatic hyperplasia (BPH)

The prostate gland begins to enlarge from the age of 45 years. By the age of 70 years the vast majority of men have some benign enlargement, making it the most common disease of the prostate gland. It is caused by nodular hyperplasia (increased cell division forming nodules) of the inner and outer periurethral glands of the central zone of the prostate. The underlying fault is believed to be an imbalance between oestrogen and androgen secretion. It does not develop into prostate carcinoma.

The enlarged prostate gland can compress the urethra, causing difficulty urinating called 'prostatism'. This only occurs in the more severely affected men and it is characterized by the following symptoms:

- Increased frequency of micturition (urinating).
- Increased urgency.
- Reduced size and force of urinary stream.
- Hesitancy and interruption.
- Dribbling at the end of micturition.

If BPH is very severe, urinary obstruction may result due to compression of the internal urethral sphincter. Chronic urine retention follows, leading to recurrent urinary tract infections or renal impairment.

BPH is diagnosed by the history and rectal examination in the absence of evidence for renal failure or carcinoma of the prostate. Mild disease can be treated medically with α-blockers to lower prostate tone. More progressive disease may be treated by transurethral resection of the prostate (TURP); however, this procedure can often cause retrograde ejaculation and occasionally impotence. The histology of the resected prostate tissue should be examined under a microscope to exclude malignancy.

Neoplastic disorders

Prostatic carcinoma is the second most common male carcinoma. It usually affects the elderly, but the incidence is currently increasing in younger men. Prostate carcinoma typically affects a different part of the prostate from BPH (Fig 14.11). The risk factors for prostate cancer are not known. Prostate carcinomas exhibit a diverse range of behaviours and some of this diversity can be explained by various molecular alterations (Figure 14.12).

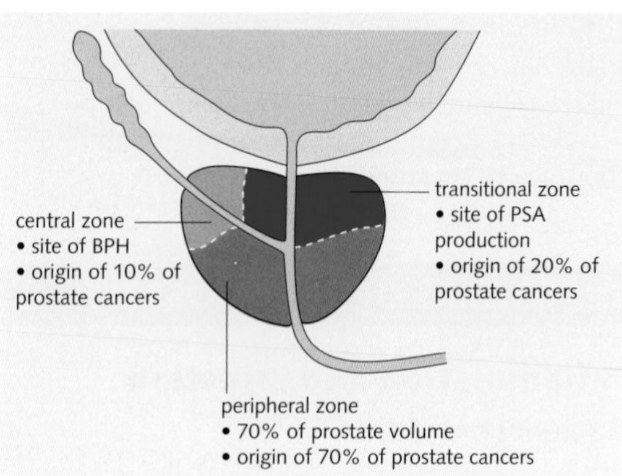

Fig. 14.11 The physical anatomy of prostate disorders. (BPH, benign prostatic hypertrophy; PSA, prostate-specific antigen.)

Presentation

Since prostate carcinoma develops in the external glands of the prostate, away from the urethra, it is initially asymptomatic. As the tumour grows it begins to compress the urethra, causing similar symptoms to those of BPH, although they tend to progress more rapidly. This is a relatively late feature. Systemic and metastatic symptoms can be the first signs in advanced disease, including:

- Weight loss.
- General malaise.
- Anaemia.
- Back pain.

Rectal examination can reveal a hard nodule on the posterior surface of the prostate gland. As the tumour grows the median groove of the gland is obliterated. The staging system of prostate tumours is shown in Fig. 14.13.

Diagnosis and investigation

The possibility of prostate cancer should be excluded in all patients with symptoms of prostatism. Raised levels of the blood-borne tumour marker called 'prostate-specific antigen' (PSA) suggest carcinoma. This marker can also be used to monitor treatment. Blood specimens for PSA measurement should be taken prior to rectal examination, since this can raise the levels. Further investigation includes:

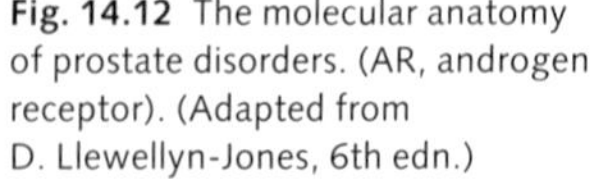

Fig. 14.12 The molecular anatomy of prostate disorders. (AR, androgen receptor). (Adapted from D. Llewellyn-Jones, 6th edn.)

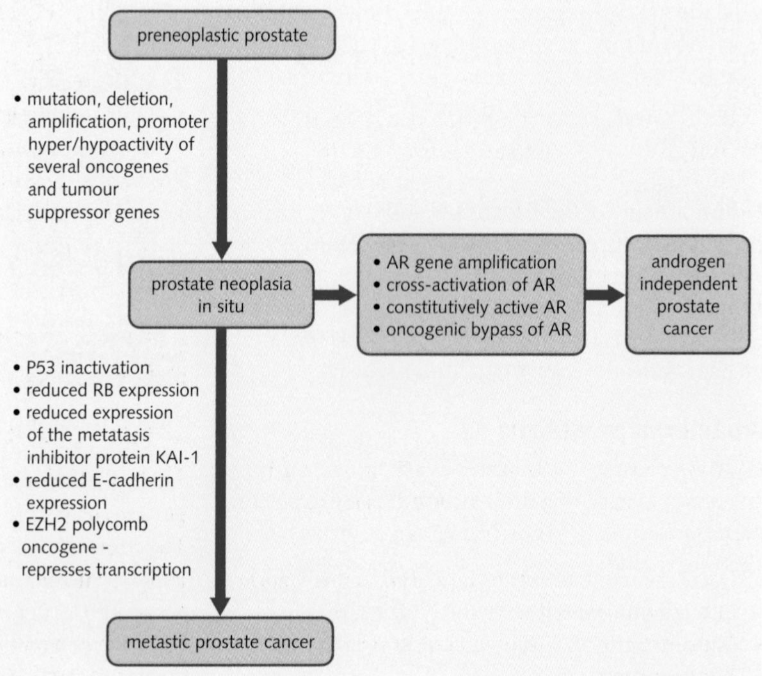

Fig. 14.13 Staging and prognosis of prostate carcinoma

Stage	Description	Symptoms	Five-year survival (%)
A1	Microscopic, focal and well-differentiated tumours	None	95
A2	Microscopic, diffuse and/or poorly differentiated tumours	None	80
B	Larger tumours that are palpable rectally	None	75
C	Tumours that involve the entire prostate gland ± local invasion	Prostatism	50
D	Metastatic spread to lymph nodes or organs including bones	Prostatism and systemic/metastatic symptoms	35

- Transrectal ultrasound.
- Rectal or transurethral needle biopsy.
- Bone X-rays to locate metastases.

Treatment

Early-stage, asymptomatic tumours are often simply observed or treated with radiotherapy, though resection is recommended by some clinicians. Radical retropubic prostatectomy is performed in early-stage disease or cancer confined to the prostate but other surgical procedures may be performed on patients with late-stage tumours. This procedure carries a high risk of urinary and erectile dysfunction.

If the patient has incurable metastatic disease then the following medical treatments may help:

- Cyproterone acetate blocks androgen receptors, which can reduce tumour size and invasion.
- Continuous GnRH analogues can inhibit LH secretion from the pituitary gland, reducing testosterone secretion.

Invasion and metastasis

Prostate cancer can remain localized or, with the appropriate molecular alterations (see Fig. 14.12), metastasize by the following routes:

- Local spread within the gland and to the bladder and seminal vesicles.
- Lymphatic spread to the pelvic and para-aortic lymph nodes.
- Blood-borne spread to the bones, especially the pelvis, spine and skull. It causes characteristic osteosclerotic lesions, i.e. bone is formed not destroyed.

Prostate cancers typically express androgen receptors which, when activated, stimulate cellular proliferation. Androgen blockade can be an effective therapy in this case. However, cancer cells can become increasingly independent of androgen and therefore blockade becomes less effective. Androgen independence can by acquired by amplification of the androgen receptor gene, cross-activation of androgen receptors by other molecules (IGF), mutations in androgen receptors (which cause constitutive activity) and activation of oncogenes, which activate cellular proliferation and bypass androgen pathways.

DISORDERS OF THE PENIS

Structural abnormalities

Congenital abnormalities

Hypospadias

The body of the penis is formed by the fusion of the urogenital folds round the urethra, as described in Chapter 11. This fusion can fail to varying degrees, resulting in hypospadias in which a meatus (opening) of the urethra forms along the ventral surface (underneath) of the penis, usually at the base of the glans; it is the most common structural abnormality of the penis.

Hypospadias is caused by a deficiency of fetal testosterone production. It is associated with undescended testes, a 'hooded' foreskin and a downward curvature of the penis called congenital chordee. It can be corrected surgically using the foreskin.

Epispadias

This is a much rarer condition than hypospadias. It is a similar abnormality except that the urethral meatus is on the dorsal (top) surface of the penis, usually at the base of the body. It can cause urinary incontinence and recurrent urinary infections; it is corrected surgically. It is often associated with other abnormalities of the genitalia or urinary tract.

Phimosis

Phimosis is the result of a taut foreskin, which cannot be retracted over the glans. It is normal after birth, but the foreskin should become retractable within a few years as the adhesions between the glans and foreskin breakdown. Phimosis can be congenital, but more commonly is caused by fibrotic changes due to chronic or recurrent *Candida* infection. Treatment is with topical steroids and foreskin stretching. Phimosis causes dyspareunia (pain on intercourse) and can obstruct urinary flow. Attempts to retract the fibrosed foreskin can cause the foreskin to get stuck behind the glans, paraphimosis. The venous drainage becomes obstructed, restricting blood flow and causing oedema.

Inflammation and infection

The penis, especially the glans and urethra, is very susceptible to the same sexually transmitted infections that affect the female reproductive tract. A summary of these infections is shown in Fig. 14.14.

Viral infection

The penis is prone to the same viral infections as the female vulva.

Herpes simplex

This is a sexually transmitted disease caused by herpes simplex virus (HSV, usually type II). It causes a recurrent, acute and itchy skin infection. This progresses to form vesicles and painful skin erosions on the glans. The inguinal lymph nodes are often enlarged and painful.

The primary infection is often subclinical, but the virus then remains latent in the dorsal root ganglion that supplies that area of skin. The virus can be reactivated causing recurrent attacks.

HSV can be diagnosed from viral culture of the fluid in the blisters. It is treated symptomatically (e.g. anaesthetic cream) but aciclovir is often used for asymptomatic contacts, the initial infection or in the immunosuppressed. The virus can be transmitted to other body parts on the hands: the eyes are particularly susceptible.

Genital warts

This is a sexually transmitted disease caused by human papilloma virus (HPV), of which there are many types. They cause benign, warty skin lesions

Fig. 14.14 Summary of infections of the male reproductive tract

Infection	Organism	Symptoms	Treatment
Herpes	Herpes simplex virus	Burning red blisters that may recur	Aciclovir if recurrent
Warts	Human papilloma virus	Growths on the penile skin	Podophyllotoxin cream
Gonorrhoea	*Neisseria gonorrhoeae*	Dysuria, white urethral discharge	Penicillin or ceftriaxone
Non-gonococcal urethritis	*Chlamydia trachomatis*	Milder dysuria, white urethral discharge	Erythromycin
Syphilis	*Treponema pallidum*	Ulcerated nodules, but may become systemic	Penicillin
Balanitis	*Candida albicans* (fungus)	Itching, white urethral discharge	Nystatin cream

called condyloma acuminata, usually on the glans or inner surface of the foreskin.

The warts are treated with cryotherapy, in which a liquid nitrogen spray freezes and kills infected cells, or with podophyllin cream, which burns the infected cells chemically. The warts often recur despite treatment. Some strains of HPV predispose to malignant change of the penile skin (see below).

Bacterial infection

Gonorrhoea

This is a sexually transmitted disease caused by the bacterium *Neisseria gonorrhoeae* (often called gonococcus) that infects the distal urethra. Symptoms include dysuria (pain on urinating) and a urethral discharge of a whitish pus. It is diagnosed by microscopy and culture of the pus to identify the organism and its antibiotic sensitivity; many gonococcus bacteria are now resistant to penicillin, in which case ceftriaxone is used.

Untreated gonorrhoea can lead to the following complications:

- Epididymo-orchitis.
- Proctitis (infection of the rectum).
- Infective arthritis.
- Septicaemia.

Non-gonococcal urethritis

More commonly, the urethra can be infected by other bacteria, particularly *Chlamydia trachomatis*. It causes similar but milder symptoms. Epididymo-orchitis can also develop, but non-gonococcal urethritis is usually cured by a single dose of erythromycin. Reiter's syndrome after gastroenteritis includes urethral discharge, balanitis, painful joints and bilateral conjunctivitis.

Syphilis

This is a sexually transmitted disease caused by the bacterium *Treponema pallidum* that initially infects the glans or the inner surface of the foreskin. Today, syphilis is a rare disease; the complications are almost never seen because of effective treatment. The untreated disease follows four stages:

- Primary syphilis—a solitary, painless ulcerated nodule appears at the infection site. The inguinal lymph nodes become enlarged but not painful.
- Secondary syphilis—2 months later, a systemic disease may develop including scaly rashes and mucosal ulcers over much of the body surface. It normally resolves after several months.
- Tertiary syphilis—rarely the disease may enter a chronic stage in which characteristic rubbery granulomas (called gummata) develop throughout the body.
- Quaternary syphilis—with time syphilis may affect the cardiovascular and central nervous system, with potentially fatal effects.

Syphilis is diagnosed by serological (antibody) tests, and it is treated with penicillin, which is also given to recent sexual contacts.

Fungal infection

Thrush is an infection of the penis with *Candida albicans*. This fungal infection is often an endogenous infection (from another body part), but can be sexually transmitted.

Thrush causes inflammation of the foreskin and glans called balanitis producing red, itchy patches and a white urethral discharge. It is diagnosed by microscopy and culture of the discharge. Treatment is with topical antifungals (e.g. nystatin). Chronic balanitis can cause phimosis when the foreskin is too tight to retract over the glans penis.

Neoplastic disorders

Benign tumours

Benign tumours of the penis take the form of warts caused by HPV. These are called condyloma acuminata; they are discussed with the other viral infections of the penis.

Malignant tumours

Carcinoma of the penis is rare, but squamous cell carcinoma can develop in the penile skin. A series of dysplastic changes from carcinoma in situ to invasive carcinoma are grouped together as 'penile intra-epithelial neoplasia' or PIN. Dysplastic change affects elderly uncircumcised men. Poor hygiene and HPV infection are predisposing factors.

DISORDERS OF THE MALE BREAST

Gynaecomastia

The male breast contains the same tissue components as the female breast in the undeveloped, prepubescent state. If the male breast enlarges, the condition is called gynaecomastia. It is caused by any condition or process that raises oestrogen or lowers testosterone levels.

It often occurs during puberty, but will usually resolve with time. The underlying cause should be treated.

Carcinoma

Breast carcinoma in men is very rare compared with that in females; it accounts for <1% of all breast cancer. The carcinoma is usually of the intraductal or infiltrating duct types (described in Chapter 13). It presents in elderly men as a breast lump or nipple discharge. The tumours have often metastasized to the axillary lymph nodes, lungs, brain, bone or liver by the time of presentation, so the prognosis is poor.

The process of reproduction

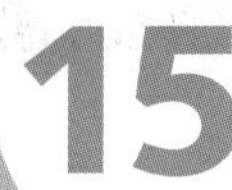

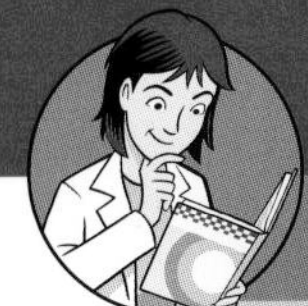

Objectives

By the end of the chapter you should be able to:

- Describe the physiology of sexual arousal.
- Describe the physical changes that occur during the male and female orgasm.
- Describe the common causes of male and female sexual dysfunction.
- Explain what is meant by fertilization and infertility.
- Describe the process of fertilization and understand the barriers to polyspermy.
- Describe the early development of the zygote and implantation.
- Discuss methods of contraception.
- List the advantages and disadvantages of different types of hormonal contraception.
- Make a table showing the common causes of infertility and their treatments.
- Describe placental development.
- Recognize the consequences of placental malfunction.
- Describe the hormonal changes which occur throughout pregnancy.
- Describe the actions of oestrogen, progesterone and hCG during pregnancy.

The previous two chapters have described the organization of the male and female reproductive systems, along with how the gametes are produced. This chapter describes how the gametes meet and the processes that occur from fertilization until the baby is born and being breastfed.

During pregnancy many processes and changes take place under hormonal control. The main hormones are:

- Progesterone.
- Oestrogens.
- Human chorionic gonadotrophin (hCG).
- Human placental lactogen (hPL).
- Prolactin.
- Oxytocin.

SEXUAL INTERCOURSE

Sexual arousal and sensation

In both men and women, sexual arousal is derived from both physical and psychological stimulation.

Sexual arousal activates the parasympathetic nerves supplying the genitalia, which cause erection of the penis or clitoris; the mechanism of erection is described in Chapter 14.

Physical stimulation

Physical stimulation of the glans of the penis in the male or the clitoris in the female results in sexual arousal; however, other parts of the body can also have this effect (erogenous zones). These structures contain an abundance of sensory receptors that are stimulated by the massaging action of sexual intercourse. Stimulation of the internal genitalia contributes to these sensations (e.g. vagina, urethra and prostate). These signals reach the spinal cord via the pudendal nerves and are transmitted to the central nervous system. In addition to feeding into higher centres and causing arousal, these signals trigger local reflexes via the lumbar and sacral spinal cord. These reflexes are capable of eliciting the physical signs of sexual arousal. Erection and ejaculation, in the absence of sensation, are possible in male patients with severed spinal cords as a result of these reflex loops.

Psychological stimulation

Psychological stimuli greatly enhance the response to physical stimuli. Erotic thoughts can activate the limbic system, causing sexual arousal including lubrication and erection.

Physiology of sexual intercourse

Stages of sexual intercourse

Sexual intercourse is also called coitus. The physiological changes which accompany sexual arousal are often described in the four stages of the EPOR model (Fig. 15.1):

- Excitement phase—initial rapid rise in the level of sexual arousal.
- Plateau phase—sexual arousal is maintained at a high level.
- Orgasmic phase—sexual arousal crosses the threshold resulting in orgasm.
- Resolution phase—the fall in sexual arousal following the cessation of coitus; physical and behavioural changes revert to normal.

Excitement and plateau phases

Sexual arousal causes stimulation of the parasympathetic nerve plexuses supplying the genitalia.

Physiological changes in the male:

- Vasocongestion of the penis (leading to erection) and scrotum.
- Secretion of small amounts of pre-ejaculatory fluid that may contain sperm.

Physiological changes in the female:

- Vasocongestion and engorgement of the clitoris (leading to erection), vagina, labia minora, and nipples.
- Secretion of lubricating fluid by the greater vestibular (Bartholin's) glands on either side of the vestibule and a fluid transudate from blood vessels in the vaginal wall.
- Smooth muscle relaxation of the vagina causes dilation of the vagina.

These physical changes are part of a positive feedback loop and increase the level of stimulation which causes further sexual arousal.

Systemic changes occur in both sexes:

- Rise in heart rate and blood pressure.
- Rise in respiratory rate.
- Rise in temperature and blood supply to the skin.
- Increase in muscle tone.

These changes reach a peak at the point of orgasm.

The male orgasm and resolution

When sexual arousal reaches the 'threshold' a reflex is initiated in the lumbar sympathetic nerves called an orgasm; it is accompanied by intense physical sensations. In the male the orgasm is accompanied by the expulsion of roughly 200 million spermatozoa in 2–4 mL of seminal fluid. The sperm are projected deep into the vagina, close to the external os of the cervix. This expulsion occurs in two phases:

- Emission—the epididymis, vas deferens, seminal vesicles and prostate begin to contract, pushing sperm and seminal fluid into the urethra. This urethral sensation heightens stimulation and contraction.
- Ejaculation—the urethra contracts rhythmically, expelling the semen in a series of pulses.

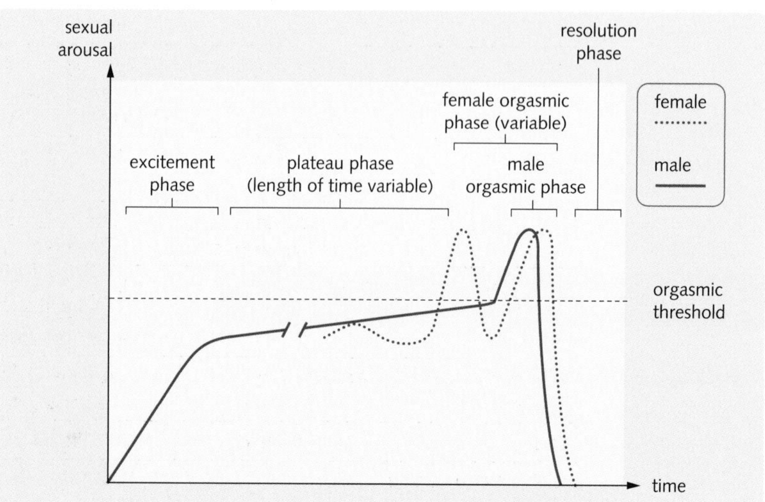

Fig. 15.1 The EPOR model of sexual arousal.

The sympathetic stimulation of male ejaculation inhibits the erection maintained by the parasympathetic input. The male enters an 'absolute refractory' period during which further arousal is not possible; resolution will follow unless there is further stimulation.

The female orgasm and resolution

The female orgasm causes intense physical sensations and muscle contraction throughout the body in a similar manner to the male orgasm. A female orgasm is not necessary for pregnancy to occur, though it may raise fertility. Following the female orgasm, sexual arousal returns to the plateau phase without an absolute refractory period. Continued stimulation can result in further orgasms, otherwise resolution will occur.

SEXUAL DYSFUNCTION

The term 'sexual dysfunction' includes any process that interferes with a normal sex life. This can be caused by stress or physical or mental illness, but the majority of conditions result from ignorance, embarrassment or poor communication between sexual partners. Any therapy should involve both partners and encourage discussion and intimacy.

Male sexual dysfunction

Reduced libido

This is a lack of sexual desire; it is less common in men than women. It can be caused by psychological reactions to a deteriorating relationship or depression. It can also be caused by physical conditions including systemic illness, medications and a decrease in testosterone levels with age.

Erectile dysfunction (impotence)

Erectile dysfunction is the inability to maintain an erection suitable for vaginal penetration despite normal sexual desire. It is the most common presentation of sexual dysfunction in men and it can be caused by many conditions (Fig. 15.2). Erectile dysfunction can be treated by the following methods according to the cause:

- Sexual counselling.
- Vacuum aids.
- Smooth muscle relaxants [phosphodiesterase 5 inhibitors including tadalafil (Cialis), vardenafil (Levitra), sildenafil (Viagra®)].
- Intracavernosal injections directly into the penis (prostaglandin E_1).
- Implants.

Fig. 15.2 Causes of male sexual dysfunction

Cause	Examples	Mechanism
Psychological	Performance anxiety, stress	Stress inhibits the parasympathetic nervous system that maintains erection
Alcohol	Brewer's droop	Acutely inhibits sensory nerves, chronically damages liver raising oestrogen levels
Medications	Antihypertensives	Reduce blood flow to the penis
	Antidepressants and antipsychotics	Antagonize sexual arousal in the CNS
Endocrine	Diabetes	Long-term complications can damage the nerves and blood vessels of the penis
Vascular disease	Atherosclerosis	Prevents sufficient blood reaching the penis to maintain erection
Neurological	Multiple sclerosis	Inhibits sexual arousal in the CNS

CNS, central nervous system.

Erection is dependant, in part, on mediators derived from the NANC system. Nitric oxide (NO) stimulates the relaxation of the smooth muscle in the corpora cavernosa and stimulates arterial dilatation, which together contribute to erection. NO operates by increasing second messenger, cGMP. cGMP is degraded by enzymes called cyclic nucleotide phosphodiesterases. Inhibitors to these enzymes, such as sildenafil (Viagra®) enhance the action of cGMP and are used in the treatment of erectile dysfunction.

Premature ejaculation

The definition of premature ejaculation depends on the expectations and desires of both partners. In severe cases ejaculation may occur prior to penetration. It is made worse by anxiety and can be treated by relaxation techniques.

Female sexual dysfunction

Reduced libido

A lack of sexual desire can be present from puberty or it can develop with time, in which case it is often a reaction to a deteriorating relationship or depression. It can be caused by physical illness that prevents the enjoyment of sexual intercourse (e.g. vaginal infection, general illness or medications).

Anorgasmia

The majority of women require more time and greater stimulation to achieve orgasm than men. Anorgasmia is the complete failure to achieve orgasm; it is not infrequent orgasms. The best treatment involves teaching both partners about the female body; encouraging masturbation may also benefit some women.

Dyspareunia

Dyspareunia is pain on intercourse. There are two kinds:

- Superficial—felt on the external genitalia.
- Deep—felt internally.

Apart from the common vaginismus (see below), dyspareunia tends to have a physical cause (Fig. 15.3).

Vaginismus

This is involuntary contraction of vaginal muscle upon attempted penetration, causing apareunia or dyspareunia. It is a common psychological condition caused by fear of penetration, sometimes resulting from previous dyspareunia.

Apareunia

This is the inability of the vagina to accept penile penetration. It can be caused by congenital malformations of the vagina or severe vaginal infections, but most commonly it is caused by vaginismus.

Fig. 15.3 Causes of female dyspareunia

Type of dyspareunia	Disease process	Symptoms and signs
Superficial	Vulval/vaginal infections	Lesions and discharge
	Previous surgery or trauma	Scars
	Cystitis and UTIs	Urinary frequency, urgency, and pain
	Oestrogen deficiency	Lack of lubrication post-menopausal
Deep	Endometriosis	Recurrent pelvic pain in time with the menstrual cycle
	Pelvic inflammatory disease	Abdominal pain
	Fibroids	Menorrhagia and pelvic pain
	Ovarian cysts/tumours	Pelvic pain and menorrhagia

UTI, urinary tract infection.

Sexual dysfunction can have vascular, neural, endocrine, muscular, psychological or multifactorial causes. Assessment of patients with sexual dysfunction should include a psychological history. An assessment of coexisting morbidities, such as diabetes mellitus (which can cause autonomic neuropathies) or trauma to the pudendal nerve should be made. A drug history is also important as drugs can interfere with each step of the sexual response. A generalized assessment of endocrine function is useful in identifying lesions in the hypothalamic–pituitary axis.

THE PROCESS OF FERTILIZATION

Oocyte

At ovulation, the oocyte is released from the mature ovarian follicle onto the surface of the ovary in the peritoneal cavity. At this stage, it has completed the first division of meiosis and has arrested at metaphase of the second meiotic division. It is surrounded by two layers:

- Zona pellucida—a glycoprotein layer.
- Corona radiata—granulosa cells from the follicle (also called cumulus oophorus).

The oocyte is wafted into the uterine tube by the action of cilia on the fimbriae. Further ciliary action and peristalsis move the oocyte along the uterine tube to the ampulla. It is capable of fertilization for less than 24 hours.

Sperm

About 200 million sperm are ejaculated deep into the vagina close to the external cervical os. They are suspended in the fructose-rich, alkaline seminal fluid; this provides the energy required by the sperm and acts as a buffer to the acidic vaginal environment. The motile sperm must cover a significant distance to reach the oocyte in the uterine tubes.

Their passage may be assisted by physiological changes brought about by the female orgasm and chemical signals directing them towards the oocyte.

Within the female genital tract, sperm are viable for less than 48 hours. The majority degenerate and are absorbed by the female, with only about 200 sperm reaching the oocyte in the ampulla of the uterine tube. The quickest sperm can arrive in just 5 minutes.

Capacitation

The ejaculated sperm cannot penetrate the oocyte until they undergo capacitation. The following changes occur in the uterus or uterine tubes:

- Removal of glycoproteins covering the acrosome.
- Reorganization of membrane phospholipids to alter the membrane potential and charge.
- Influx of calcium that increases flagellar activity and motility.
- Activation of the acrosome allowing the release of enzymes.

Capacitation must be mimicked during in-vitro fertilization (IVF) by incubation in a suitable medium.

Fertilization

Fertilization normally occurs in the ampulla of the uterine tube. The sperm must penetrate the layers surrounding the oocyte and, in the process, prevent other sperm from fertilizing the oocyte a second time. This process requires several steps:

1. *Penetration of the corona radiata* The acrosome membrane begins to perforate, releasing the enzyme hyaluronidase, which disrupts the cell matrix and enables sperm to push through the remaining granulosa cells.
2. *Penetration of the zona pellucida* Receptors on the acrosome bind to ZP3 molecules causing the release of acrosin, an enzyme that digests the glycoprotein chains of the zona pellucida. The sperm can then push through the weakened structure.
3. *Fusion of the plasma membranes* The membranes of the sperm and oocyte bind via integrin receptors and fuse. The sperm nucleus enters the oocyte cytoplasm leaving its tail and membrane behind. (NB No sperm mitochondria enter the oocyte.)
4. *Fast block* The membrane fusion causes the oocyte to depolarize, preventing other sperm from binding for about a minute.
5. *Slow block* The fusion also causes calcium to enter the oocyte resulting in the release of cortical granules containing hydrolytic enzymes. These enzymes break down the ZP3 molecules of the zona pellucida, permanently preventing other sperm from binding.
6. *Second meiotic division* The calcium influx also causes the oocyte to complete the second meiotic division. This produces two haploid cells:

- Female pronucleus with the majority of the cytoplasm.
- Second polar body with almost no cytoplasm.

7. *Formation of the pronuclei* The nucleus of the sperm enlarges to form a pronucleus that is indistinguishable from the female pronucleus. The DNA within each pronucleus is replicated.
8. *Mixing of the chromosomes* The nuclear membranes surrounding the pronuclei break down and the maternal and paternal chromosomes mix producing a diploid (46 chromosomes) zygote.
9. *First mitotic division* The zygote immediately begins to divide by mitosis and a copy of the replicated DNA enters each cell. This division takes about 30 hours to complete.

DEVELOPMENT AND IMPLANTATION

Early development

The zygote divides into two cells called blastomeres as the embryo is transported along the uterine tube. The blastomeres continue to divide mitotically, becoming smaller with each division. The cells then reorganize to form a tighter ball held together by tight junctions; a process called compaction. When the embryo reaches the 12- to 16-cell stage it is called a morula.

The morula enters the uterus about 3 days after fertilization. Glands in the endometrial lining secrete a glycogen-rich fluid under the influence of progesterone from the corpus luteum. Glycogen can cross the zona pellucida to nourish the morula.

Soon after the morula enters the uterus, a cavity develops forming an inner and outer layer of cells:

- Trophoblast—the outer cell layer that will form the placenta.
- Embryoblast—the inner cell mass that will form the embryo.

The conceptus is now called a blastocyst. Over the next 2 days the zona pellucida breaks down, allowing the blastocyst to increase in size. It is now ready for implantation. These changes are shown in Fig. 15.4.

Implantation

About 6 days after fertilization, the blastocyst binds to the endometrial lining. This usually occurs in the

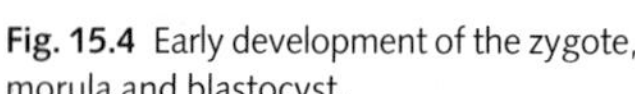

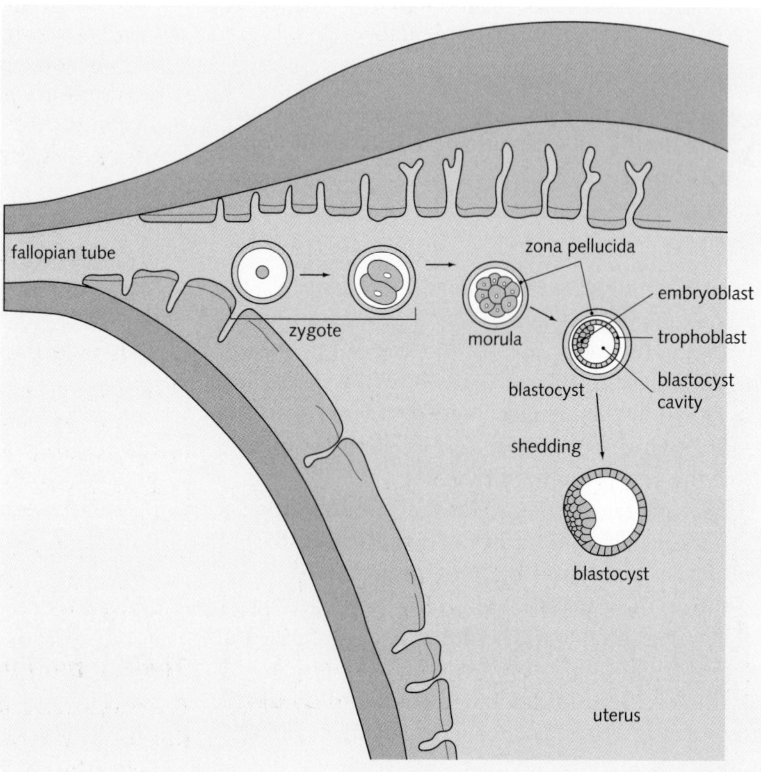

Fig. 15.4 Early development of the zygote, morula and blastocyst.

The fast and slow blocks do not always prevent multiple fertilizations. Triploid (three sets of chromosomes) zygotes are formed, but they usually die within the uterus; the mechanism for this abortion is unknown.

body of the uterus with the embryoblast nearer to the endometrium and the cavity closer to the uterus lumen. The trophoblast layer grows rapidly and differentiates to form two layers:

- Cytotrophoblast—the layer nearest the embryoblast, composed of dividing cells that join the syncytiotrophoblast.
- Syncytiotrophoblast—the layer nearest to the endometrium; it is composed of cytoplasm containing many nuclei without cell boundaries.

The syncytiotrophoblast develops finger-like projections that invade the surrounding endometrium to hold the blastocyst in place. It releases enzymes that break down the glycogen-rich endometrial stroma to release nourishment for the developing embryoblast. This entire process is called implantation (Fig. 15.5).

CONTRACEPTION

Humans are most unusual animals, since neither the female nor the male is aware of the time of ovulation.

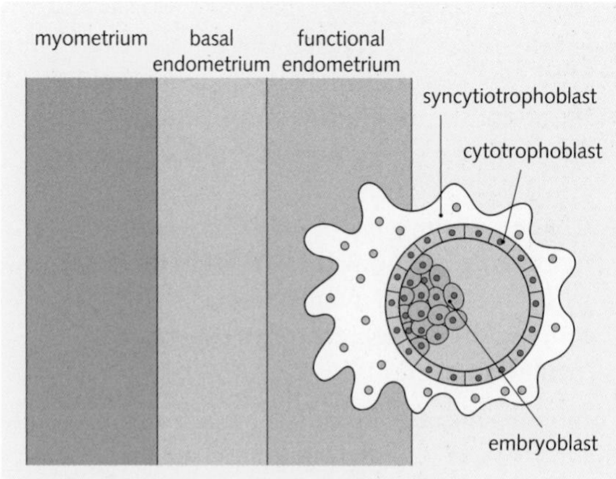

Fig. 15.5 Implantation of the blastocyst.

The majority of female animals display ovulation with dramatic changes in colour, smell and behaviour, to which the male responds appropriately. On the good side, this allows humans to engage in sex at any time throughout the year. However, it makes pregnancy very difficult to avoid.

A wide range of reliable contraceptive methods are now available, allowing people to choose a method that suits their lifestyle and beliefs. This is achieved either by control of ovulation or by methods that prevent fertilization. No method of contraception can prevent pregnancy 100% of the time in 100% of women. The failure rate is measured as the percentage of women who become pregnant during 1 year of use. This percentage varies widely between contraceptive methods and the reliability of the user; the lower the figure the more effective the contraception. Fig. 15.6 shows examples of common contraceptive methods and Fig. 15.7 shows where their contraceptive actions take place.

Natural contraception

None

The average age of first contraceptive use is 8 months later than the average age of first sexual intercourse. Many adolescents have disproved the myth that you cannot get pregnant the first time you have sex. Without any form of contraception around 80% of women become pregnant during 1 year of regular, frequent, unprotected sex.

Postcoital douche

Since the sperm are deposited in the vagina, washing the vagina out after sex reduces fertility. This method is very ineffective: it has a failure rate of 45% because the sperm are rapidly transported through the cervix.

Coitus interruptus

This is also called the withdrawal method; the man withdraws his penis from the vagina just before ejaculation. While the theory is good, in practice the sympathetic system hijacks the body to propagate the species. Even with successful withdrawal, pregnancy can still result since sperm is also present in the male pre-ejaculatory secretions. The failure rate of 20% speaks for itself.

Rhythm method (natural family planning)

The oocyte can only survive for 24 hours without fertilization, whereas the sperm can survive for 48 hours or longer. In theory, fertilization can only

Fig. 15.6 Examples of methods of contraception

Method	Rhythm method	Condoms	COCP	IUD	Mirena® (IUS)	Vasectomy
Action	Natural	Barrier	Hormonal	Prevents implantation	Hormonal	Surgical sterilization
Failure rate (%)	2.5–30	1.5–7	1	2	0.1	0.05 per lifetime
Advantages	Free, approved by Catholic church	Cheap, easy, portable and protects from STDs	Cheap, effective, light periods	Lasts up to 5 years	Very effective, light periods, minimal effort	Very effective, simple operation
Disadvantages	Requires high motivation and control	Reduces spontaneity and may affect sensitivity	Several side effects including risk of cardiovascular disease and breast cancer	Must be fitted by doctor, risk of PID and heavy menstrual bleeding	Must be fitted by doctor, risk of PID	Irreversible

Fig. 15.6 Examples of methods of contraception. (COCP, combined oral contraceptive pill; IUD, intrauterine device; IUS, intrauterine system; PID, pelvic inflammatory disease; STDs, sexually transmitted diseases.)

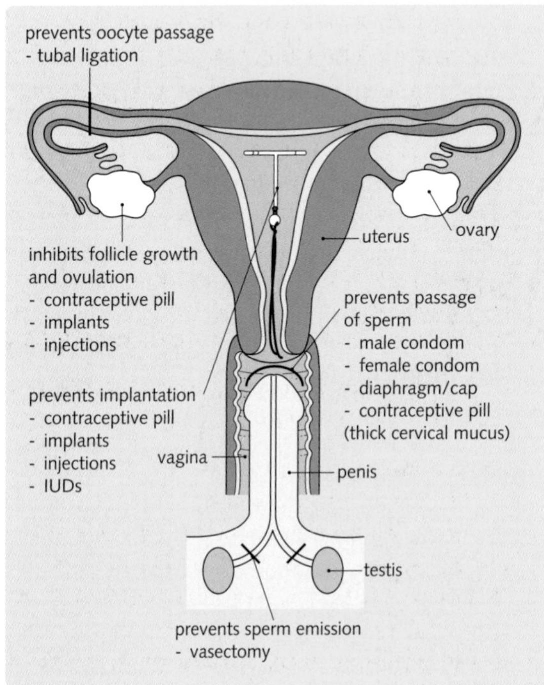

Fig. 15.7 Locations of contraceptive actions. (IUDs, intrauterine devices.)

occur following sexual intercourse in the 3 days around ovulation. By determining the exact date of ovulation and avoiding sex before and after this date pregnancy can be avoided. In practice, a wider period of sexual abstinence is used, usually about 9 days per cycle. There are a number of methods for detecting the date of ovulation:

- Keeping a calendar of the menstrual cycle and changes.
- Changes in cervical mucus; it becomes clear, sticky, and stretchy at ovulation.
- Changes in temperature; there is a rise of about 0.3°C after ovulation. Note that after ovulation basal body temperature drops slightly then rises and stays high until just before the next period.
- Changes in the types of oestrogens and luteinizing hormone (LH) levels in the urine using over-the- counter kits.
- Mittelschmerz; rarely, women experience 'ovulation pain'.

Combining the primary indicators such as temperature and mucus and secondary indicators such as ovulation pain, the failure rate ranges from 2.5 to 30%, depending on the motivation of both partners and the regularity of the menstrual cycle. No further follow-up is needed once the methods have been learnt and this method is acceptable to all religions.

Breastfeeding lactational amenorrhoea method (LAM)

Breastfeeding induces a reduction in GnRH, LH and FSH and results in amenorrhoea. This offers 98% protection against pregnancy when a woman is fully breastfeeding, the baby is less than 6 months old and menstruation has not returned.

Barrier contraception

The aim of barrier protection is to prevent the sperm from reaching the oocyte, thus preventing fertilization. All barrier methods offer some protection against sexually transmitted diseases including human immunodeficiency virus (HIV) infection. The failure rate ranges from 1.5 to 7%, depending on the motivation of both partners.

Male condom

Condoms are currently the only method of contraception where the responsibility is entirely on the part of the man. Condoms are sheaths of lubricated latex that fit over the erect penis to prevent sperm from entering the vagina. After intercourse the penis should be withdrawn as soon as possible whilst holding the condom in place. Modern condoms do not interfere with sensation significantly, but they may reduce spontaneity. They are readily available, cheap, portable and offer good protection against many sexually transmitted diseases (STDs), including HIV. They require no medical supervision and have no side effects unless sensitive to the latex, but should not be used with oil-based lubricants. They can slip off and break if not used properly.

Female condom

These are larger versions of male condoms that fit into the vagina. There is a risk of the penis 'missing' the condom, but a large ring at the open end aims to prevent this by holding it against the vulva. They do not need to be fitted by a specialist. The main disadvantage is the rustling noise, similar to a plastic bag, which accompanies intercourse.

Diaphragm

Diaphragms are reusable circular latex devices that fit in the vagina (or caps that fit over the cervix); they are used with a covering of spermicidal cream to kill the sperm. They can be inserted a couple of hours before sex, but they must not be removed for at least 6 hours afterwards. They must initially be fitted by a medical professional and require teaching and practice for reliable use. Disadvantages are increased incidence of cystitis and *Candida* vaginal infections.

Spermicides

Spermicides act to kill sperm.The only spermicide in use in UK is nonoxynol 9. This method is not an effective contraceptive when used alone.

Hormonal contraception

Hormonal contraception is the artificial administration of oestrogens and/or progestogens to reduce fertility. They mimic the hormonal changes of pregnancy to prevent further ovulation. Oestrogens act in the following ways:

- Strongly suppress FSH to prevent follicle development.
- Suppress LH release to prevent ovulation.
- Weakly inhibit implantation.

Progestogens have slightly different effects:

- Thicken the cervical mucus so that sperm cannot pass.
- Inhibit development of the endometrium to prevent implantation.
- Weakly suppress FSH to prevent follicle development.
- Weakly suppress LH release to prevent ovulation.

The use of oestrogen-containing contraception has a number of beneficial effects:

- Lighter, shorter periods.
- Regular, controllable periods.
- Reduces symptoms of premenstrual syndrome (PMS).
- Reduces the risk of ovarian and endometrial cancer.
- Controls the symptoms of endometriosis.

Unfortunately, oestrogens also increase the risk of two serious diseases:

- Thromboembolism—the hormones increase the levels of many clotting factors so the blood is prone to coagulate, causing deep vein thrombosis (DVT) and a risk of pulmonary embolus (PE). There is also a risk of hypertension.
- Cancer—there may be a small and temporary increase in the incidence of breast cancer in young women. This is offset by the reduction in risk of ovarian and endometrial cancer.

Since both these diseases are rare in the younger age groups that use hormonal contraception, the overall risk remains very small. In fact, it is less than the risk of childbirth or abortion. Smoking greatly increases these risks.

A number of less serious side effects are occasionally experienced:

- Break-through bleeding—irregular menstrual bleeding is common in the first few months of use.
- Slight weight gain—this is usually temporary.
- Headaches and migraine.
- Acne—caused by oestrogen.
- Dry eyes—a concern for contact lens users.
- Loss of libido due to androgen inhibition.

The side effects do result in a number of contraindications for oestrogen-containing contraception; in most cases, progestogen-only contraception can be used instead. These are similar to the contraindications for hormone replacement therapy (HRT) and, likewise, are frequently asked in exams:

- Oestrogen-dependent cancer (including breast cancer).
- Cardiovascular and thromboembolic disorders.
- Liver disease with abnormal liver function tests (LFTs).
- Undiagnosed vaginal bleeding.
- Pregnancy or breastfeeding.
- Smokers aged over 35 years.
- Severe migraines.

Combined oral contraceptive pill (COCP)

The 'Pill' is the most common method of contraception used by young women. It contains low doses of both oestrogen and progestogen giving a failure rate of 1%. It is taken for 21 days followed by a 7-day break, during which withdrawal bleeding occurs; this is not real menstruation. Originally the pill was designed to be taken continuously, and this can still be done without risk; the break has been added for the reassurance of the user. The side effects are described above. Failure of oral contraception is due to user compliance, incomplete absorption due to gastrointestinal problems, drug interaction due to changes in gut flora resulting from antibiotic use which may interfere with enterohepatic recirculation

Progestogen-only pill (POP)

As the name suggests, this oral contraceptive only contains progestogen. It has a higher failure rate (2%), especially in younger women, but it can be used in women in whom COCPs are contraindicated or not tolerated. It must be taken continuously at the same time (within 3 hours) every day. The main side effect is the menstrual irregularity that occurs in 25% of users.

Depot progestogen

Long acting progestogens can be injected intramuscularly to give 2–3 months of contraception. It has similar side effects and failure rate to POPs, but it carries a risk of amenorrhoea and temporary infertility for several months after discontinuation.

Subdermal implants

A progestogen-containing tube (Implanon®) can be implanted in the upper arm to give 3 years of contraception. The side effects and failure rate are similar to POPs. It must be removed after 3 years, but it can be removed earlier to rapidly restore fertility.

Intrauterine system (IUS or Mirena®)

This is a type of plastic intrauterine device (IUD) that releases progestogen; it does not contain copper. The progestogen acts locally to give excellent contraception; it reduces menstrual bleeding and prevents side effects. IUSs last 5 years and the failure rate is about 0.1%. There are some cases emerging where bleeding recommences after 2 years even though the implant is still releasing progestogen, but this is currently under investigation.

Prevention of implantation

Intrauterine devices

These are small plastic devices surrounded by copper wire that are inserted into the uterus lumen. The copper inactivates sperm to prevent fertilization. The device inhibits implantation. Threads are attached to the device to allow insertion and removal, which must be performed by a trained medical professional. Insertion can be difficult in young or nulliparous women (i.e. women who have never given birth). The woman can check the IUD remains in place by feeling for these threads at the cervix os. The IUD can be left in place for 5 years, throughout which the failure rate is about 1%. There are several side effects and risks:

- Expulsion—especially in the first 2 months.
- Cramping and menstrual bleeding—usually diminishes with time.
- Pelvic inflammatory disease (PID)—caused by bacterial infection at insertion.
- Increased risk of ectopic pregnancy.

An IUD can be used as emergency contraception to prevent implantation and, therefore, pregnancy if it is inserted within 5 days of unprotected sexual intercourse.

Postcoital medication (emergency contraception)

The progestogen 'morning-after' pill is available in the UK. This pill contains higher doses of the steroids that are used for contraception. The high levels of steroids act to make the endometrium unfavourable for implantation and prevents or delays ovulation if given early enough in the cycle. The emergency hormonal contraception is between 98 and 100% effective if it is taken within 72 hours (3 days) of unprotected sexual intercourse. Side effects may include nausea and vomiting, so an antiemetic is sometimes prescribed.

Irreversible contraception

Sterilization is the most popular form of contraception in older men and women. It involves surgery to prevent the sperm or oocyte from reaching the site of fertilization. Since the male operation is simpler and more effective it should be considered the preferred technique in stable couples who have completed their family. Both techniques should be considered a permanent form of contraception, although microsurgery can successfully reverse sterilization in about 50% of cases.

Vasectomy

This is a quick operation performed under local anaesthetic in which a section of each vas deferens is removed. The cut ends are tied or burnt closed by diathermy to prevent sperm from reaching the urethra. It does not interfere with testosterone production or sensation. The man is potentially fertile for 3 months after the operation due to sperm within the proximal vas deferens; during this time other contraception should be employed. There is a risk of postoperative bruising and bleeding. It is the most effective form of contraception with a failure rate of about 0.05% per lifetime.

Tubal ligation

This is the equivalent operation in the female. It is usually performed under general anaesthetic using a laparoscope to cut, burn or clip both uterine tubes. The woman becomes infertile after her next period and the failure rate is low at 0.5% per lifetime. The major complications are due to the general anaesthetic.

INFERTILITY

Infertility is defined as the inability to conceive after 2 years of regular unprotected sex (NICE guidelines 2004). It is a common problem, affecting about 1 in 6 couples. 84% of couples will be pregnant within 12 months, rising to 92% in the second year. Infertility is caused by:

- Abnormalities in the male (30%).
- Abnormalities in the female (45%).
- Unexplained (25%).

Male infertility

Male infertility is usually caused by abnormalities in sperm production; these include:

- Azoospermia—no sperm.
- Oligospermia—also called a low sperm count (less than 20 million/mL; the average is about 60 million/mL).
- Asthenozoospermia—this is decreased sperm quality due to reduced motility or abnormal morphology (shape).

Some of the conditions that can cause these abnormalities are shown in Fig. 15.8. Less commonly, male sexual dysfunction can prevent normal sexual intercourse.

Female infertility

The causes of female infertility are more varied:

- Ovulation problems—oligomenorrhoea or amenorrhoea (45%).
- Structural abnormalities of the uterine tubes—blocked tubes commonly due to pelvic inflammatory disease in the past (45%).
- Structural abnormalities of the uterus and cervix (5%).
- Disorders of the cervical mucus (5%).

Fig. 15.8 Causes of male infertility

Abnormality	Cause
Azoospermia	Blockage of genital tract
Oligospermia	Testosterone deficiency
	Hyperprolactinaemia
Asthenozoospermia	Raised scrotal temperature, e.g. varicocoele
	Antisperm antibodies
Oligospermia or asthenozoospermia	Genetic disorders, e.g. Klinefelter's
	Genital tract infection (current or previous with scarring)

The main conditions that cause these abnormalities are shown in Fig. 15.9. Some clinicians believe that an inadequate luteal phase can also cause infertility because the blastocyst does not have time to implant successfully before the corpus luteum regresses. Infertility can also be caused by sexual dysfunction.

Investigation

Counselling and reassurance are extremely important in the management of infertility. Many of the questions and procedures can be very embarrassing so the couple must feel they can trust the practitioner. The investigations should be aimed at diagnosing and treating the cause of infertility, not finding which partner is 'at fault'. Infertility is investigated by:

- Examination of sperm under a microscope.
- Hormone investigations—FSH, LH, prolactin, progesterone, oestrogen, testosterone and thyroid hormone.
- Pelvic ultrasound—looks for gross abnormality and can detect the presence of correctly developing ovarian follicles.
- Hysterosalpingography or laparoscopy and dye test—contrast media/dye is injected into the uterus to image the uterine tubes by X-ray or visually (see Fig. 19.9).
- Postcoital test—checks cervical mucus and sexual technique.

Fig. 15.9 Causes of female infertility

Abnormality	Cause
Oligomenorrhoea or amenorrhoea	Weight loss
	Post COCP pituitary insensitivity
	Polycystic ovaries
	Hyperprolactinaemia
Abnormal fallopian tube	Pelvic inflammatory disease (Chlamydia)
	Endometriosis
	Pelvic surgery
Abnormal cervix	Cervical stenosis
Abnormal cervical mucus	Immunological reaction against sperm

Treatment

Infertility is rarely absolute; it is usually caused by the reduced fertility (subfertility) of one or both partners. Where possible, treatment is aimed at the underlying cause. Medical treatment includes:

- Bromocriptine—which treats hyperprolactinaemia.
- Clomiphene—an antioestrogen, which stimulates FSH release and follicle development.
- hCG—which can trigger ovulation by acting like LH.
- LH and FSH injections—follicle stimulants, if clomiphene fails.
- GnRH analogues—follicle stimulants, if clomiphene fails.

Medications that stimulate follicle development may induce multiple pregnancies.

If these simpler treatments fail, assisted fertilization techniques can be used. These are both expensive and emotionally draining, though they have a 20–30% success rate (live births per cycle); this is compared with a rate of about 15% in fertile couples without assisted fertilization. Assisted fertilization techniques require hyperstimulation of the ovaries using the medications described above. The ovary responds by producing several eggs that are harvested using a transvaginal needle under ultrasound control. The techniques then differ:

- In-vitro fertilization (IVF)—oocytes are fertilized in vitro and re-introduced into the uterus. This is the only treatment for blocked uterine tubes.

- Intracytoplasmic sperm injection (ICSI)—this is used alongside IVF if the sperm are abnormal and are incapable of fertilization.
- Gamete intrafallopian transfer (GIFT)—oocytes are re-introduced into the uterine tubes along with sperm for in-vivo fertilization.

THERAPEUTIC ABORTION

Worldwide, about 25 million abortions are performed each year. It is one of the safest clinical interventions. It is referred to as therapeutic abortion where it is performed to preserve the health of the mother, though 95% are performed for social or psychiatric reasons. In the UK, induced abortion is legal until 24 weeks gestation, though it is rarely performed beyond 20 weeks. It is a relatively safe procedure with no risk of subsequent reduced fertility if performed without complications before 13 weeks gestation. In developing countries without legalized abortion, fatality rates are much higher. An appropriate method of contraception is usually included as part of the treatment.

The method used for abortion depends in part on gestational age, mother's decision and local policy.

Early medical termination of pregnancy is preferred during the first 49 days from the last menstrual period. Oral mifepristone (an anti-progestogen) is administered first; it causes separation of the trophoblast from the endometrial wall and raises the sensitivity of the uterus to prostaglandins. Prostaglandin analogues (e.g. misoprostol) are given 48 hours after mifepristone; they can be taken orally or applied vaginally and they induce uterine contractions.The fetus is usually expelled vaginally within 12 hours of the prostaglandin treatment. Medical termination often causes bleeding and pain, but pain relief is available. Alternatively, dilation and extraction of the intact fetus can be performed. After 13 weeks a 'late' medical termination of pregnancy is advocated.

Surgical termination of pregnancy (STOP) is a day-case procedure performed under general anaesthetic in which the products of conception are removed using suction curettage. It is performed on women too far into their pregnancy for early medical termination. Rare complications include tissue retention, haemorrhage and acute haematometra (accumulation of blood in the uterus). After 12–14 weeks gestation fetal parts cannot be readily aspirated, but with adequate dilatation they can be removed piecemeal from the uterus.

THE PLACENTA

Development

The placenta develops partly from the trophoblast surrounding the developing fetus. The development of the trophoblast is described in the section 'Implantation' (p. 178). The placenta also develops partially from the maternal endometrium; the development is shown in Fig. 15.10.

Lacunar phase

Eight days after fertilization, the syncytiotrophoblast (SCT) begins to erode endometrial capillaries. Cavities called lacunae develop within the syncytiotrophoblast; they are continuous with the maternal capillaries and fill with maternal blood. This supplies oxygen and nutrition to the blastocyst through diffusion and it represents the early maternal circulation in the developing placenta. The lacunae link together to form a network, whilst the capillaries enlarge to form sinusoids.

Chorionic villi

The chorionic villi are branching projections from the blastocyst into the syncytiotrophoblast and functional endometrium. They increase the surface area in contact with maternal blood. Development progresses in three stages:

- Primary villi—2 weeks after fertilization, swellings in the cytotrophoblast (CT) extend into the syncytiotrophoblast and begin to branch.
- Secondary villi—at the start of the third week, mesenchyme from the embryo invades the cytotrophoblast of the primary villi.
- Tertiary villi—the mesenchyme forms blood vessels that link up with the newly formed fetal circulation by the end of the third week.

At this stage, the placenta has a blood supply from the mother and fetus, allowing more efficient exchange of nutrients, gases and waste products. The placenta

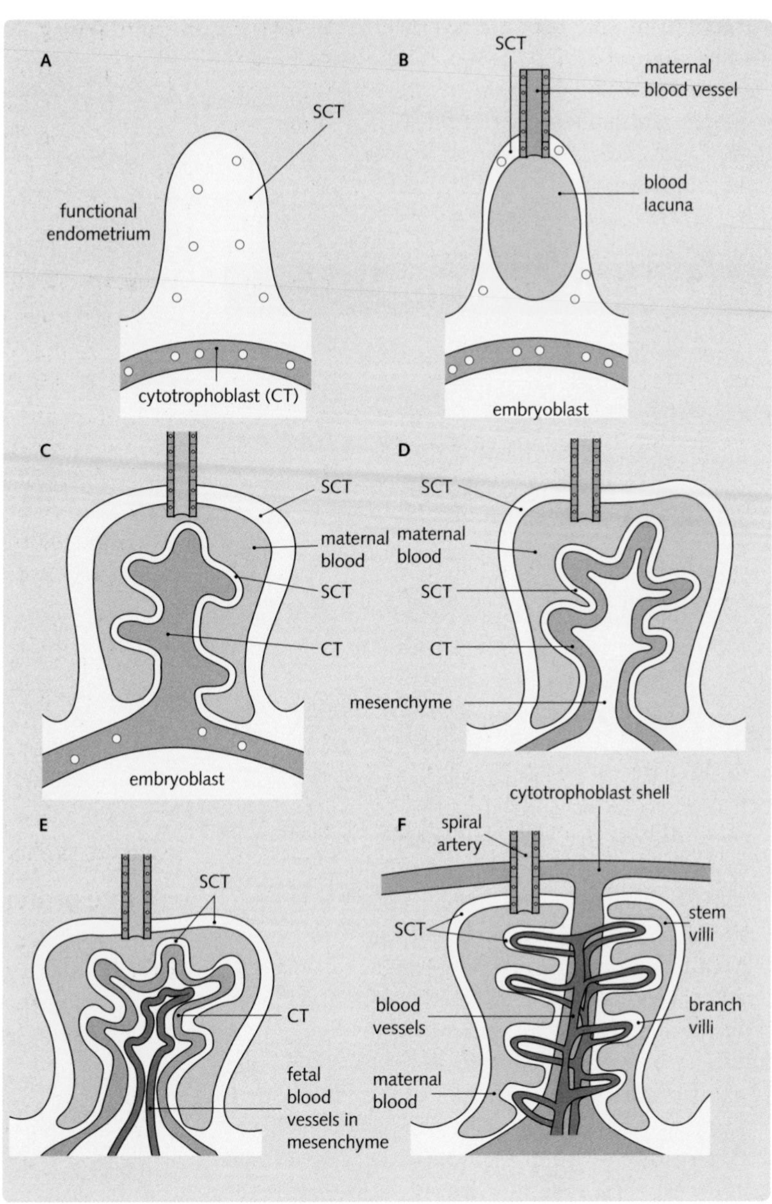

Fig. 15.10 Development of the placenta: (A) syncytiotrophoblast invasion; (B) lacunar phase; (C) primary chorionic villi; (D) secondary chorionic villi; (E) tertiary chorionic villi; (F) mature chorionic villi. See text for details. (CT, cytotrophoblast; SCT, syncytiotrophoblast.)

continues to develop throughout pregnancy, in advance of the growing needs of the fetus.

Further development of the villi

As the tertiary villi form, the cytotrophoblast extends through the syncytiotrophoblast at the tip of each villus. These cells are now in direct contact with endometrial cells, and they form a cytotrophoblast shell that holds the embryo in place. This shell remains directly connected at the top of chorionic villi that are now called stem villi.

Branching villi at the sides of the stem villi are called branch villi. These are surrounded by maternal blood in the lacunae, and they are the site of exchange between fetal and maternal blood. The cytotrophoblast lining of the branch villi breaks down to reduce the distance molecules must diffuse between the two circulations. As the placenta continues to grow, the lacunae become supplied by the spiral arteries and endometrial veins. Deoxygenated fetal blood reaches the placenta via the two umbilical arteries and oxygenated blood returns to the fetal circulation via the umbilical vein.

During this time, extravillous cytotrophoblast cells invade into the decidua basalis, the spiral arteries and the inner third of the myometrium. Remodelling of the spiral arteries during placental development is responsible for creating the high-flow, low-resistance system, ensuring an adequate maternal blood flow. Several pregnancy complications including pre-eclampsia, fetal growth retardation and late sporadic miscarriage are associated with inadequate spiral artery remodelling.

Further growth of the placenta occurs at the embryonic pole (the side to which the umbilicus is attached) by widening and lengthening; it does not penetrate further into the endometrium. This forms the familiar plate-like shape on one side of the uterus. The endometrium on the same side also changes to form the decidua basalis; this grows into the placenta forming incomplete septa that divide it into sections called cotyledons.

Babies that are small for gestational age (SGA) can be constitutionally small, incorrectly dated or they can be suffering from fetal growth retardation (FGR). This is a cause of perinatal mortality and morbidity and carries an increased risk of degenerative disease when the child reaches adulthood. Early-onset FGR is caused by maternal vascular disease, chromosomal abnormalities or intrauterine infection. Late-onset FGR is usually caused by uteroplacental insufficiency. Early onset is associated with proportionately small babies, whereas late onset is associated with a relatively large head.

Structure

It is important to remember that maternal and fetal blood do not mix within the placenta. Maternal blood enters large lacunae (cavities) from spiral arteries and is drained by endometrial veins. Fetal circulation in the branch villi is separated from the maternal circulation by two layers:

- Thin syncytiotrophoblast layer.
- Single-cell layer of endometrium in the fetal capillary.

This allows for rapid diffusion between the two circulations. A diagram of the fully developed placenta is shown in Fig. 15.11.

Functions

The placenta supplies all the requirements of the developing fetus whilst maintaining an environment in which the fetus can grow. The metabolic rate of the placenta is very high due to protein synthesis, active transport and growth. The many actions involved in this task fall into four categories and are described below.

Gaseous transport

Oxygen and carbon dioxide cross the placenta by passive diffusion. The rapid metabolism of the fetus uses up oxygen, so blood in the umbilical arteries has less oxygen than the maternal blood. This forms a concentration gradient that allows oxygen to diffuse across the placenta into the fetal blood. This process is also aided by fetal haemoglobin, which binds oxygen more strongly than adult haemoglobin. High levels of CO_2 are generated, crossing the placenta in the opposite direction.

Nutrient transport

Nutrients cross the placenta by passive facilitated diffusion and by active transport.

Towards the end of pregnancy, an excess of nutrients is transported so the fetus can develop energy stores such as glycogen and fat. These stores include brown adipose tissue that is broken down within the first few days after birth to create heat.

Immune protection

The fetus inherits codominantly paternal major histocompatibility complex (MHC) gene products and causes the maternal immune system to recognize the fetus as foreign or non-self. The placenta acts as a barrier to prevent immunological rejection; the syncytiotrophoblast cells at the fetal maternal interface lacking MHC class 1 and class 2 antigens.

Fetal alcohol syndrome: Alcohol can cross the placenta and enter the fetal circulation. Activity of the enzyme ethanol dehyrodgenase is lower in fetuses than in adults. As such, the fetus relies on maternal liver detoxification. Elevated alcohol impairs DNA synthesis and protein synthesis and inhibits differentiation. Nutrient transport across the placenta is also impaired. The severe outcome of fetal alcohol syndrome is characterized by growth retardation, impaired CNS development and dysmorphology. Tobacco can cause intrauterine growth restriction and increased perinatal mortality.

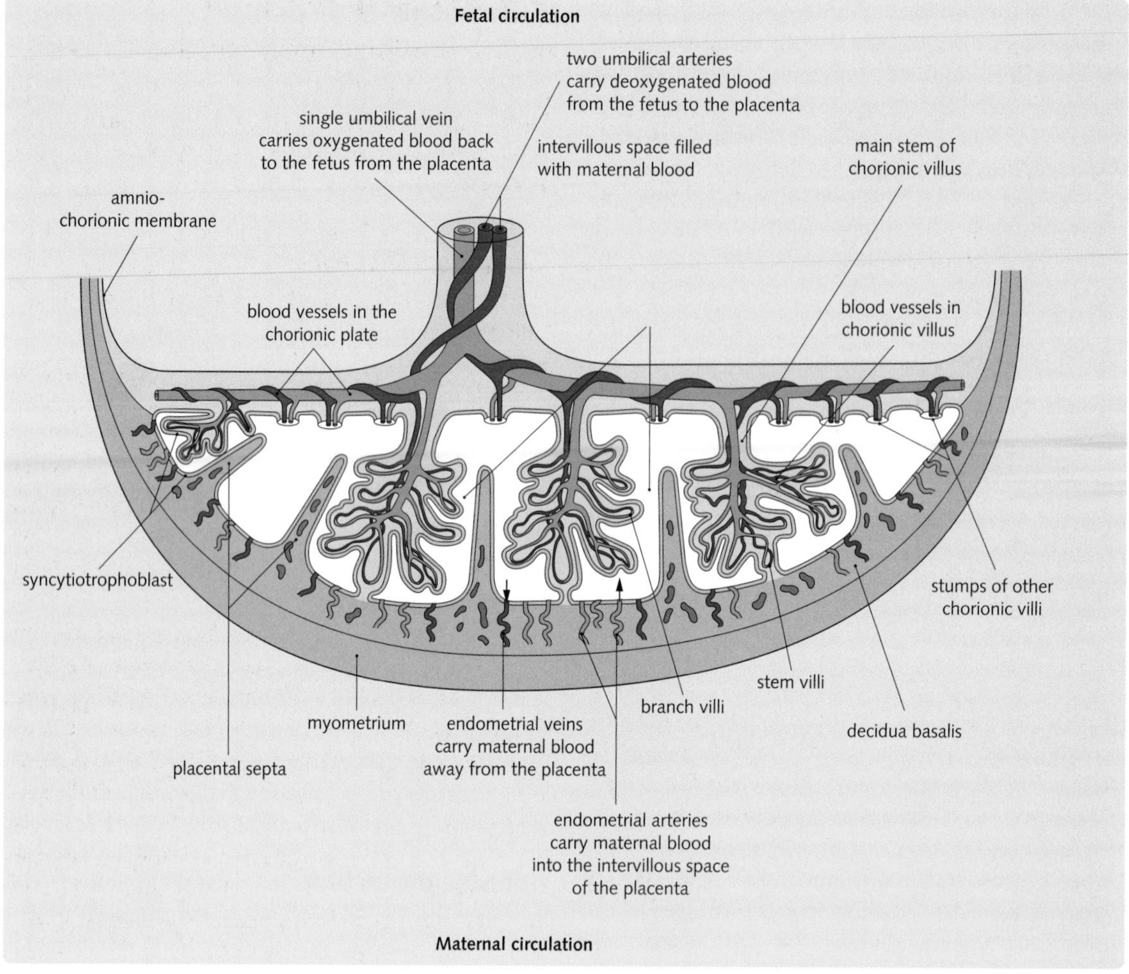

Fig. 15.11 Structure of the mature placenta. (Adapted from Moore & Persaud, 5th edn.)

Secretion of hormones

The placenta secretes high levels of steroid and protein hormones that regulate and maintain pregnancy. It also allows maternal and fetal hormones to cross. These hormones are described in the next section.

REPRODUCTIVE HORMONES IN PREGNANCY

Sources of reproductive hormones

Endocrine signals are essential for implantation and the maintenance of pregnancy. As the pregnancy progresses, the hormone levels change as shown in Fig. 15.12. There are two phases of hormonal secretion during pregnancy:

- Corpus luteum phase—the corpus luteum secretes hormones to maintain the endometrium and the developing placenta.
- Placental phase—the placenta takes over hormonal secretion to allow maternal adaptation to pregnancy, birth and lactation.

Corpus luteum phase

In the normal menstrual cycle, the corpus luteum secretes progesterone and oestrogen for about 10 days following ovulation, after which it regresses. The dramatic fall in progesterone levels causes degeneration and shedding of the endometrium resulting in menstruation. The blastocyst must prevent the next

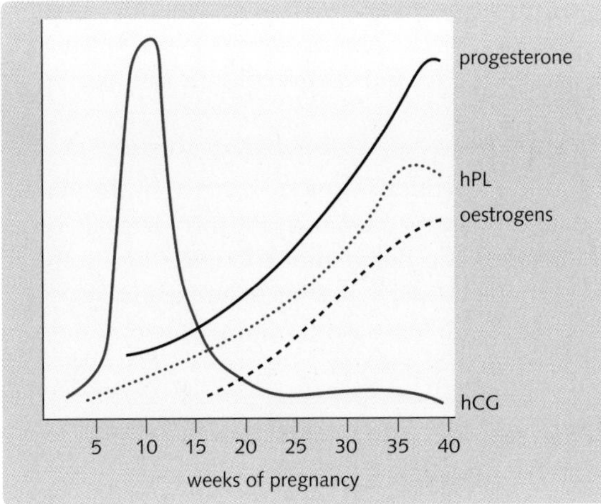

Fig. 15.12 Changes in the maternal blood levels of hormones during pregnancy. (Adapted from D Llewellyn-Jones, 6th edn.)

menstruation by maintaining the corpus luteum and its steroid secretion.

Soon after implantation, around day 6, the syncytiotrophoblast (outer layer of cells) secretes the hormone human chorionic gonadotrophin (hCG). This hormone is equivalent to LH, and it acts on the corpus luteum to prevent regression. Progesterone levels continue to rise and the functional endometrium is maintained. The corpus luteum continues to be the main source of progesterone and oestrogen for the first 6 weeks of development.

Placental phase

The placenta secretes the following hormones:

- hCG.
- Progesterone.
- Oestrogens.
- Human placental lactogen (hPL).
- Relaxin.

Other hormones include placental GnRH, placental CRH, placental TRH, placental ACTH, placental inhibin and placental GH.

By the sixth week the placenta is the main source of progesterone and oestrogens, which help the mother's body adapt to pregnancy. hPL helps regulate nutrient levels and metabolism; it also causes the glandular tissue of the breast to develop. Relaxin is secreted towards the end of pregnancy to prepare the body for birth.

Reproductive hormones

Human chorionic gonadotrophin

hCG is a peptide hormone secreted by the syncytiotrophoblast of the conceptus from implantation. It has a similar structure and actions to LH. These actions include:

- Maintenance of the corpus luteum.
- Regulation of placental oestrogen secretion.
- Stimulation of testosterone secretion in the male fetus.

The corpus luteum is initially formed and maintained by the ovulatory LH surge and hCG simply replaces the falling levels of LH to prevent regression. hCG is secreted for the first 10 weeks of pregnancy until the placenta is capable of secreting sufficient sex steroids to maintain the pregnancy. After 8 weeks the corpus luteum is no longer needed for hormone production and hCG levels begin to fall.

The β-subunit of hCG can be detected in the urine just before the first day of a missed period, usually about 6–8 days after potential fertilization. This allows time for the blastocyst to implant and hCG levels to rise. This principle is used for the urine pregnancy testing available in hospitals and over the counter in pharmacies. Since hCG levels fall after the corpus luteal phase these tests no longer work after 20 weeks. False positives may rarely indicate underlying disease (see the section on placental disorders).

Progesterone

The synthesis of progesterone is described in Chapter 12. Plasma levels of progesterone rise throughout pregnancy, secreted initially by the corpus luteum then by the placenta. It is the single most important hormone in the maintenance of pregnancy. Actions include:

- Maintenance and development of the functional endometrium.
- Inhibition of smooth muscle in the uterus to prevent premature expulsion.
- Metabolic changes, including fat storage.
- Physiological adaptation to pregnancy (this is described in the Chapter 16).
- Relaxation of smooth muscle throughout the body, which may cause some side effects (e.g. constipation and oesophageal reflux).

Oestrogens

The structure and synthesis of oestrogens are described in Chapter 12. Plasma levels of oestrogens (especially oestriol) rise throughout pregnancy, secreted initially by the corpus luteum then by the placenta. Like the granulosa cells, the placenta lacks several key enzymes for the synthesis of oestrogen from cholesterol. These steps must be performed by the fetal adrenal gland allowing the fetus to regulate placental oestrogen secretion. This does not affect progesterone secretion, which is formed from cholesterol in just two steps.

The actions of oestrogen prepare the body for birth and lactation. They include:

- Growth of the smooth muscle of the uterus (myometrium).
- Increased blood flow to the uterus.
- Softening of the cervix and pelvic ligaments.
- Stimulation of breast growth and development directly.
- Stimulation of pituitary prolactin secretion.
- Inhibition of pituitary LH and FSH secretion.
- Stimulation of synthesis of oxytocin receptors in the myometrium in late pregnancy.
- Water retention.

Human placental lactogen

hPL is a peptide hormone secreted by the syncytiotrophoblast; levels rise throughout pregnancy. It is sometimes called human chorionic somatomammotropin because its actions are similar to growth hormone and prolactin. These actions include:

- Maternal lipolysis (fat breakdown) and fatty acid metabolism sparing glucose.
- Maternal insulin resistance sparing glucose for the fetus.
- Enhancing active amino acid transfer across the placenta.
- Stimulating the growth and development of the breasts.
- Increasing cell growth and protein synthesis.

Relaxin

Relaxin is a peptide hormone secreted by the placenta late in pregnancy. It relaxes the myometrium, cervix and the pelvic ligaments, allowing the uterus to enlarge and the pelvis to stretch during birth. It acts by stimulating collagenase enzymes, which breakdown collagen in these tissues.

Reproductive hormones from other sources

Inhibin

Inhibin is a peptide hormone secreted by the ovary in the pregnant and non-pregnant state. It may suppress pituitary FSH secretion and stimulate progesterone production during pregnancy.

Prolactin

The structure, synthesis and control of prolactin is described in Chapter 2. Prolactin secretion from the pituitary gland rises throughout pregnancy due to stimulation by oestrogens. It has a similar action to hPL in that it stimulates the growth and development of the breasts and regulates fat metabolism.

During pregnancy the high levels of placental oestrogens prevent the secretion of milk. After birth the fall in oestrogen levels allows prolactin to act on the breast. If the mother breastfeeds the baby, sensory signals from the nipple cause further prolactin secretion after pregnancy. The high prolactin levels have two effects:

- Secretion of milk, though it is oxytocin that causes the milk to be ejected.
- Inhibition of pituitary FSH and LH, which has a contraceptive effect.

Pregnancy and birth

16

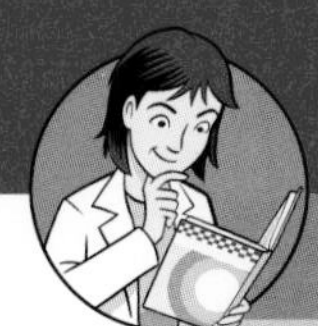

Objectives

By the end of the chapter you should be able to:

- List the maternal adaptations to pregnancy.
- Describe the three stages of birth and list the factors that stimulate labour.
- Describe the breast changes which occur during pregnancy and lactation.
- Describe the presentation, aetiology and treatment of ectopic pregnancies.
- Describe the presentation, aetiology and treatment of pre-eclampsia and eclampsia.
- Describe the presentation, aetiology and treatment of hydatidiform moles and choriocarcinoma.

MATERNAL ADAPTATIONS TO PREGNANCY

Throughout pregnancy the mother's body is undergoing changes that achieve three main purposes:

- Maintenance of a suitable environment for fetal growth.
- Preparation of the mother for childbirth.
- Preparation of the mother for lactation.

A summary of these changes is shown in Fig. 16.1.

Symptoms and signs of pregnancy

Presentation

The diagnosis of pregnancy may be a joyful or disastrous moment, depending on the situation and beliefs of the mother. There is also a wide range of knowledge and experience between women of different backgrounds and age groups. The earliest signs of pregnancy are:

- A missed period.
- Nausea, possibly with vomiting.
- Temporarily increased frequency of urination.
- Fuller breasts and larger nipples, possibly with tenderness.

A positive urine β-hCG test confirms the diagnosis, and many patients will have done this test at home before presenting to a doctor. Further confirmation can be obtained using ultrasound, but this is not normally necessary.

Side effects

In addition to the early signs mentioned above, the maternal adaptations to pregnancy can cause symptomatic side effects; the common side effects are shown in Fig. 16.2.

Genital tract

Placental hormones cause changes mainly in the lower genital tract:

- Uterus—expands dramatically through pregnancy; the muscle layer hypertrophies massively in preparation for birth.
- Cervix—softens and becomes more readily dilated.
- Vagina—hypertrophy of muscle and becomes more readily dilated.

Cardiovascular system

The effectiveness of the cardiovascular system must increase to cope with:

- Increased oxygen demands of the fetus and placenta—about 130% of normal.
- Extravascular space created by the expanding uterus and placenta.

The early adaptations are mostly caused by an increase in stroke volume with a slight increase in heart rate by 15 bpm. Together these factors raise cardiac output to about 140% of normal by the sixth month. Cardiac output then begins to fall because pressure from the enlarged uterus inhibits venous return. Blood pressure falls slightly during mid-pregnancy

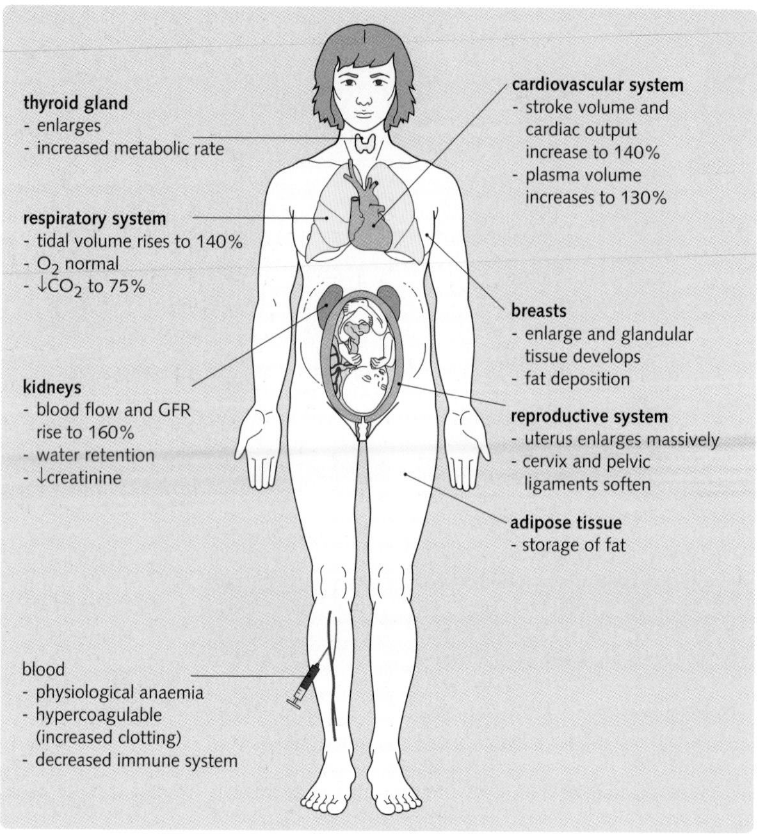

Fig. 16.1 Maternal adaptations to pregnancy. (GFR, glomerular filtration rate.)

because of peripheral vasodilation and decreased peripheral resistance to nearly 50% of non-pregnant values caused by increased production of vasodilator prostaglandins. It then begins to rise until birth.

Blood volume rises in the latter half of pregnancy to about 130% of normal, though there is a slight rise throughout pregnancy. Aldosterone and oestrogen cause renal water retention, so the plasma volume increases. There is also an increase in red blood cells, but this is less than the fluid retention so the blood becomes diluted with a fall in haemoglobin concentration and haematocrit causing a physiological anaemia. The excess blood volume fills the placental vasculature and also protects the mother from haemorrhage during birth. Pregnancy is a state of increased coagulability with increased risk of thrombosis and embolism leading cause of maternal mortality. This is potentiated by a decrease in plasma fibrinolytic activity which disappears within 1 hour of delivery.

Respiratory system

The increased oxygen demands of the fetus and placenta also require adaptations in the respiratory system causing pregnant women to overbreathe. Progesterone makes the chemoreceptors more sensitive to CO_2, causing the tidal volume to increase to 140% of normal while the respiratory rate remains the same. This maintains arterial oxygen saturation at normal levels whilst arterial CO_2 levels are about 75% of normal. These adaptations often give a sensation of breathlessness during pregnancy.

Renal system

Blood flow to the kidney increases during early pregnancy and then remains high. This causes the glomerular filtration rate (GFR) to rise to about 160% of normal. This would normally result in sodium loss, but increased secretion of renin, angiotensin II and aldosterone counteract these changes.

Progesterone causes the smooth muscle of the collecting ducts and ureters to become dilated. This slows the excretion of urine, making urinary tract infections (UTIs) more common. The urethra is also relaxed and the fetus exerts pressure on the bladder, so urinary incontinence is relatively common in late pregnancy.

Fig. 16.2 Common symptoms of pregnancy

Symptom	Cause	Stage of pregnancy
Morning sickness (nausea ± vomiting)	Rising oestrogen levels	From 4 weeks but then declines
Increased pigmentation	Raised levels of melanocyte-stimulating hormone (MSH) from the pituitary causing pigmentation of the face (chloasma) and abdominal striae	Gets progressively worse through pregnancy
Breathlessness	Changes in the cardiorespiratory system	
Gestational diabetes	Impaired glucose tolerance due to cortisol and hPL	
Constipation	Relaxation of smooth muscle caused by progesterone	
Heartburn and reflux		
Carpel tunnel syndrome	Water retention caused by oestrogen	
Ankle oedema		
Goitre	Raised thyroid-stimulating hormone (TSH) acting on the thyroid gland	
Severe abdominal distension	Fetus developing inside the uterus	Late
Prurigo of pregnancy	Itchy rash over abdomen and limbs	
Back ache	Softening of ligaments due to oestrogen	
Urinary frequency	Fetal head presses on the bladder	

Endocrine system

The secretion of the anterior pituitary hormones is altered during pregnancy (Fig. 16.3):

- FSH and LH secretion is almost completely stopped.
- Prolactin secretion rises throughout pregnancy.
- Thyroid-stimulating hormone (TSH) secretion initially falls then increases.
- Adrenocorticotrophic hormone (ACTH) secretion increases.
- Melanocyte-stimulating hormone (MSH) secretion increases.

The anterior pituitary gland enlarges as a result of these changes.

The rise in secretion of most hormones is caused by direct actions of placental hormones and an increase in plasma binding proteins (caused by the action of oestrogens on the liver) that reduces negative feedback.

Thyroid glands

hCG is structurally similar to TSH and inhibits TSH secretion in the 1st trimester but, as the hCG levels fall in the 2nd and 3rd trimesters, TSH then rises above normal. The increase in TSH, together with a reduction in iodine from the overactive kidneys, causes the thyroid gland to enlarge to trap sufficient iodine. Pregnancy is a state of relative maternal iodine deficiency. Thyroid hormone synthesis also increases but so does the synthesis of thyroid-hormone binding proteins stimulated by oestrogen. Overall, maternal active/free thyroid hormone levels remain normal. The fetal thyroid secretes thyroxine from 12 weeks; this is independent of maternal control as TSH does not cross the placenta.

Fig. 16.3 Changes that occur in pituitary hormone secretion during pregnancy and the effects caused by these changes

Secretion of anterior pituitary hormone	Hormone secretion in pregnancy (compared with non-pregnancy)	Effect of altered plasma hormone level in pregnancy
Prolactin ↑↑↑	Enhanced by placental oestrogens	Promotes growth and development of the breasts and regulates fat metabolism
FSH ↓ and LH ↓	FSH secretion is suppressed by inhibin and placental oestrogens LH secretion is suppressed by the combined effect of progesterone and oestrogen	Prevents further follicular development and ovulation during pregnancy
GH ↓	Suppressed by hPL	Unknown (hPL has similar effect to GH)
ACTH ↑	Rise	Stimulates increased cortisol secretion from the adrenal cortex
TSH	Falls in first trimester but then rises in second and third	Changes in thyroid hormone secretion are counteracted by changes in plasma protein synthesis

ACTH, adrenocorticotrophic hormone; FSH, follicle-stimulating hormone; GH, growth hormone; hPL, human placental lactogen; LH, luteinizing hormone; TSH, thyroid-stimulating hormone.

Adrenal glands

In contrast, free cortisol levels do rise, despite the increase in plasma binding proteins. This raises amino acid and glucose levels in the blood to improve fetal growth.

Aldosterone secretion from the adrenal cortex also rises slowly in response to the rising ACTH levels. It helps prevent the sodium loss caused by the raised GFR in the kidney.

Changes in metabolism

The mother usually gains 9–15 kg during pregnancy though the majority of this is caused by the fetus, placenta and fluid retention. Six months after birth, maternal weight is usually just 1 kg higher than before the pregnancy. Women have a larger appetite during pregnancy to supply the developing fetus, placenta and breasts. The excess of nutrients is regulated by changes in metabolism.

Carbohydrates

The hormone hPL causes insulin resistance to develop by stimulating insulin-like growth factor and this effect is enhanced by the raised cortisol. Insulin production is nearly doubled. The renal threshold for glucose falls and most pregnant women will lose glucose in the urine (glycosuria). As a result, the maternal metabolism uses a higher proportion of fatty acids and glucose use decreases. Pregnancy is a state of progressive insulin resistance due to hPL. This glucose is spared for the growing fetus.

If the mother already has a degree of impaired glucose tolerance (e.g. obesity) then diabetes mellitus can result. The glucose levels should be strictly controlled because hyperglycaemia predisposes to large babies, difficult births and other paediatric complications. After birth, this gestational diabetes mellitus usually resolves.

Amino acids

Progesterone inhibits the breakdown of amino acids in the liver to increase their availability for the fetus. The raised cortisol also increases the blood levels while hPL aids transport across the placenta.

Fat

Fat stores are initially broken down through the action of hPL to drive maternal metabolism. Towards the end of pregnancy, fat is stored in the breasts and subcutaneous tissues. Fat only accounts for a fraction of weight gain through pregnancy.

Other changes

Other minor changes occur during pregnancy:

- Immune system is regulated to prevent rejection of the fetus and this can predispose to some infections and altered autoimmune disease conditions eg rheumatoid arthritis tends to improve but systemic lupus flares up.
- Pelvic ligaments soften to allow the fetus to pass during birth.
- Venous congestion in lower limbs due to the pressure of the fetus on venous return; it can cause varicose veins.

Many birth defects can be detected prior to parturition, including neural tube defects, chromosomal abnormalities and other genetic conditions. Perinatal screening enables mothers to prepare for the birth of a baby with disabilities or to opt for pregnancy termination. Down syndrome is detected by a combination of nuchal fold thickness detected on ultrasound (week 10) and the triple test of maternal serum alpha feto-protein, oestriol and hCG (week 15–20). Follow-up with amniocentesis (0.5% risk of miscarriage) or chorionic villus sampling (1% risk of miscarriage but can be performed earlier in pregnancy) is advocated.

PARTURITION AND LABOUR

Position of the fetus

It is important to determine the position of the fetus before the onset of labour so that potential problems can be identified and preparations made. The position is assessed through palpation and ultrasound scans. There are three aspects to the fetal position, described below.

Lie

The lie describes the orientation of the baby's long axis; in simple terms, it is the orientation of the back. It can be:

- Longitudinal—this is the normal position with the back lying along the uterus.
- Oblique—the back is at an angle across the uterus.
- Transverse—the back lies across the uterus.

Palpation can also reveal which side the back is on, in a longitudinal lie.

Presentation

This is simply the part of the fetus that is nearest the cervix and, therefore, most likely to come out first. There are three main presentations:

- Cephalic—head first; this is normal.
- Breech—the bottom or feet first.
- Shoulder—associated with a transverse lie.

Cephalic presentations are further divided according to which part of the head is presenting. The term 'denominator' is used to describe the foremost part of the head. This is important because it affects the widest part of the head that must be born. The different types of cephalic presentation are shown in Fig. 16.4; occipitoanterior is the normal presentation. Fig. 16.5 shows some important points on the fetal skull along with the widest diameters of each presentation.

Clinically the presentation is described along with the extent to which the presenting part is palpable; this is described in fifths so that a fully palpable head scores 5/5, which decreases as the head descends, e.g. 3/5.

Position

The position of the fetus describes the direction that the denominator is facing compared with the pelvis. This is divided into two sections, which are then subdivided.

Fig. 16.4 Comparison of the four variations of cephalic presentation

Presentation	Vertex (occipitoanterior)	Deflexed (occipitoposterior)	Brow	Face
Position of the neck	Flexed	Deflexed	Extended	Very extended
Denominator	Occiput	Vertex	Bregma	Chin
Widest diameter	Suboccipito-bregmatic	Occipitofrontal	Mentovertical	Submento-bregmatic
Width	9.5 cm	11.5 cm	13.5 cm	9.5 cm

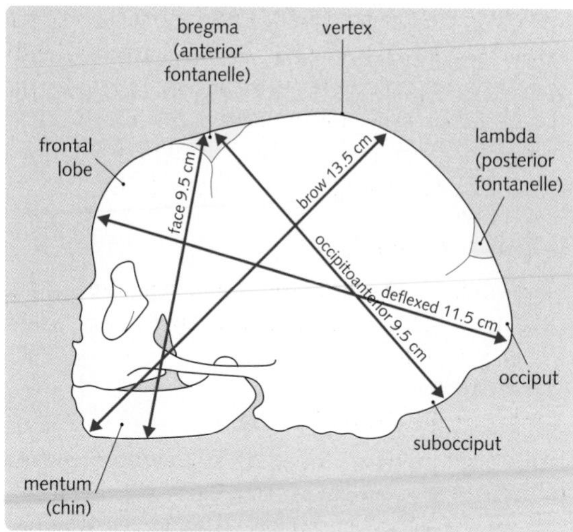

Fig. 16.5 Anatomy of the fetal skull and the widest diameters in the four types of cephalic presentation.

Firstly:

- Left (L)—faces the mother's left.
- Right (R)—faces the mother's right.
- Straight—faces the pubic symphysis or sacrum directly.

Secondly:

- Anterior (A)—faces the pubis bone.
- Transverse (T)—across the pelvis.
- Posterior (P)—faces the sacrum.

These two sections are combined with the name of the denominator to describe the position, e.g. left occipitoanterior (LOA) or occipitoposterior (OP). The occipitoposterior position is often associated with a deflexed presentation.

Sequence of labour

Labour is the sequence of actions leading to childbirth (parturition), including the expulsion of the placenta. In normal pregnancies, childbirth occurs after 37–42 weeks; the average is 40 weeks (280 days). Labour begins with regular, painful uterine contractions accompanied by cervical dilatation. It is often preceded by several weeks of false labour with irregular, painful contractions (called Braxton Hicks contractions) and no cervical dilatation. True labour is divided into three stages: first, second and third.

First stage

This is from the onset of true labour until full cervical dilatation (10 cm). The length of the stage varies widely between women; however, the cervix should dilate at a rate of 1 cm/h:

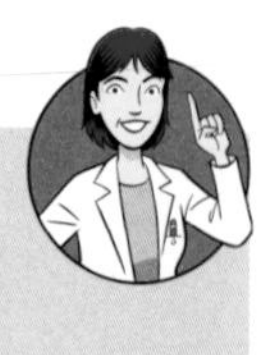

Trimesters—the development of the fetus in the uterus is divided into three periods of equal length (about 13 weeks) each called a trimester.

- 8–10 hours in first labour (nulliparous women, known as 'primips').
- 2–6 hours in subsequent labours (multiparous women or 'multips').

As labour progresses, the uterine contractions become stronger and more frequent. The contractions push the fetal head into the pelvis towards the cervix. The pain experienced is due to hypoxia of the uterus caused by occlusion of the blood vessels during the muscular contractions. The amniotic membrane often ruptures during this stage, resulting in the loss of amniotic fluid (breaking of the waters). The baby performs two actions before or during the first stage:

1. Engagement of the head into the pelvis.
2. Descent of the head through the pelvis, usually in left occipitoanterior (LOA) position.

The first stage is subdivided into two phases:

- Latent phase—the cervix dilates slowly from 0 to 4 cm.
- Active phase—the cervix dilates more rapidly from 4 to 10 cm.

Second stage

This is from full cervical dilatation until the birth of the baby. It usually lasts 40–60 minutes in primips and 10–15 minutes in multips. The baby must perform eight actions for normal birth to occur:

1. Flexion of the neck so its chin is on its chest and the occiput will be presented.
2. Internal rotation of the head so that it faces the sacrum.
3. Crowning of the occiput (when the baby is visible between contractions).
4. Extension of the neck as the head is born (support the head and check for the umbilical cord at the back of the neck).
5. Restitution as the head rotates back to the normal position outside of the mother.

6. External rotation of the head towards the mother's thigh as the shoulders rotate.
7. Birth of the anterior (top) shoulder (push the baby's head down).
8. Birth of the posterior (bottom) shoulder and body (pull the baby's head up and support the body).

Uterine contractions continue and are assisted by voluntary 'pushing' by the mother (contractions of the diaphragm and abdominal muscles). Once the head has crowned, the mother is asked to stop pushing so that the head can pass the vaginal opening smoothly to prevent tearing.

The pain is most severe during the second stage; it is caused by stretching of the cervix, vagina and perineum. The pain is conducted by normal somatic sensory nerves.

Third stage

This is from birth of the baby until the delivery of the placenta and membranes. Naturally, it lasts between 10 and 45 minutes though current practice is to actively manage this stage. This involves:

- Intramuscular injection of Syntometrine® (5 units oxytocin and 500 μg ergometrine) during the birth of the body.
- Pulling the umbilical cord once there are signs of placental separation (lengthening of the cord, contraction of the uterus or a gush of blood).

The uterus shrinks to the 20-week size and contractions continue. The entire placenta and decidua basalis detach from the uterus and are expelled, causing haemorrhage from the ruptured blood vessels. The haemorrhage is stopped by the muscle fibre arrangements within the uterus; this is more effective using active management. The contractions slowly subside once the afterbirth has been expelled. The placenta is inspected carefully to ensure that no sections remain in the uterus.

Initiation of parturition

The myometrium of the uterus becomes more excitable toward the end of gestation causing false labour that blends into the coordinated contractions seen in true labour. The exact mechanism that initiates this increase in excitability and onset of labour are not known, though several factors have been identified.

Oestrogen:progesterone ratio

Progesterone inhibits contractions and promotes uterine quiescence during pregnancy, but its secretion stabilizes or drops towards the end. Oestrogens promote excitation and stimulate contractions by stimulating increased gap junctions, prostaglandin synthesis, oxytocin receptors and local oxytocin production and secretion continues to increase until birth. The balance of these hormones moves in favour of oestrogen, causing increased excitability.

Uterine distension

Stretching the muscle of the uterus increases contractility, so fetal growth and movement may have a stimulatory effect.

Cervical distension

Irritation and stretching of the cervix causes oxytocin release, which stimulates contractions. The fetal head activates this release by pressing against the cervix.

Fetal hypothalamus maturation

At full term, the fetal hypothalamus and pituitary secrete more CRH, ACTH and oxytocin. This oxytocin may cross the placenta to act on the uterus.

Fetal adrenal activity

Cortisol secretion from the fetal adrenal glands increases as fetal ACTH rises. This stimulates placental oestrogen secretion and prostaglandin synthesis in the uterine muscle, which raises myometrial contractility.

Hormonal control of parturition

Oxytocin

Oxytocin is a peptide hormone synthesized in the hypothalamus and secreted by the posterior pituitary gland (it is described in Chapter 2).

During labour, oxytocin levels rise due to cervical stimulation by the head. It stimulates uterine contractions that push the fetus against the cervix, stimulating further oxytocin release. A positive feedback mechanism develops called the Ferguson reflex.

Oxytocin receptors in the uterine muscle are increased during late pregnancy by the action of oestrogen. Oxytocin binding stimulates prostaglandin production, which causes the increased contractility (especially PGE_2) and potentiates ion channels, which allow the reflux of Ca^{2+} and Na^+. Stimulation of receptors by oxytocin may also lead to an increase in intracellular Ca^{2+} from sarcoplasmic reticulum.

Prostaglandins

Prostaglandins are locally acting eicosanoids that regulate many processes throughout the body (see Chapter 1). During labour, the prostaglandin PGE_2

is synthesized in the uterine muscle cells in response to oxytocin. It increases gap junctions and stimulates the release of calcium ions, which cause muscle contractions in a similar fashion to oxytocin.

PGE_2 is also synthesized in the cervix, where it stimulates cervical softening and dilatation, known as ripening.

Relaxin

Relaxin promotes the relaxation of the pelvic ligaments and softens the cervix prior to parturition. This allows both structures to stretch so the fetus can pass through the pelvis.

Induction of labour

Labour can be induced using three methods that can be used in combination or alone:

- Prostaglandins (PGE_2) by vaginal pessary or gel, which acts within a few hours.
- Intravenous oxytocin, which takes about 12 hours to act.
- Rupture of the amniotic membrane (amniotomy), which can only be performed if the cervix is more than 4 cm dilated.

DISORDERS OF LABOUR

Prolonged labour

The progress of labour is plotted on a partogram that records measurements including the frequency and strength of contractions, dilatation of the cervix and descent of the presenting part. The pattern on the partogram can be used to distinguish between two types of prolonged labour (Fig. 16.6).

Primary dysfunctional labour

Primary dysfunctional labour describes slow dilatation of the cervix or descent of the presenting part. It is a common condition, especially in primips. It is usually due to inefficient uterine contractions and it can be treated using intravenous oxytocin to improve the strength of contractions. Alternatively, artificial rupture of the membranes (if they have not already ruptured) using an 'amnihook' can have a similar effect.

Secondary arrest of labour

Secondary arrest describes a labour that 'gets stuck' after progressing normally. The head fails to descend and the cervix remains at the same dilatation. This is less common than primary dysfunctional labour though it is often difficult to distinguish the two patterns. Secondary arrest should be suspected when prolonged labour occurs in a multip; it can also occur in primips. It is caused by:

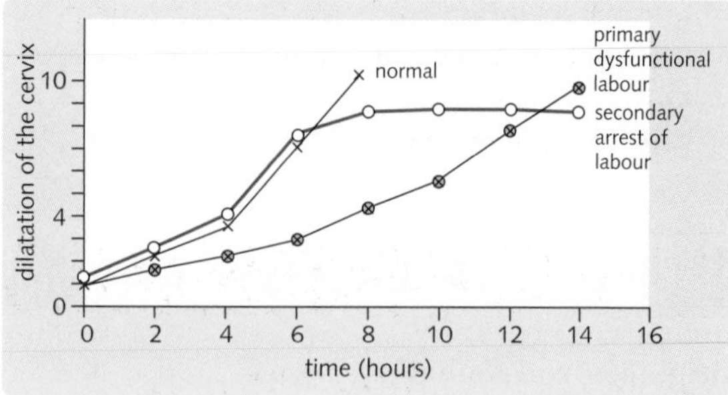

Fig. 16.6 Dilatation of the cervix in normal, primary dysfunctional and secondary arrested labour.

- Inefficient uterine contractions.
- Cephalopelvic disproportion (the head is too large for the pelvis).
- Malposition of the fetus (e.g. breech).

Since inefficient uterine contractions are the most common cause, intravenous oxytocin is used. If the labour still fails to progress, or if fetal distress is detected, then caesarean section is needed.

Assisted delivery

The second stage of labour is a critical period for the fetus and mother. If the second stage progresses slowly (beyond 1 h in multips or 1.5 h in primips) or fetal compromise is suspected, then an assisted delivery may be considered. There are four main types of assisted delivery:

- Kjelland's forceps—these are rotational forceps used to correct a malposition; they are rarely used in developed countries.
- Neville–Barnes forceps—the most common forceps used for mid pelvic-cavity deliveries.
- Wrigley's forceps—short forceps used for low pelvic-cavity deliveries and caesarean sections.
- Ventouse extraction—a suction device that fits onto the fetal vertex.

All assisted deliveries carry the risk of increased trauma to the fetus and mother. There are a number of criteria that must be met before an assisted delivery can be attempted:

- Fetal position known, with cephalic presentation.
- Presenting part descended to the ischial spines or below with $<1/5$ palpable abdominally.

- Cervix fully dilated and membranes ruptured.
- Maternal bladder empty (to limit trauma).
- Adequate analgesia.
- Consent of the mother.

LACTATION

Mammary development

During pregnancy the breast undergoes hormone-induced adaptations in preparation for lactation after birth. This section describes these changes together with the control and process of lactation. The development of the breast is described along with the other organs of reproduction in Chapter 11. The structure and disorders of the adult breast can be found in Chapters 12 and 13.

Changes during pregnancy

After puberty the female breast is composed of 15–20 lobes divided into secretory lobules, each with 10–100 acini. These acini are surrounded by fatty connective tissue; they drain into the lactiferous ducts. The breast remains in this state until pregnancy.

Development of the breasts during pregnancy is caused by the rising levels of four hormones:

- Oestrogens—cause the ductal system to grow and branch and fat to be stored in the stroma; inhibit milk production.
- Progesterone—causes growth and an increased number of acini.
- hPL—causes development of the acini cells so they are capable of milk secretion.
- Prolactin—causes development of the acini similar to hPL.

In the last few weeks of pregnancy, oestrogen fails to inhibit breast secretion completely so small quantities of a yellowish fluid called colostrum are secreted. Colostrum contains virtually no fat, is low in lactose and has high concentrations of protein and antibodies.

After birth the oestrogen, progesterone and hPL levels fall because the placenta is expelled. Prolactin secretion continues if the mother breastfeeds the baby; this maintains the breast changes brought about by the other hormones. The lack of oestrogen allows prolactin to stimulate production of milk instead of colostrum, though it takes a few days for the change to occur.

The breast changes caused by oestrogens and progesterone occur to a lesser degree towards the end of each menstrual cycle. The breasts often become swollen and tender.

Hormonal control

Lactation is caused by the effects of two hormones:

- Prolactin—causes milk secretion.
- Oxytocin—causes milk ejection.

Both hormones are secreted by the pituitary gland in response to nipple stimulation. Prolactin is secreted by the anterior pituitary gland with production increased by frequent suckling and oxytocin is secreted by the hypothalamus and released from the posterior pituitary. The synthesis and secretion of these hormones are described in Chapter 2.

Prolactin

Prolactin secretion increases throughout pregnancy causing the acinar cells of the breast to develop. During pregnancy, milk production is inhibited by high oestrogen levels. After childbirth, oestrogen levels fall dramatically and prolactin stimulates the secretion of milk.

During breastfeeding, stimulation of the nipple causes prolactin secretion, resulting in milk secretion and maintenance of the breast. The milk accumulates within the breast causing swelling unless oxytocin triggers the milk to be ejected. This neuroendocrine reflex is shown in Fig. 16.7. Once breastfeeding is stopped, nipple stimulation diminishes so prolactin secretion and milk production cease.

The high levels of prolactin during lactation inhibit LH and FSH secretion giving breastfeeding a contraceptive effect. This is only effective while the baby is suckling regularly. Once lactation ceases, the normal ovarian cycle and fertility return within 4–5 weeks.

Oxytocin

Milk is ejected from the breast by the action of hormonal, rather than neural, signals on the smooth muscle in the breast. Oxytocin induces the smooth muscle cells surrounding the acini to contract so milk is squeezed out of the nipple. Suckling stimulates this oxytocin release causing milk ejection within about 30 seconds. The reflex is shown in Fig. 16.7. Even the sound of the baby crying can stimulate the release of oxytocin and the ejection of milk. On the other hand, emotional stress can inhibit this reflex and this can be a particular problem if the woman is worried about her ability to breastfeed.

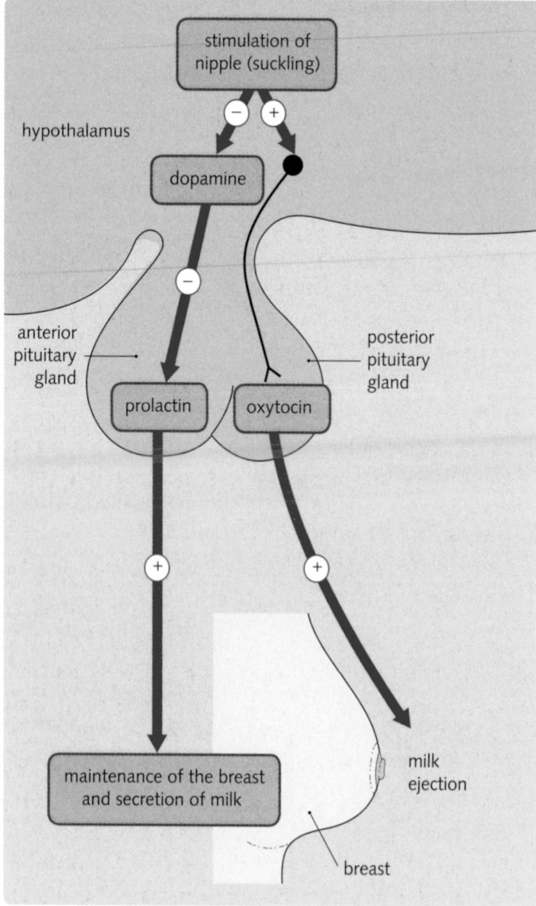

Fig. 16.7 Regulation of lactation by prolactin and oxytocin.

Colostrum and milk

Colostrum is a pale yellow fluid that lacks the fat content of milk. It is richer in antibodies so it protects the neonate against early infection; this is called passive immunity. Stable milk production occurs after 5 days.

Breast milk is a mixture of essential nutrients in water, the main constituents are:

- Lipids (fat).
- Casein (protein).
- Lactose (sugar).

It also contains vitamins, minerals and antibodies. Milk produced by other mammals has a different composition, making it unsuitable for human babies. For example, cow's milk contains less lactose but more casein than human milk. Special formula milks are available for women who choose not to breastfeed.

It is important to consider whether a woman is breastfeeding when prescribing medications. A number of chemicals can enter breast milk and affect the baby, including oestrogen (e.g. combined oral contraceptive pill) and alcohol. HIV-positive mothers are advised not to breastfeed, since there is a risk of the virus infecting the baby through the milk.

Lactation is a very energy-intensive process, even more so than pregnancy. The woman will require about 120% of her normal energy usage. This extra energy is derived from stored fat and the diet.

DISORDERS OF PREGNANCY AND THE PLACENTA

Ectopic pregnancies

It is important to consider the possibility of an ectopic pregnancy in any woman presenting with abdominal or pelvic pain. A pregnancy is described as 'ectopic' if the blastocyst implants in any location other than the endometrium of the uterus. Ninety-nine per cent of the time this means the uterine tubes, but it can also occur on the ovary or in the abdomen. The incidence is about 1 in 100 pregnancies in developed countries; the risk is increased by factors that slow the transport of the oocyte:

- Pelvic inflammatory disease.
- Previous pelvic surgery.
- Previous ectopic pregnancy.
- Pregnancy despite progesterone-only pill or IUD use.
- Pregnancy from assisted fertilization (e.g. IVF).

Once the blastocyst has implanted, the trophoblast attempts to form a placenta by invading the surrounding structures. Initially this allows the embryo to grow, but the pregnancy usually terminates after 6–10 weeks due to a lack of space and nutrients.

There is a high risk of complications following ectopic pregnancy, the most serious of which is tubal rupture. The trophoblast erodes through the wall of the uterine tube, causing intraperitoneal bleeding. In a minority of cases this can be severe and life threatening.

Symptoms and signs

Subacute

The majority of patients with ectopic pregnancy present following intra-abdominal haemorrage or mild rupture. The most common symptoms are:

- Unilateral abdominal pain and tenderness.
- Recent amenorrhoea.
- Vaginal bleeding.

On vaginal examination there may be a tender mass in a uterine tube. The abdominal pain may be so mild that it is ignored until vaginal bleeding occurs.

Acute

In severe tubal rupture the patient presents with severe abdominal pain and sudden collapse. She will have hypovolaemic shock and an acute abdomen (tender with guarding).

Investigations

Diagnosis of subacute ectopic pregnancy from the history and examination alone is very difficult due to the non-specific symptoms. Blood tests for hCG will be positive indicating a pregnancy (if measured over a couple of days it may rise slower than expected). An ultrasound scan will show an empty uterus and may reveal the mass in the uterine tube. If the embryo is not found then a laparoscopy is performed to examine the tubes directly.

Acute tubal rupture is a surgical emergency. It is investigated and treated by laparotomy to remove the entire affected uterine tube as soon as possible.

Treatment

If ectopic pregnancies are diagnosed before abortion or rupture occurs, they are treated surgically using laparoscopy ('keyhole' techniques) or laparotomy (opening the abdomen); there are three treatment options:

- Removal of the entire uterine tube that contains the embryo.
- Removal of just the embryo through an incision in the tube.
- Injection of methotrexate (cytotoxic drug) into the embryo to induce early abortion.

Since there is a high risk of recurrence or infertility following ectopic pregnancy, any further pregnancies need careful monitoring.

Miscarriage

Miscarriage (spontaneous abortion) is the expulsion of a fetus from the uterus before it is capable of independent survival; clinically, this is before 24 weeks or below 500 g. After 24 weeks, it is termed a premature delivery. Miscarriage is very common, affecting about 10% of pregnancies, usually between the 6th and 10th weeks, though more may occur before the mother realizes she is pregnant. It is caused by:

- Fetal abnormalities, often due to chromosomal disorders (60%).
- Abnormal implantation or placenta.
- Uterine abnormality.
- Maternal illness.
- Idiopathic (unknown).

Symptoms and investigations

Miscarriage is suspected if a pregnant woman experiences vaginal bleeding. Ultrasound is used to visualize the fetus and this normally shows the fetus is alive and well.

If the bleeding is associated with cervical dilatation and uterine contractions (which may be described as pelvic pain) then miscarriage becomes inevitable. The woman must be admitted to hospital to ensure that the entire fetus and placenta are expelled. This is performed by inspecting the expelled material and performing a further ultrasound scan of the uterus. Any retained material must be extracted surgically through the cervix.

Placenta praevia

If the placenta is located over the lower uterine segment (sometimes including the cervix) the condition is called placenta praevia; the incidence is about 1 in 200 pregnancies. It is important not to perform a vaginal examination if placenta praevia is suspected. The severity of placenta praevia is graded 1–4 according the distance from the cervix (1 being the furthest). The placenta is prone to bleeding as the uterus grows or when the cervix dilates in labour. The bleeding is usually painless and the uterus remains soft and non-tender; it may also present with the fetus in an abnormal position due to the location of the placenta. The risk of placenta praevia is increased by multiple pregnancies and previous caesarean sections. It is diagnosed and monitored by ultrasound. Delivery is performed by caesarean section at 37 weeks (or earlier if bleeding is severe), except grade 1, which may allow normal vaginal delivery.

Placental abruption

Placental abruption occurs when the placenta separates from the uterine wall before the fetus has been delivered, resulting in bleeding. Vaginal bleeding is usually overt, but blood is concealed within the uterus in about 20% of cases. The bleeding ranges from mild to life threatening. It is a common disorder (about 1 in 80 pregnancies) with several predisposing factors; hypertension, smoking, multiple pregnancies and polyhydramnios (excess amniotic fluid). Abruption can present with:

- Vaginal bleeding.
- Abdominal pain and tenderness.
- Rigid uterus.
- Evidence of fetal compromise.

Ultrasound is used to identify concealed collections of blood and to distinguish abruption from placenta praevia. The extent of bleeding is determined according to clinical signs of shock and blood tests, which reveal haemoglobin and platelet concentration. Fetal compromise is detected and monitored using a fetal heart monitor. The mother should be resuscitated and stabilized; induced delivery or emergency caesarean section may be indicated.

Pre-eclampsia and eclampsia

Eclampsia is the presence of seizure activity in pregnant woman with pre-eclampsia and usually presents in third trimester. The precedent condition of pre-eclampsia is characterized by the hypertension and proteinuria during pregnancy.

Pre-eclampsia

Pre-eclampsia affects about 5% of women during pregnancy to varying degrees. Treatment is needed if the blood pressure rises above 140/100 or if urine protein is consistently greater than 300 mg/L. Pre-eclampsia is largely asymptomatic though generalized oedema can occur at any stage. If the following symptoms and signs develop, an eclamptic convulsion is likely:

- Severe headache.
- Irritability.
- Blurred vision.
- Epigastric pain.
- Vomiting.
- Brisk reflexes.

Eclampsia

Careful blood pressure and urine monitoring aims to prevent pre-eclampsia progressing to eclampsia; in developed countries eclampsia is very rare. The woman experiences a brief period of disorientation followed by a tonic–clonic seizure. The initial seizure can be followed by further seizures, coma or haemorrhagic stroke. There is a risk of death for both the mother and fetus, but this is usually prevented by early detection and treatment of pre-eclampsia.

Aetiology

The exact underlying cause is unclear. It is believed that poor placental invasion results in uteroplacental ischaemia, which in turn results in endothelial damage and a hypertensive inflammatory response. In normal placentation, the trophoblast invades the maternal spiral arteries and stimulates their distension. When this fails the arteries remain high-resistance with a resultant paucity of placental perfusion. The precipitating event may be low levels of placental growth factor (PlGF). Women with low levels of PlGF in their urine are likely to develop pre-eclampsia. These women also have high levels of soluble fms-like tyrosine kinase 1 (sFlt-1) in blood, which binds PlGF with the result that the low levels of PlGF are unable to foster growth of new blood vessels in the placenta. Both the placenta and fetus become ischaemic, leading to poor development, and an association of fetal growth retardation with pre-eclampsia. Cells from the ischaemic placenta can be carried (embolize) into the maternal circulation where they trigger the release of thromboplastins. The thromboplastins cause vasoconstriction and poor renal perfusion resulting in:

- Hypertension.
- Proteinuria.
- Oedema.

These signs characterize pre-eclampsia. If the condition continues, cerebral hypoxia and oedema can result, causing the tonic–clonic convulsions of eclampsia. Symptoms of eclampsia also include: right upper quadrant pain, visual disturbances, hyperactive reflexes, headache, proteinuria and oedema. There is also a high risk of blood clots forming in the blood vessels (disseminated intravascular coagulation; DIC) that can produce tissue infarctions. The aetiology of pre-eclampsia is shown in Fig. 16.8.

Death can occur from:

- Cerebral haemorrhage (stroke) or oedema.
- Cardiac failure.
- Cardiorespiratory arrest.
- Organ failure following DIC.

Treatment

Even mild pre-eclampsia requires frequent blood pressure checks. If the blood pressure exceeds 140/100 or there is significant proteinuria then admission and treatment are required. Investigations include full blood count, platelet count, liver enzymes, glucose, U&Es and 24-hour urine. The best management plan for pre-eclampsia and eclampsia is delivery of the baby, often by caesarean section, although eclamptic fits can still occur up to 48 hours later. Several medications may slow the rise in blood pressure so that the baby has more time to mature. Diuretics cannot be used as they lower the blood volume making the placental ischaemia worse. Magnesium sulphate is used

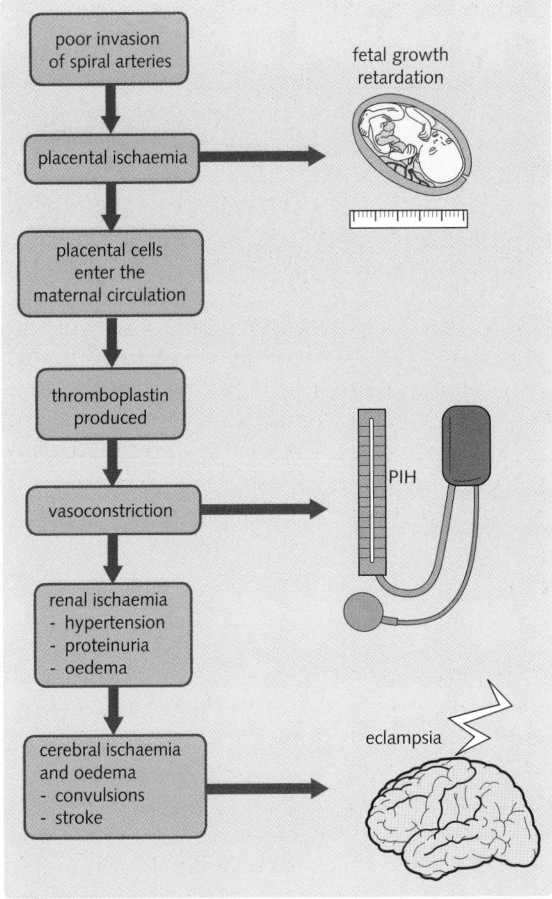

Fig. 16.8 The aetiology of pregnancy-induced hypertension (PIH; pre-eclampsia).

in severe pre-eclampsia or eclampsia. It causes the arteries to relax, restoring blood flow to the brain and inhibits coagulation. Treatment must be monitored as it can depress breathing.

Transmission of the HIV virus from mother to child is referred to as vertical transmission. Untreated, the risk of transmission is around 25% and is dependent on maternal viral load. Antiviral therapy should be given during the pregnancy; intravenous antivirals should be given during labour, and the newborn should be treated with antivirals for 6 weeks. Breastfeeding carries a significant risk of transmission. Unfortunately, where appropriate replacement feeds are not available the risks of malnutrition often outweigh the risk of HIV. Where safe surgical practices are available, elective caesarean is advocated.

Neoplasia of trophoblastic origin

During implantation, the trophoblast normally invades the endometrium. If this process is disrupted there is a high chance of the trophoblast forming an invasive tumour.

Hydatidiform mole

Hydatidiform moles are benign tumours of the chorion that forms the placenta. Chorionic villi enlarge to form grape-like vesicles that secrete hCG and progesterone. They are usually caused by major abnormalities of fertilization. There are two types: partial and complete (Fig. 16.9).

Hydatidiform moles occur in about 1 in 2000 of UK pregnancies. The secretion of hCG and progesterone causes exaggerated symptoms of pregnancy:

- Severe morning sickness.
- Early pre-eclampsia.
- Abnormally large and doughy uterus.
- Vaginal bleeding.

Fig. 16.9 Comparison of partial and complete hydatidiform mole

Feature	Partial mole	Complete mole
Extent of placental involvement	Only a section	Entire placenta
Fetal tissue	Present but fetus is normally non-viable	Not present
Usual cause	Two sperms fertilizing the oocyte (polyspermy)	Two sperms entering an oocyte that has lost its nucleus
Risk of developing malignancy	Low	High

Moles produce the following results on investigation:

- Absence of fetal heart sounds.
- 'Snowstorm-like' appearance on ultrasound scans.
- Extremely high hCG levels.

They are treated by suction evacuation of the uterus followed by hCG level monitoring to detect the recurrence that occurs in 10%, often in a malignant form called choriocarcinoma.

Invasive mole

This represents the middle ground between a hydatidiform mole and choriocarcinoma. The tumour invades the myometrium, but it does not spread outside of the uterus. There is a higher risk of recurrence and further invasion.

Choriocarcinoma

This is a highly malignant tumour of the trophoblast without recognizable chorionic villi. It is usually preceded by the recurrence of a hydatidiform mole. It can also occur following pregnancies (1 in 50,000) or miscarriages (1 in 5000). The cancer contains many areas of haemorrhage and necrosis; while villi are not formed, it does secrete high levels of hCG.

It presents in the same manner as a hydatidiform mole or with symptoms and signs of metastasis. Histological examination is used to determine the degree of malignancy.

The prognosis is excellent despite the early blood-borne metastasis to the brain, liver and lungs. It responds to chemotherapy very well and hCG levels can be monitored to guide treatment. Fertility is often not affected.

CLINICAL ASSESSMENT

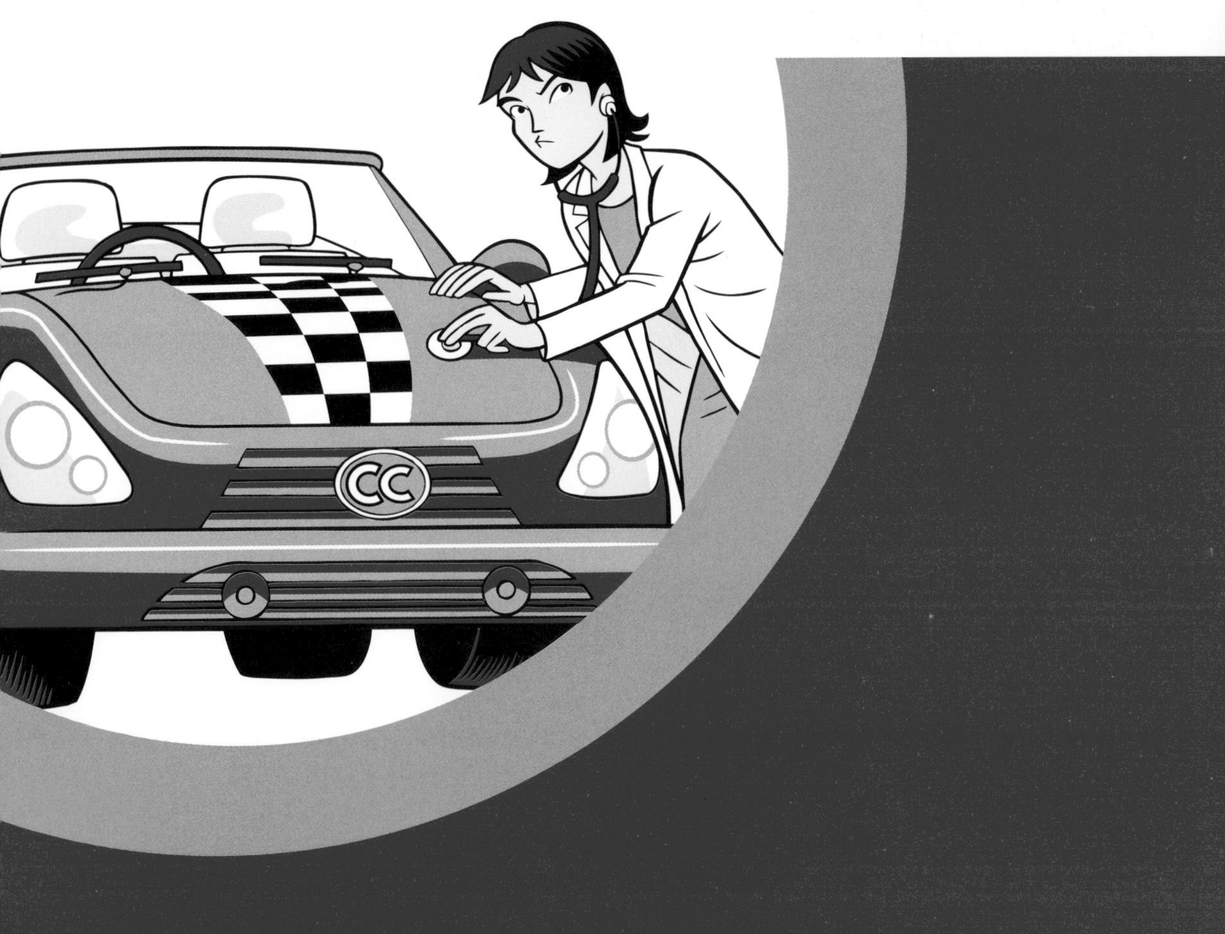

17 Common presentations of endocrine and reproductive disease

Medicine can be learnt empirically on a disease-by-disease basis. However, patients do not usually present with a disease but with a collection of symptoms and signs. Upon encountering patients with symptoms suggestive of endocrine disease, you must be able to construct a differential diagnosis. Only at this stage can appropriate investigations be conducted and a definitive diagnosis given. The next three chapters highlight the presentations, examination findings and investigations pertinent to making the diagnosis of endocrine and reproductive pathologies. Where possible, try to think why a disease should cause a particular symptom or sign and why particular investigations might reveal something about the underlying pathology.

Since the disorders of these two systems have a substantial overlap, the disorders are presented together in alphabetical order. The important questions in the history are outlined along with a guide to differential diagnosis. The following disorders are included:

- Amenorrhoea.
- Breast lumps.
- Galactorrhoea.
- Gynaecomastia (male).
- Hirsutism (female).
- Loss of consciousness and coma.
- Menorrhagia and intermenstrual bleeding (female).
- Polyuria.
- Scrotal lumps.
- Sexual dysfunction (male and female).
- Thyroid lumps and goitre.
- Weight gain and obesity.
- Weight loss.

Amenorrhoea (Fig. 17.1)

This is failure of menstruation to occur at the expected time; there are two types:

- Primary—failure to start menstruating by 16 years of age.
- Secondary—no menstruation for 6 months after starting menstruation during puberty.

Important questions in history taking are shown in Fig. 17.1. Primary amenorrhoea is usually just late puberty, while secondary amenorrhoea is most commonly caused by low body weight. A number of endocrine disorders can also be responsible, including hyperprolactinaemia.

Breast lumps (Fig. 17.2)

Breast lumps are a common presentation, especially since breast self-examination is encouraged. While breast cancer is very common and can occur at any age, the majority of breast lumps are benign. Despite this every lump needs careful examination and further investigation.

Galactorrhoea (Fig. 17.3)

This is the inappropriate production of milk from the breasts (i.e. without a recent birth). It usually affects women, but rarely can affect men.

Hyperprolactinaemia is the most common cause, but the reason for this excess is often not found.

Gynaecomastia (Fig. 17.4)

This is growth of the breasts in men caused by an abnormal balance between testosterone and oestrogen. It is not the same as simple fat deposition caused by obesity or old age. It is a normal finding during puberty, but otherwise medications or drugs are the most common cause.

Hirsutism (Fig. 17.5)

This is when a woman develops a male pattern of facial and body hair. It should not be confused with excessive hair growth (hypertrichosis) or development of male secondary sexual characteristics (virilism). Polycystic ovary disease is the most common cause, but in many cases a cause is never found (idiopathic hirsutism).

Fig. 17.1 Important questions and causes of amenorrhoea

Find out	Findings	Differential diagnosis
Age	>50 years	Menopause, can also be premature
Weight	Low	Low weight is a very common cause
Growth and sexual development	No secondary sexual characteristics, short stature	Turner syndrome
	Minimal pubic hair	Testicular feminization
Sexual history and contraception	Recent intercourse, no contraception	Pregnancy
	Recently started a progestogen-only form of contraception	May cause amenorrhoea
	Recently came off the Pill	Pituitary insensitivity
Systems review	Galactorrhoea, previous sparse periods, weight gain	Hyperprolactinaemia
	Weight gain, hirsutism, acne	Polycystic ovarian syndrome
	Weight loss, irritability, sweating	Hyperthyroidism
Social and medical history	Recent stress or illness	Pituitary insensitivity

Fig. 17.2 Important questions and causes of breast lumps

Find out	Findings	Differential diagnosis
Age	Young	Fibroadenoma
	Pre-menopause	Fibrocystic change, duct ectasia or duct papilloma
	Elderly	Fibrocystic change, fat necrosis, breast cancer or phyllodes tumour
Obstetric history	No pregnancies	Slightly higher risk of breast cancer
	Recent pregnancy	Breast abscess
Systems review	Bone pain or jaundice	Metastasis from breast cancer
	Creamy nipple discharge and nipple retraction	Duct ectasia
	Bloody nipple discharge and nipple retraction	Breast cancer
	Eczema round the nipple	Paget's disease (breast cancer)
Family history	Strong family history of breast or ovarian cancer	Breast cancer (*BRAC* genes)

Fig. 17.3 Important questions and causes of galactorrhoea		
Find out	**Findings**	**Differential diagnosis**
Sexual history and contraception	Recent intercourse, no contraception	Pregnancy
Obstetric history	Recent miscarriage or termination	The hyperprolactinaemia of pregnancy takes time to return to normal
Systems review	Female: amenorrhoea, weight gain	Hyperprolactinaemia
	Male: impotence, less facial hair, visual disturbance, gynaecomastia	Hyperprolactinaemia
	Visual disturbance, headache	Pituitary tumour loss of dopamine inhibition
	Weight gain and lethargy	Hypothyroidism is a rare cause
Medical history	Chronic renal failure	Can cause hyperprolactinaemia
Drug history	Methyldopa, oestrogens, tricyclic antidepressants, haloperidol	Drug-induced hyperprolactinaemia

Fig. 17.4 Important questions and causes of gynaecomastia		
Find out	**Findings**	**Differential diagnosis**
Age	10–16 years	Puberty
Medical history	Testicular torsion, infection or maldescent	Testosterone deficiency
	Chronic renal failure	Excess oestrogen
Systems review	Small genitalia, tall stature, female fat distribution	Klinefelter syndrome
	Impotence, less facial hair, visual disturbance	Hyperprolactinaemia
Drug history	Spironolactone, tricyclic antidepressants, oestrogens, griseofulvin	Induce gynaecomastia
Family history	Very strong history of breast or ovarian cancer	Male breast cancer (*BRAC* genes)
Social history	Frequent use of amphetamines or cannabis	Induce gynaecomastia
	Chronic alcoholism	Liver disease, excess oestrogen

Fig. 17.5 Important questions and causes of hirsutism

Find out	Findings	Differential diagnosis
Age of onset	Childhood	Congenital adrenal hyperplasia
	>50	Menopause
Systems review	Associated virilism	Androgen-producing tumours or congenital adrenal hyperplasia
	Amenorrhoea, weight gain, acne	Polycystic ovarian syndrome
	Weight gain, skin bruising, muscle weakness	Cushing's syndrome
Family history	Other relatives affected	Familial hirsutism
Drug history	Use of high-dose steroids	Induces hirsutism in the same manner as Cushing's syndrome
	Danazol for endometriosis	Androgenic effects
Social history	Use of androgens to enhance sporting ability	Excess androgens

Fig. 17.6 Important questions and endocrine/reproductive causes of loss of conciousness and coma

Find out	Findings	Differential diagnosis
Age	Young	IDDM (diabetic ketoacidosis)
Obstetric history	Over 20 weeks pregnant	Eclampsia
Sexual history	Recent intercourse, no contraception	Ruptured ectopic pregnancy
	Current use of combined contraceptive pill	Thromboembolism
Systems review	Weight loss, sweating, palpitations, cardiac arrhythmia	Thyrotoxicosis (hyperthyroidism)
	Weight gain, hypothermia, lethargy, recent illness	Myxoedema coma (hypothyroidism)
	Weight loss, polyuria, thirst for several months	NIDDM (HONK)
	Recent weight loss, polyuria, thirst and sweet-smelling breath	IDDM (diabetic ketoacidosis)
	Pigmentation, weight loss, anorexia, nausea and vomiting	Addison's disease
	Headache, visual disturbances, gynaecomastia	Raised intracranial pressure following pituitary adenoma

HONK, hyperosmolar non-ketotic state; IDDM, insulin-dependent diabetes mellitus; NIDDM, non-IDDM.

Loss of consciousness and coma (Fig. 17.6)

Loss of consciousness can be caused by many disorders and endocrine and reproductive disturbance are not the most common. Other causes are excluded from this table.

Menorrhagia and intermenstrual bleeding (Fig. 17.7)

Menorrhagia is excessive bleeding during menstruation (>80 mL per period). Intermenstrual bleeding is blood discharged from the vagina between periods. The most common cause of both conditions is dysfunctional uterine bleeding, especially at the extremes of reproductive age.

Polyuria (Fig. 17.8)

A number of endocrine disorders can upset the kidneys to cause polyuria. This is the excretion of an excess volume of dilute urine causing dehydration and thirst (polydipsia). It is not the same as frequency, in which only small amounts of urine are passed frequently so the total volume is not great.

Scrotal lumps (Fig. 17.9)

Lumps in the scrotum are common presenting complaints and self-examination is being encouraged. Scrotal lumps can arise from the testis, other structures in the scrotum or from the abdominal cavity. There is a wide variety of underlying causes including tumours, infections and trauma. Testicular cancer is the most common malignancy in young adult males.

Sexual dysfunction

Female (Fig. 17.10)

In women the presenting complaints are:

- Lack of sexual desire (decreased libido).
- Failure to reach orgasm (anorgasmia).
- Pain on intercourse (dyspareunia).

Decreased libido and anorgasmia often stem from psychological causes or difficulties within the relationship. Dyspareunia tends to have more physical causes.

Male (Fig. 17.11)

In men the presenting complaints are decreased libido and impotence. Medications and alcohol are the most common causes.

Thyroid lumps and goitre (Fig. 17.12)

A goitre is an enlarged thyroid gland. The enlargement may be caused by the entire gland or by a nodule; any lumps must be investigated to exclude malignancy. Thyroid lumps are often associated with disorders of the thyroid hormones and they are especially common in women.

Weight gain and obesity (Fig. 17.13)

Obesity is defined as a body mass index (BMI) (see box) greater than 30, while 25–30 is classified as overweight. The cause of obesity is unknown in the vast majority of patients, though current research into the regulation of eating may change this. Currently, obesity alone does not warrant investigation, whereas unexplained weight gain does. The causes of weight gain can lead to obesity so the two are considered together.

Weight loss (Fig. 17.14)

Weight loss is often a sign of fairly severe disease, so it must be taken seriously. It can be caused by the failure of the heart, kidneys, or liver, but also by several endocrine disorders.

BMI is calculated from the weight in 'kg' and height in 'm'. The weight is divided by the height squared. For example, a man weighing 85 kg with a height of 1.65 m has a BMI of $85/(1.65 \times 1.65) = 31.2$.

Fig. 17.7 Important questions and causes of menorrhagia and intermenstrual bleeding

Find out	Findings	Differential diagnosis
Age	Young	Dysfunctional uterine bleeding
	Pre-menopause	Dysfunctional uterine bleeding, fibroids, uterine polyps, ovarian cysts, endometriosis
	Post-menopause	Endometrial or cervical carcinoma
Sexual history	Recently started using the Pill	Breakthrough bleeding is common for a few months
	Use of copper IUD	Causes menorrhagia
	Risk of pregnancy	Ectopic pregnancy, miscarriage
	Pregnant	Miscarriage, placenta previa, placental abruption
Systems review	Pelvic pain, dyspareunia	Fibroids, polyps, endometriosis and adenomyosis
	Fever, malaise, pelvic pain	Pelvic inflammatory disease
	Hirsutism, weight gain, acne	Polycystic ovarian syndrome
	Weight loss, irritability, sweating	Hyperthyroidism
	Weight gain and lethargy	Hypothyroidism
Drug history	Oestrogen (e.g. HRT)	Endometrial hyperplasia

HRT, hormone replacement therapy; IUD, intra-uterine device.

Fig. 17.8 Important questions and causes of polyuria

Find out	Findings	Differential diagnosis
Age	Young	IDDM
	Middle-aged or elderly	NIDDM
Medical history	Renal disease	Nephrogenic diabetes insipidus
	Trauma or surgery to the head	Cranial diabetes insipidus
Fluid intake	Excess intravenous fluids	Iatrogenic diabetes
Systems review	Tiredness, thirst, weight loss	Diabetes mellitus
	Bone pain, muscle weakness, headaches, confusion	Hypercalcaemia
Drug history	Any diuretic	Iatrogenic diabetes
	Opiates	Cranial diabetes insipidus
	Lithium, demeclocycline	Nephrogenic diabetes insipidus
	Anticholinergics	Cause a dry mouth and excessive fluid intake
Family history	Diabetes mellitus	Especially NIDDM
	Diabetes insipidus	X-linked inheritance (rarely)
Social history	Psychological problems, abuse	Psychogenic polydipsia

IDDM, insulin-dependent diabetes mellitus; NIDDM, non-IDDM.

Fig. 17.9 Important questions and causes of scrotal lumps

Find out	Findings	Differential diagnosis
Age of onset	Congenital	Indirect hernia, hydrocoele, varicocoele
	Puberty	Testicular torsion, epididymo-orchitis
	Young	Teratomas are common
	Middle-aged	Epididymal cyst or may be a seminoma
	>50 years	Hydrocoele, chronic epididymitis or lymphoma
Medical history	Recent trauma	Haematoma, haematocoele
	Recent vasectomy	Sperm granuloma, haematocoele
	Tuberculosis or syphilis	Infectious granuloma
Systems review	Infertility	Varicocoele
	Fever, malaise, scrotal pain, UTI	Epididymo-orchitis
	Weight loss, scrotum feels heavy	Testicular tumour
Social history	Intensive exercise	Testicular torsion
	Recent lifting, e.g. moved house	Indirect hernia

UTI, urinary tract infection.

Fig. 17.10 Important questions and causes of sexual dysfunction in females

Find out	Findings	Differential diagnosis
Age	Post-menopause	Oestrogen deficiency causing a lack of lubrication
Sexual history	Muscles of the vagina tense on attempted intercourse	Vaginismus causing dyspareunia
	Never achieved orgasm	Anorgasmia
Medical history	Previous surgery or trauma	Dyspareunia
Systems review	Fever, malaise, dyspareunia	Infections of the urethra, vulva, vagina or pelvic inflammatory disease
	Menorrhagia, pelvic pain, deep dyspareunia	Ovarian cysts and tumours, endometriosis, fibroids
	Amenorrhoea, galactorrhoea and decreased libido	Hyperprolactinaemia
Social history	Lack of communication with partner	Decreased libido and anorgasmia
	Lack of sexual awarenes	Anorgasmia

Fig. 17.11 Important questions and causes of sexual dysfunction in males

Find out	Findings	Differential diagnosis
Medical history	Diabetes mellitus	Impotence is a chronic complication of diabetes mellitus
	Multiple sclerosis	Inhibits sexual arousal
Systems review	Gynaecomastia, visual disturbance	Hyperprolactinaemia
	Small testes, deficient male pattern hair	Hypogonadism
Drug history	Antihypertensives and diuretics	Iatrogenic impotence
	Antidepressants, antipsychotics, oestrogens	Decreased libido
Social history	Lack of communication with partner	Psychological impotence and decreased libido
Social history	Excessive alcohol intake	Causes acute and chronic impotence

Fig. 17.12 Important questions and causes of thyroid lumps and goitre

Find out	Findings	Differential diagnosis
Age	10–16	Temporary physiological goitre
	Young	Papillary carcinoma
	Middle-aged	Autoimmune causes, medullary or follicular carcinoma
	Elderly	Multinodular goitre, medullary, anaplastic carcinoma or lymphoma
Obstetric history	Pregnancy	Temporary physiological goitre
Systems review	Weight loss, sweating, palpitations, irritability, heat intolerance	Graves' disease, multinodular goitre, toxic adenoma
	Weight gain, cold intolerance, tiredness, lethargy, dry skin and hair	Hashimoto's thyroiditis, de Quervain's thyroiditis
	Fever, malaise and painful neck	Infectious goitre (e.g. de Quervain's thyroiditis)
	Bone pain	Metastases from thyroid cancer
Family history	Thyroid disease	Autoimmune thyroid disease
	Medullary carcinoma	MEN IIa and IIb syndromes
Social history	Unusual diet or immigration from inland developing country	Iodine deficiency

MEN, multiple endocrine neoplasia.

Fig. 17.13 Important questions and causes of weight gain and obesity

Find out	Findings	Differential diagnosis
Systems review	Abnormal fat distribution, easy bruising, muscle weakness, hirsutism	Cushing's syndrome
	Lethargy, depression, cold intolerance	Hypothyroidism
	Amenorrhoea, acne, hirsutism	Polycystic ovarian syndrome
Drug history	Steroids, antidepressants	Stimulate eating
Family history	Other obese members	Genetic or environmental causes
Social history	Stress or history of binge eating	Psychological cause
	Recently gave up smoking	Often slight weight gain

Fig. 17.14 Important questions and causes of weight loss

Find out	Findings	Differential diagnosis
Age	Elderly	Malignancy or organ failure are most likely
Systems review	Increased appetite, sweating, palpitations, heat intolerance	Hyperthyroidism
	Reduced appetite, malaise, vomiting	Addison's disease, malignancy or organ failure
	Polyuria, thirst, tiredness	Diabetes mellitus
	Light-coloured chronic diarrhoea, large appetite	Malabsorption
Social history	Perception of weight	Eating disorders (e.g. anorexia nervosa)
	Unprotected sexual intercourse or intravenous drug use	HIV infection

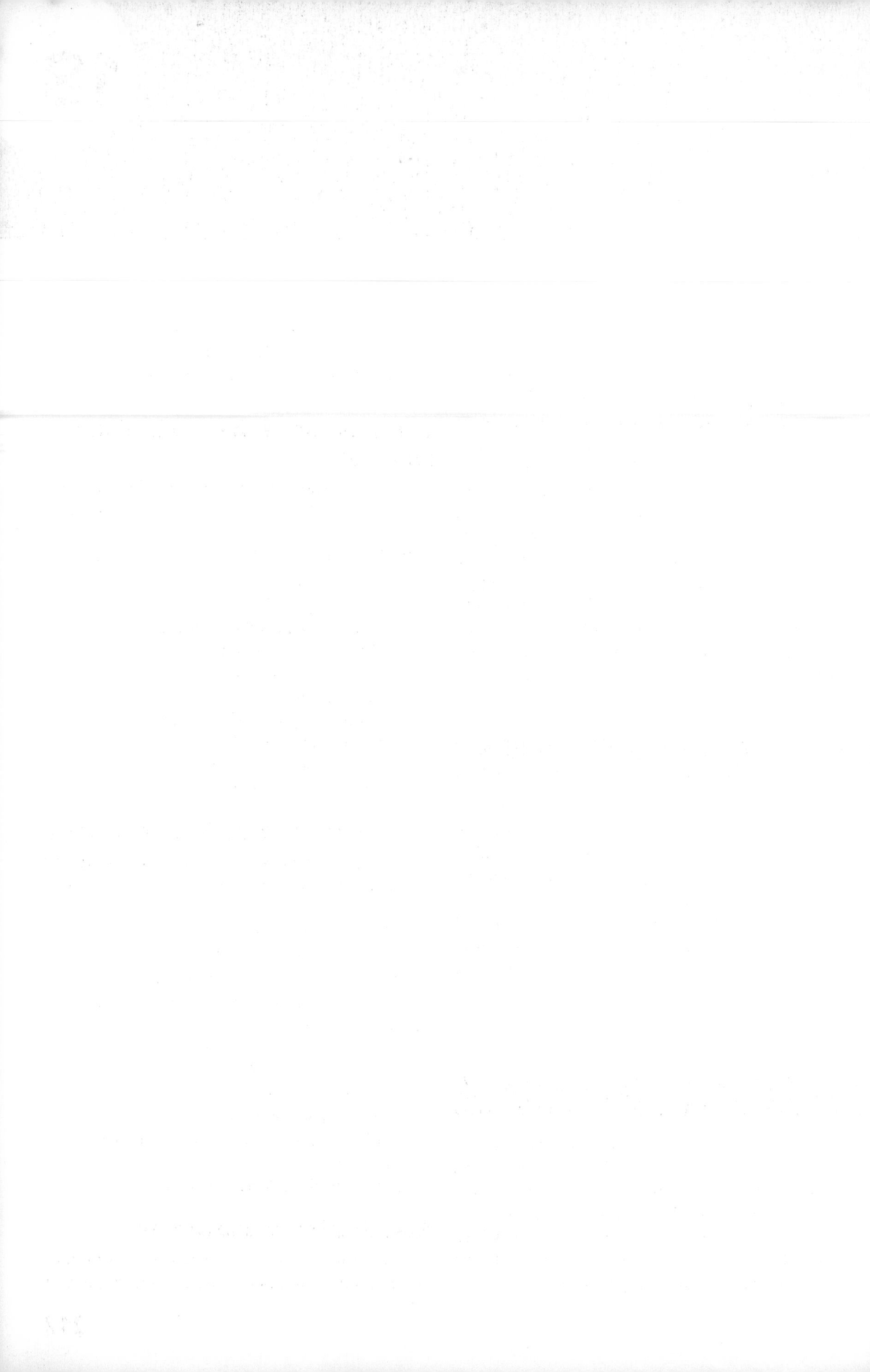

Clinical examination of the endocrine and reproductive systems

18

Endocrine dysfunction can manifest in all organs, as demonstrated by the varied symptomatic presentations discussed in the preceding chapter. The same is true of the signs of endocrine disorders and extensive endocrine examination therefore necessitates a general examination of all systems. Some endocrine disorders require more specific examinations. These include examination for evidence of thyroid dysfunction, examination of the female reproductive system and the female breast, examination of the pregnant abdomen, and examination of the male reproductive system. This chapter will first highlight the findings, pertinent to endocrine disease, which are revealed by systematic examination. This will be followed by description of the specific examinations of the reproductive systems that are common exam questions.

HISTORY

History-taking for endocrine disease should follow the same general pattern as all other histories; presenting complaint, history of presenting complaint, past medical history, drug history, social history, family history, systems review and summary. The full history information for the myriad of different endocrine pathologies is given throughout the individual chapters in this book. A separate crash course is available for a more detailed look at history-taking and examination.

GENERAL INSPECTION

When meeting a patient and taking a history, it is important to be aware of signs that give information about the patient's condition. These can include their surroundings (e.g. walking sticks), speech and mental state. Some physical signs can also be seen whilst taking the history, with particular relevance to the endocrine and reproductive systems are:

- Facial features and external eye signs (Fig. 18.1).
- Skin complexion (Fig. 18.2).
- Body physique and posture (Fig. 18.3).

Examination of the hands, limbs and feet

The features of endocrine disease to look for in the nails, hands, limbs and feet are outlined in Figs 18.4–18.7.

Examination sequence

1. Inspect the nails.
2. Test capillary refill.
3. Inspect the hand and skin creases.
4. Feel and count the pulse.
5. Take the blood pressure.
6. Inspect the limbs and feet.
7. Test tone and power of the limbs.
8. Test reflexes of the limbs.
9. Test sensation of the limbs.
10. Test coordination of the limbs.

Examination of the head and neck

Signs found in the head, eyes and neck that suggest endocrine disorders are shown in Figs 18.8–18.11.

Examination sequence

1. Inspect the face, eyes and neck.
2. Test the visual acuity and visual fields.
3. Test the eye movements and look for lid lag.
4. Inspect the fundi.
5. Test the sensation and power of the face.
6. Listen to their speech.
7. Feel for lymph nodes.
8. Examine any lumps present.
9. Look for the height of the jugular venous pressure (JVP).
10. Feel for tracheal deviation or tug.

Examination of the thorax

Examine the thorax as you would in a combined examination of the cardiovascular and respiratory

Fig. 18.1 Common findings on inspection of the face

Findings	Diagnostic inference
Harsh facial features, large nose, protruding jaw and large hands	Acromegaly
Infant with a broad flat face, widely spaced eyes and a protruding tongue	Cretinism (resulting from hypothyroidism)
Eyes that appear to be bulging out of their sockets, i.e. exophthalmos	Graves' disease (not in other forms of hyperthyroidism)

Fig. 18.2 Common findings on inspection of the skin

Findings	Diagnostic inference
Generalized pigmentation of the skin	Addison's disease, Cushing's disease (not in Cushing's syndrome)
Flushed, red skin with excessive sweating	Thyrotoxicosis, phaeochromocytoma
Boils/skin infections	Undiagnosed or poorly controlled diabetes mellitus

systems. Signs found in the thorax suggestive of endocrine disorders are shown in Fig. 18.12

Examination of the abdomen

Examine the abdomen as you would in a GI exam. Signs found in the abdomen which suggest endocrine and reproductive disorders are shown in Figs. 18.13 and 18.14.

EXAMINATION OF A LUMP OR MASS

If a lump is detected during the examination, it must be assessed for the features shown in Fig. 18.15. This is a very common presentation and it applies to lumps found in all locations.

SPECIFIC EXAMINATION OF THE ENDOCRINE AND REPRODUCTIVE SYSTEMS

Examination of the thyroid gland and the clinical manifestations of thyroid disorder

Signs of thyroid disease are elucidated by examining the energetic state of the patient. Then the hands are assessed for temperature, sweatiness, thyroid nail

Fig. 18.3 Common findings on inspection of the body

Findings		Diagnostic inference
Short stature	Failure to grow	Dwarfism
	Infant with flat face	Hypothyroidism (cretinism)
	Bone deformities	Rickets (vitamin D deficiency)
	Female with masculine body shape and webbing of the neck	Turner syndrome (45 chromosomes, X0)
Tall stature	Male with female fat distribution (breasts and hips)	Kleinfelter syndrome (47 chromosomes, XXY)
	Child with excess growth	Gigantism
Overweight	Abnormal fat distribution, wasted arms and legs	Cushing's syndrome
	Purely abdominal	Pregnancy
	Lethargic	Hypothyroidism
Underweight	Young with recent weight loss and wasting	Diabetes mellitus (IDDM)

IDDM, insulin-dependent diabetes mellitus

Fig. 18.4 Common findings on examination of the hands

Findings	Diagnostic inference
Hands are enlarged, greasy, spade-like, with thickened skin	Acromegaly
Palms are warm and moist ± tremor	Thyrotoxicosis
Palms are cold and dry	Hypothyroidism
Palmar creases are pigmented	Addison's disease, Cushing's disease, ectopic ACTH syndrome
Note the extent of the areas where the patient complains of 'pins and needles' (paraesthesia) or numbness (anaesthesia) in the fingers and hands	Diabetes mellitus (complication), hypocalcaemia
Trousseau's sign, showing neuromuscular irritability–test by occluding the blood flow to the hands, using an inflated blood pressure cuff around the upper arm, which causes a typical contraction of the hand (thumb adducts, fingers extend) within 2 minutes	Hypocalcaemia
Tinel's sign, showing carpal tunnel syndrome diagnosed by tapping over the flexor retinaculum and causing paraesthesia in the medial fingers	Hypothyroidism, acromegaly
Decreased skin turgor, signifying dehydration–present if skin on the back of the hand does not return to normal immediately after being pinched	Uncontrolled diabetes mellitus, diabetes insipidus, hypercalcaemia

ACTH, adrenocorticotrophic hormone.

Fig. 18.5 Common findings on inspection of the nails

Findings	Diagnostic inference
Separation of the nail from its bed (onycholysis) and nail tips appear white	Thyrotoxicosis
Clubbing of the fingertips, caused by swelling of the soft tissue at the base of the nail	Graves' disease (not in other forms of thyrotoxicosis)
Nails look broken and weak (fragile nails)	Hypocalcaemia
Deformed nails with inflammation of the surrounding skin is a sign of infection (often caused by *Candida albicans*)	Uncontrolled diabetes mellitus

Fig. 18.6 Common findings on examination of the limbs

Feature	Findings	Diagnostic inference
Pulse rate and rhythm	Rapid pulse rate of >100 beats per minute (tachycardia)	Thyrotoxicosis, phaeochromocytoma
	Slow pulse rate of <60 beats per minute (bradycardia)	Hypothyroidism
	Irregular pulse rhythm (signifying cardiac arrhythmias)	Thyrotoxicosis and hypercalcaemia
	Reduced or absent pulses in the feet and legs (caused by peripheral vascular disease)	Diabetes mellitus (complication)
Skin, muscle and bone structure of the limb	Infected or ulcerated skin (look especially on the lower leg and ankles)	Diabetes mellitus (complication), Cushing's syndrome (both cause poor wound healing)
	Multiple bruising over the skin, with no history of trauma	Cushing's syndrome
	Thickened skin over the tibia, with elevated dermal nodules and plaques (pretibial myxoedema)	Graves' disease (not in other forms of thyrotoxicosis)
	Proximal muscle wasting (observe and feel the biceps and quadriceps muscles)	Cushing's syndrome, hypothyroidism, thyrotoxicosis
	Bone deformity, e.g. 'bow-legs' or 'knock-knees' (observe when the patient is standing)	Rickets (vitamin D deficiency; rare in UK)
	Pitting oedema at the ankles (caused by salt and water retention)	Cushing's syndrome (SIADH does not cause oedema)
Blood pressure	High blood pressure (hypertension)	Cushing's syndrome, diabetes mellitus (complication), acromegaly
	Low blood pressure whilst moving from lying to standing position (postural hypotension)	Addison's disease, diabetic autonomic neuropathy

SIADH, syndrome of inappropriate autidiuretic hormone secretion.

signs (onycholysis) and dryness. The lower leg is examined for pretibial myxoedema. The eyes are then examined (see Fig. 18.10). Refer back to Chapter 3 to recall which signs reflect over-activity as opposed to under-activity of the thyroid gland.

Examination of the thyroid gland involves anterior and lateral inspection for enlargement and nodules. The patients should be asked to swallow as thyroid masses will move. Palpation from behind the patient involves identification of the thyroid isthmus between the cricoid cartilage and the suprasternal notch. Palpation is continued laterally over the two thyroid lobes feeling for enlargement and nodules. The thyroid should be palpated on swallowing. Complete the exam by palpating the surrounding lymph nodes.

Examination of the female reproductive system

It is essential to carefully explain the examination you wish to perform when it involves intimate body parts. A chaperone must be present at every examination for medico-legal reasons and to reassure the patient. Prior to examination, ensure the patient has emptied the bladder and is wearing a gown. Have the patient lie supine.

Fig. 18.7 Common findings examination of the feet

Findings	Diagnostic inference
Feet are large and wide and patient's shoe size has recently increased	Acromegaly
Skin ulcers and/or gangrene	Diabetes mellitus
Dry, cold, hairless skin of the feet and weak or absent foot pulses may signify ischaemia caused by peripheral vascular disease (check by testing capillary refill)	Diabetes mellitus (complication)
Note the extent of the areas where the patient complains of 'pins and needles' (paraesthesia) or numbness (anaesthesia) in the feet and lower legs	Diabetes mellitus (complication), hypocalcaemia

An enlarged thyroid gland can be distinguished from a thyroglossal cyst by asking the patient to swallow and stick out the tongue. The thyroid gland will move with the trachea on swallowing, whereas a thyroglossal cyst rises when the tongue is protruded.

Examination of the vulva (external genitalia)

The vulva should be examined with the patient lying on her back with the legs apart and knees bent. The common signs of vulval disease are shown in Fig. 18.16.

Examination sequence

1. Inspect the entire vulva for redness, infestations, swelling, masses.
2. Look for vaginal discharge.
3. Ask the patient to cough or push down.
4. Look for vaginal prolapse and urinary incontinence.

Internal examination with a speculum

A warmed vaginal speculum can be used to visualize the cervix and obtain swabs or a cervical smear.

Speculum insertion

1. Warm and lubricate the speculum.
2. Warn the patient.
3. Insert speculum with handle perpendicular to perineum, inspect vaginal walls.
4. Rotate speculum 45 degrees upon insertion and open the bills so that the cervix falls between.
5. Lock open bills.
6. Inspect cervix for lesion, redness or discharge.
7. Take swabs
8. Withdraw slightly to free the cervix
9. Close the bills carefully whilst rotating and withdrawing the speculum.

Swabs routinely taken:

- High vaginal swab for *Trichomoniasis*, *Streptococcus* and *Staphylococcus*.
- Endocervical swab for *Chlamydia* and *Neisseria gonorrhoeae*.
- Cervical swab for cytological smear.

If a smear is required then the speculum should be inserted without lubricant. A wooden spatula is used to sample the cells of the cervix; the sample is smeared onto a slide and fixed immediately, before being sent for analysis.

Bimanual examination of the vagina and uterus

This examination often follows examination with a speculum. The signs of disease of the internal female reproductive system are shown in Fig. 18.17.

Examination sequence

1. Lubricate your index and middle finger.
2. Insert gently into the vagina.
3. Rotate upwards.
4. Palpate the cervix for mobility, consistency, size and shape. Note any tenderness on movement of the cervix
5. Press above the pubis with the other hand to feel the uterus–estimate uterine size.
6. Palpate laterally (adnexal structures; may include ovarian cysts, inflamed uterine tubes and tubal pregnancy); the ovaries are usually palpable in slender, relaxed women.

Breast examination

Breast examination is usually aimed at finding and describing a lump (see Fig. 18.15). If a lump is found, further investigation is always required to exclude the possibility of malignancy. This cannot be determined from the history and examination alone.

Fig. 18.8 Common findings on examination of the head

Feature	Findings	Diagnostic inference
Bone structure, facial features and complexion	Increased head circumference, protruding jaw, coarse facial features, nose and jaw enlarged, malaligned teeth with spaces between them in the lower jaw, thickened facial skin folds	Acromegaly
	Protruding forehead	Rickets (vitamin D deficiency; rare in UK)
	Pale, puffy face with coarse features	Hypothyroidism
	Round 'moon-face'	Cushing's syndrome
	Acne on face, neck and chest	Cushing's syndrome, acromegaly and polycystic ovarian syndrome
	Chvostek's sign, showing neuromuscular irritability—diagnosed by gently tapping the facial nerve where it passes through the parotid gland and causing the facial muscles to twitch briskly on the same side of the face	Hypocalcaemia
Hair distribution	Lack of normal beard growth in postpubescent males	Delayed puberty, hypopituitarism causing gonadotrophin deficiency
	Excessive facial hair (hirsutism) in females	Polycystic ovarian syndrome
Mouth	Hyperpigmented buccal mucosa	Addison's disease, Cushing's disease (not in Cushing's syndrome)
	Malaligned teeth, enlarged tongue (possibly causing dysarthria, i.e. difficulty in pronunciation)	Acromegaly
	Swollen tongue and a hoarse, croaky voice	Hypothyroidism

The potential findings of breast examination are shown in Figs 18.18 and 18.19. Always examine both breasts and explain that you need to make a comparison.

Examination sequence

1. Inspect sitting up for asymmetry, lumps.
2. Inspect sitting forwards.
3. Inspect with arms lifted for tethering, lumps.
4. Inspect with hands pressed on hips.
5. Palpate both breasts with the patient's ipsilateral arm behind the head. Using circular motions, press breast tissue against the thoracic wall. Describe any lumps.
6. Fix nipple between thumb and index finger and examine for discharge.
7. Lower arm and examine axillary and supraclavicular lymph nodes.

Examination of the pregnant abdomen (Fig 18.20)

Fetal heart sounds can be heard over a pregnant uterus using Doppler ultrasound at 10 weeks gestation and with a stethoscope at 25 weeks.

Examination of the male genitalia

The common abnormalities of the male external genitalia found on examination are shown in Figs 18.21 and 18.22.

Examination of a scrotal mass

The possible causes of lumps and swellings in the scrotum are illustrated in Fig. 18.23. The exact location of a lump relative to the testes and abdomen is especially important.

Examination sequence

1. With the patient standing, inspect the inguinal and femoral areas for hernias or varicocoeles. Inspect skin colour and texture and pubic hair. May reveal scars, nodules, ulcers, infestation or abnormal development.
2. Inspect the ventral and dorsal sides of the penis – lesions (syphilis), fibrosis (Peyronie's disease).
3. Locate the urethral meatus (look for discharge, stricture, hypospadias). Retract foreskin and examine glans for lesions or phimosis.
4. Inspect the scrotum for undescended testes, hernia, and varicocoeles.
5. Palpate the testes (lumps, torsion, orchitis), epididymis (cysts, epididymitis, tumours) and spermatic cords ('bag of worms'; varicocoeles).
6. Describe any abnormal lumps present.
7. Determine the location of any lumps.
8. Try to transluminate any lumps.
9. Palpate the surrounding lymph nodes.

Examination of the prostate gland

The prostate gland can be examined by rectal palpation. The prostate is located on the anterior wall of the rectum, which can be palpated with a gloved and lubricated index finger. The patient is positioned in the left lateral position. There are usually two lobes separated by a median longitudinal groove called the median sulcus. Assess the size, consistency, tenderness and nodularity of the prostate. Normal seminal vesicles cannot be felt. The common findings are shown in Fig. 18.24.

Fig. 18.9 Common findings on examination of the eyes

Findings	Diagnostic inference
Lid lag—slow descent of the upper lid, lags behind the descent of the eyeball	Hyperthyroidism
Lid retraction—at rest, the superior limbus of the iris and possibly even some sclera above it (white of the eye) is visible (see Fig.18.10)	Hyperthyroidism
Exophthalmos—the eye appears to bulge out of its socket and it is possible to see the whole of the iris and sometimes even sclera surrounding its circumference (see Fig. 18.10)	Graves' disease (not in other forms of thyrotoxicosis)
Anaemia—the inner surface of the lower lid looks pale if anaemia is present	Menorrhagia
Retinal disease—look for ischaemic change and neovascularisation using an ophthalmoscope (appearance of 'dots' and 'blots' signify presence of microaneurysms and microhaemorrhages,respectively)	Diabetes mellitus (complication)
Papilloedema (caused by raised intracranial pressure)—both optic discs appear convex and their margins appear blurred	Pituitary tumour
Impaired visual acuity—test the visual acuity in both eyes separately using an eye chart	Diabetes mellitus (complication
Bitemporal hemianopia visual field deficits—test the visual fields in each eye separately	Pituitary tumour

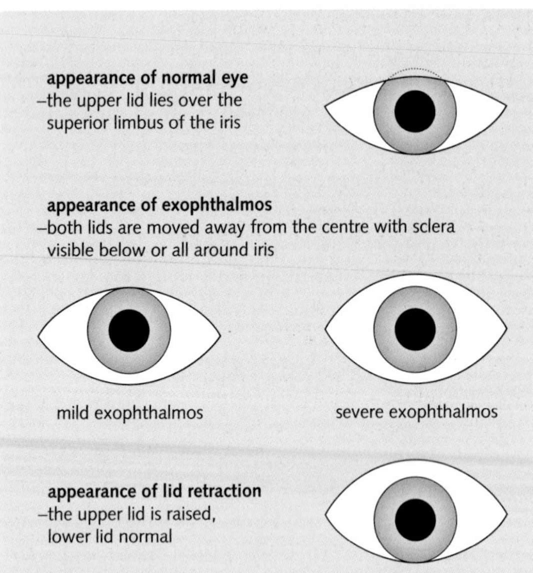

Fig. 18.10 Appearance of the eyes indicating hyperthyroidism.

Fig. 18.12 Common findings on examination of the thorax

Findings	Diagnostic inference
A 'pigeon chest' or 'rickety rosary' (outward bowing and thickening of the costochondral junctions)	Rickets (vitamin D deficiency; rare in UK)
Truncal obesity (abnormal fat distribution) and increased chest hair in men and women	Cushing's syndrome
Respiratory distress—deep, rapid hyperventilation ('air-hunger'), called Kussmaul's breathing	Diabetic ketoacidosis

Fig. 18.11 Common findings on examination of the neck

Findings	Diagnostic inference
Anterior neck swelling in the thyroid position which ascends during swallowing	Goitre
Swelling in the neck between the chin and the 2nd tracheal ring which rises when the tongue is stuck out	Congenital thyroglossal cyst

Fig. 18.13 Common findings on inspection of the abdomen

Findings	Diagnostic inference
Scars	Previous surgery possibly to treat an endocrine or reproductive system disorde
Wide purple striae (linear wrinkled 'stretch' marks) in both sexes and increased abdominal hair (hirsutism) in women	Cushing's syndrome
Abdominal distension (can be caused by fat, fluid, fetus, flatus, faeces or large solid tumours)	Cushing's syndrome (fat), hypothyroidism (fat), pelvic mass (e.g. fibroids, ovarian disease or pregnancy)
Excessive outward curvature of the spine (kyphosis) or excessive inward curvature o the spine (lordosis) can be caused by vertebral collapse	Osteoporosis secondary to menopausal hormone failure, Cushing's syndrome or thyrotoxicosis

Fig. 18.14 Common findings on palpation and percussion of the abdomen

Findings	Diagnostic inference
Enlarged liver, spleen and kidneys (organomegaly)	Acromegaly
Mass with impalpable lower border	Pelvic mass (e.g fibroids, pregnancy)
Body tenderness	Osteoporosis secondary to menopause, Cushing's syndrome or thyrotoxicosis
	Bony metastases
Lower abdominal tenderness	Pelvic inflammatory disease, ectopic pregnancy
Shifting dullness	Ascites following malignancy

Fig. 18.15 Examination and description of a lump

Feature	Findings
Skin changes	Colour, scarring, ulceration, oedema
Temperature	Hot, cold
Tenderness	Is it painful when touched?
Location	Accurate anatomical description
Size and shape	Estimates of diameter
Surface	Irregular, lobular, smooth
Edge	Sharp, rounded, indistinct
Consistency	Firm, hard, soft
Translucency	Cysts allow light to pass through
Relations	What structures is it attached to?

Fig. 18.16 Common findings on inspection of the vulva

Findings	Diagnostic inference
Rashes (redness, swelling or white thickened areas called leucoplakia)	Often caused by infections, dermatological conditions (e.g. lichen sclerosus), chemical irritants or allergies
Injury or scars	Can be due to trauma (e.g. childbirth, female circumcision or sexual abuse)
Enlarged clitoris (clitoromegaly)	Congenital adrenal hyperplasia (excessive androgen secretion)
Red painful cystic lump beneath the posterior part of the labium majus	Bartholin's cyst or abscess
Bloody vaginal discharge	Menstruation, miscarriage, cancer, cervical polyp or erosion
Purulent vaginal discharge	Infection, e.g. vaginitis, cervicitis, endometritis
Frothy, watery, pale, yellow–white or purulent discharge and pruritus	Infection caused by *Trichomonas vaginalis*
Thick, white, cottage-cheese-like discharge and inflammation of the skin and mucous membranes	Infection caused by *Candida albicans*

Fig. 18.17 Common findings on examination of the female internal genitalia

Findings	Diagnostic inference
Difficult to insert a lubricated finger	Vaginismus
Impalpable uterus	Retroverted uterus
Palpable mass laterally	Mass in the ovary or fallopian tube
Enlarged, nodular uterus	Fibroids
Enlarged, smooth uterus	Pregnancy or cancer

Fig. 18.18 Common findings on inspection of the breast

Findings	Diagnostic inference
Scar due to mastectomy (removal of breast)	Previous breast carcinoma
Breast size decreased bilaterally in women	Hypopituitarism
Enlargement of the female breast (unilateral or bilateral)	Benign hyperplasia of the breast, breast infection/ inflammation, breast neoplasia
Enlargement of the male breast (unilateral or bilateral)	Gynaecomastia (see Fig. 17.4), breast carcinoma
Skin appears pulled in and puckered	Underlying breast carcinoma
Skin has an 'orange peel' appearance (peau d'orange) because of oedema-induced widening of the orifices of sweat glands and hair follicles	Breast carcinoma that is blocking the lymphatic drainage and causing oedema
Skin nodules, abnormal skin texture and colour	Skin infiltrated with tumour cells from a breast carcinoma
Skin is erythematous (reddened) and hot	Infection of the breast or the overlying skin
Skin ulceration (determine its position, size, shape, colour, edge and base)	Advanced breast carcinoma
Nipple and surrounding skin is thickened, red, encrusted and oozy, with an underlying breast lump	Paget's disease of the nipple (breast carcinoma)
Recent nipple pigmentation increased	Addison's disease or pregnancy
Nipple asymmetry and/or retraction	Underlying breast carcinoma
Nipple discharge	Infection, benign or malignant breast tumours, lactation
Nipple duplication—can occur anywhere along the line from the axilla to the groin	Supernumerary nipples
Redness and swelling of the axilla and arm (caused by lymphadenopathy and oedema)	Metastases in the axillary lymph nodes from a breast carcinoma

Fig. 18.19 Common findings on examination of the breast

Findings	Diagnostic inference
A solitary, stony-hard, painless lump with an irregular surface and an indistinct edge, which may involve the skin, underlying muscle and regional lymph nodes	Breast carcinoma
A young patient with a solitary, firm, painless lump with a spherical (or knobbly) surface, which tends to be highly mobile and no lymphadenopathy	Fibroadenoma – but further investigations must be performed
In a pregnant woman with a lump or diffuse swelling that is tender, soft/solid and spherical with hot overlying skin and lymphadenopathy	Breast abscess
Palpable regional lymph nodes	Breast infection, breast carcinoma

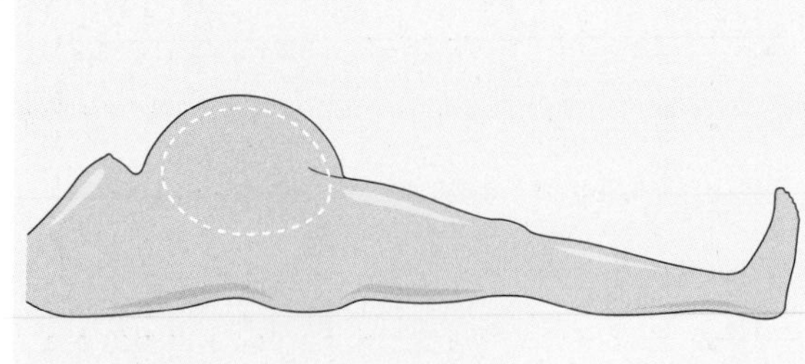

Fig. 18.20 Examination of the pregnant abdomen.

Fig. 18.21 Common findings on inspection of the male genitalia

Findings	Diagnostic inference
Skin/mucosal rashes or ulceration	Infection, inflammation, connective tissue disease, squamous cell carcinoma
Decreased pubic hair	Hypogonadism, hypopituitarism
Small penis	Hypogonadism
Abnormal position of the external urethral meatus ± hooded foreskin	Hypospadias

Fig. 18.22 Common findings on examination of the male genitalia

Findings	Diagnostic inference
Urethral discharge	Infection or inflammation
Empty scrotum (unilateral or bilateral)	Undescended or retractile testis, previous excision
Small firm testes (bilateral)	Hypogonadism, testicular atrophy due to alcohol or drugs
Small firm testis (other testis normal)	Mumps, orchitis
Exquisitely tender testis with oedematous swelling of the entire scrotal contents	Torsion of the testis (epididymo-orchitis)

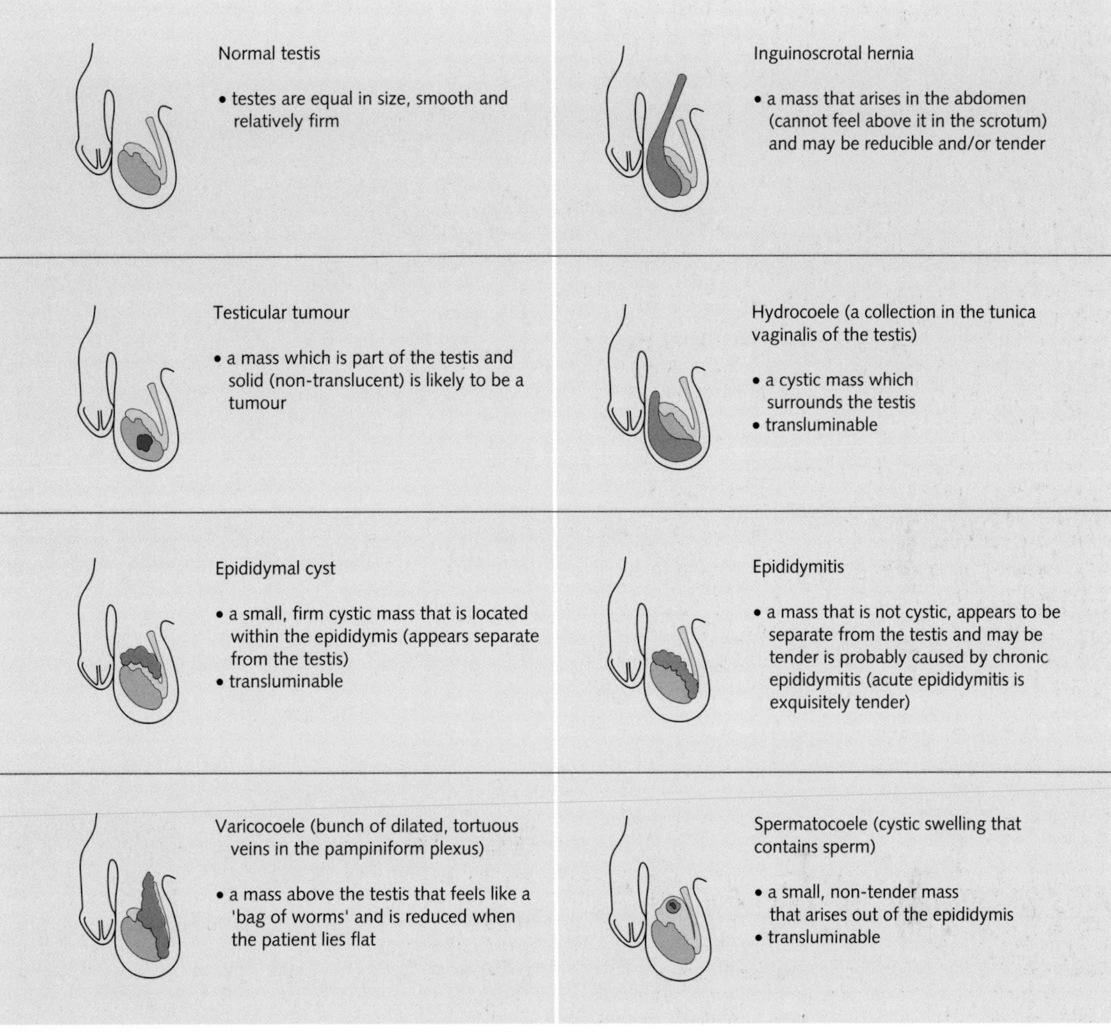

Fig. 18.23 Common findings on examination of a lump in the scrotum.

Fig. 18.24 Common findings on examination of the prostate

Findings	Diagnostic inference
Smooth, firm gland, 2–3 cm across, with two lobes separated by narrow sulcus	Normal prostate
Enlarged and mobile gland with lobules	Benign hypertrophy
Large, irregular and hard gland fixed to the rectal mucosa with a distorted central sulcus	Prostatic carcinoma

Investigations and imaging

19

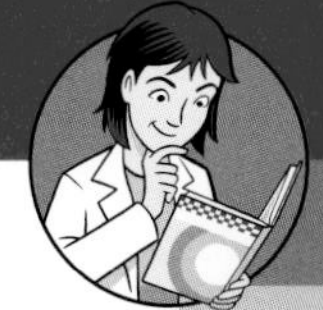

Objectives

By the end of this chapter you should be able to:

- Describe the ELISA technique and its use in endocrinology.
- Recognize which hormones are measured indirectly and why.
- With an example, describe the situations in which a suppression test is used.
- With an example, describe the situations in which a stimulation test is used.
- Describe the triple stimulation test of pituitary function and explain why all these hormones are tested together.
- With examples, describe how laboratory-based investigations other than for hormone levels can aid diagnosis.
- Describe the use of plain and contrast-enhanced radiography in diagnosis of endocrine and reproductive disorders.
- Describe the use of ultrasound in diagnosis of endocrine and reproductive disorders.
- Describe the use of CT and MRI scans in diagnosis of endocrine and reproductive disorders.
- Describe the use of radioisotope scans in diagnosis of endocrine and reproductive disorders.

Following the history and examination, an endocrine or reproductive disorder may be suspected. Many tests can be used to investigate endocrine function; however, the results can be misleading unless the appropriate test is used.

Proper investigation of a suspected endocrine disorder takes the following steps:

- Measure the level of hormone in the blood/urine or its biological effects.
- If a deficiency is suspected use a stimulation test.
- If an excess is suspected use a suppression test.
- If an abnormality is confirmed, image the suspected gland.

INVESTIGATING HORMONES

Measuring methods

This section outlines the tests used to measure hormone levels and how they change upon stimulation or suppression. These tests are performed if a hormone excess or deficiency is suspected from the history and examination; they aim to confirm the diagnosis and investigate its cause. The four main methods of investigating hormones are described below.

Direct measurement

The levels of hormones in the plasma and urine can be measured using enzyme-linked immunosorbent assays (ELISA). The sample is mixed with a known concentration of hormone bound to fluorescent markers. Monoclonal antibodies specific to the hormone are added and the hormone–antibody complexes formed are separated from the solution. The degree of fluorescence is inversely proportional to the original hormone concentration because the native hormone competes with the labelled hormone for antibodies to bind to (Fig. 19.1). In the past, radioimmunoassay (RIA) was used, but this is less sensitive. The normal concentrations of commonly measured hormones are shown in Fig. 19.2.

Indirect measurement

Some hormones produce metabolic changes that are easier to measure than the hormone itself. There are two main examples:

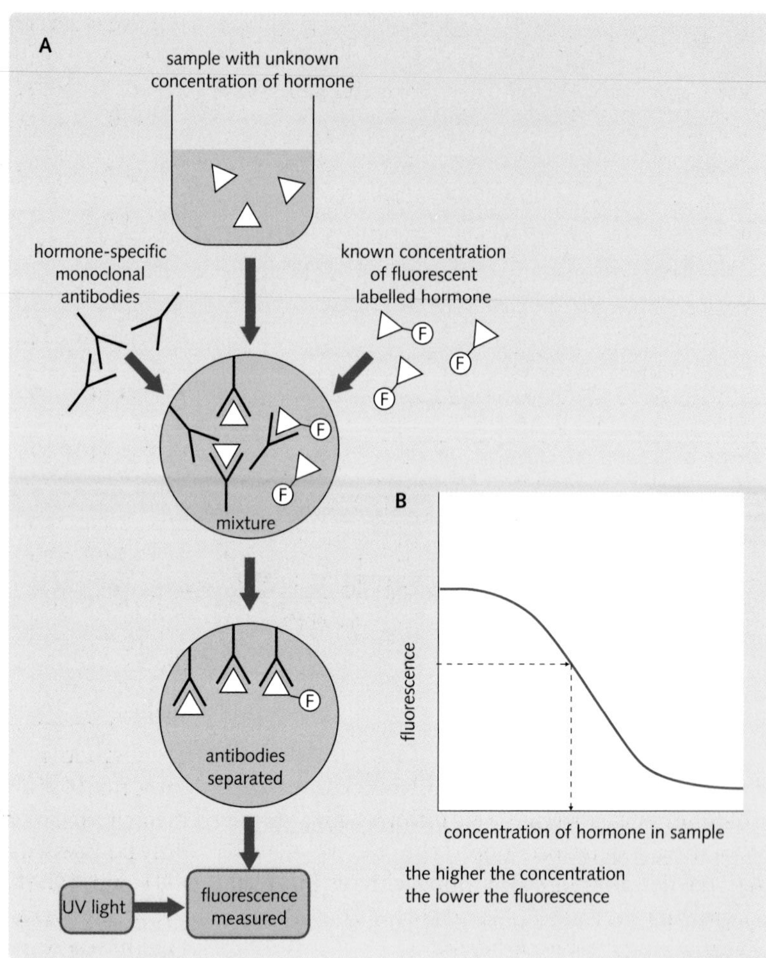

Fig. 19.1 (A) Measuring hormone levels by enzyme-linked immunosorbent assay (ELISA). (B) Interpretation of the results.

- Blood glucose is used to determine insulin levels.
- Urine vs blood osmolality is used to determine antidiuretic hormone (ADH) levels.

Stimulation tests

If a hormone deficiency is suspected then secretion is stimulated to record the response. Blood levels are measured before and after stimulation.

Suppression tests

If a hormone excess is suspected then the hormone secretion is suppressed to record the response. Blood levels are measured before and after suppression.

Hypothalamic function

The quantities of hormones secreted by the hypothalamus are generally too low to be measured clinically. Hypothalamic dysfunction is investigated by measuring the relevant pituitary hormones and their response to stimulation or suppression.

Anterior pituitary function

Hormone assays

Pituitary adenomas can affect the secretion of all the anterior pituitary hormones. For this reason, a suspected abnormality in one anterior pituitary hormone prompts investigation of all the others.

Hormones secreted by the anterior pituitary gland are measured along with the hormones that they stimulate. The tests for the following hormones are usually available:

- Thyroid-stimulating hormone (TSH), along with tri-iodothyronine (T_3) and thyroxine (T_4).

Fig. 19.2 Normal ranges of commonly measured hormones

Hormone	Normal levels
Prolactin	Male: <450 μL Female: <600 μL
Adrenocorticotrophic hormone (ACTH)	<80 ng/L
Growth hormone (GH)	<20 mU/L
Thyroid stimulating hormone (TSH)	0.5–5.7 mU/L
Thyroxine (T_4)	70–140 nmol/L
Tri-iodothyronine (T_3)	1.2–3 nmol/L
Calcitonin	<0.1 μg/L
Cortisol (morning)	450–700 nmol/L
Aldosterone	100–500 pmol/L
Renin (standing)	2.8–4.5 pmol/mL/h
Testosterone	10–35 nmol/L

- Luteinizing hormone (LH) and follicle-stimulating hormone (FSH), along with oestrogen or testosterone.
- Growth hormone (GH), along with insulin-like growth factor 1 (IGF-1) and glucose; circadian variation must be considered.
- Adrenocorticotrophic hormone (ACTH), along with cortisol; this is not performed commonly and the circadian variation must be considered.
- Prolactin.

Triple stimulation test

The combined pituitary test (CPT) stimulates the anterior pituitary gland to secrete the six major hormones. It is used to investigate hypopituitarism, usually caused by a pituitary adenoma. Three stimulatory substances are injected intravenously:

- Insulin—causes hypoglycaemia that stimulates ACTH, GH and prolactin secretion (Fig. 19.3).
- Thyrotrophin-releasing hormone (TRH)—stimulates TSH and prolactin secretion.
- Gonadotrophin-releasing hormone (GnRH)—stimulates LH and FSH secretion.

The levels of all six hormones and the hormones they stimulate are measured before and several times after the stimulation.

Individual tests for secretion

Stimulation and suppression tests are especially important for measuring GH and ACTH because of their circadian variation. Hypothalamic function can only be assessed by these tests. The tests for TSH, LH, FSH and ACTH are described under the relevant endocrine organ. There is no further test for prolactin and the tests for GH are described below.

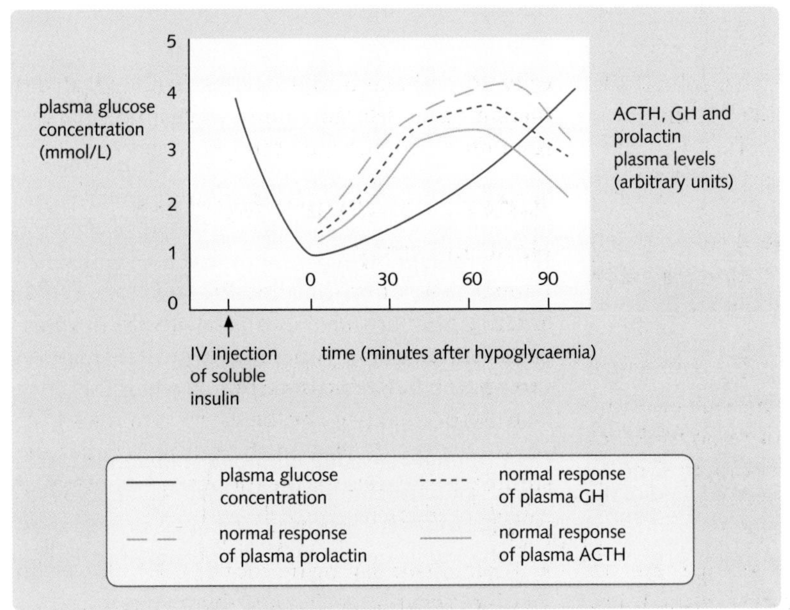

Fig. 19.3 Normal response of adrenocorticotrophic hormone (ACTH), growth hormone (GH), and prolactin to insulin-induced hypoglycaemia. (Adapted from *Lecture Notes on Endocrinology*, 5th edn by WJ Jeffcoate. With permission from Blackwell Science, 1993.)

Stimulation test

Used for GH deficiency; GH can be stimulated by:

- Insulin-induced hypoglycaemia (Fig. 19.3).
- Oral clonidine.

Blood samples are measured for glucose and GH before the test and several times over the following 2 hours. To create a suitable stimulus, blood glucose must fall below 2.2 mmol/L, causing symptoms of hypoglycaemia. Sugar may need to be given if blood glucose falls too low. GH deficiency is confirmed if secretion does not rise by >20mU/L.

Suppression test

Used for GH excess; GH is measured every 30 minutes for 2 hours following administration of glucose, i.e. an oral glucose tolerance test (see p. 236). Increased blood glucose normally suppresses GH secretion, but in acromegaly or gigantism GH levels fail to decrease.

Posterior pituitary function

Hormone assays

Oxytocin

Since abnormal plasma levels do not cause any recognized pathology, secretion is not tested.

Antidiuretic hormone

Plasma levels of antidiuretic hormone (ADH) can be measured by ELISA, but they are of little value unless combined with stimulation tests. The comparison between urine and blood osmolality is a more useful clinical measure:

- Dilute urine, concentrated blood: ADH excess (diabetes insipidus).
- Concentrated urine, dilute blood: ADH deficiency (syndrome of inappropriate ADH secretion; SIADH).

Water deprivation test

This is a stimulation test used for suspected ADH deficiency (i.e. diabetes insipidus). ADH release is stimulated by high plasma osmolality caused by water deprivation.

After a night's sleep and fasting, the patient is deprived of food and water for 8 hours, during which plasma and urine osmolality is measured repeatedly. The patient is also weighed and the test is abandoned if the patient loses >3% body weight. At the end of the test desmopressin (an ADH analogue) is given, and urine and plasma osmolality continue to be measured. This section of the test is described below under the desmopressin test.

Diabetes insipidus is diagnosed if urine osmolality is <400 mosmol/kg, the normal range is >600 mosmol/kg. The plasma osmolality should have risen to >295 mosmol/kg to induce this fall.

Desmopressin test

This is a suppression test that identifies the cause of diabetes insipidus (DI) once it has been confirmed by a water deprivation test. It can be caused by:

- Cranial DI—deficient pituitary secretion of ADH.
- Nephrogenic DI—failure of the kidney to respond to ADH.

The ADH analogue desmopressin is injected intramuscularly and the patient is allowed to drink water. Plasma and urine osmolality are measured 1 and 2 hours later. If DI is caused by ADH deficiency (i.e. cranial DI) then this should return urine osmolality to normal:

- Cranial DI—urine osmolality increases to >750 mosmol/kg.
- Nephrogenic DI—urine osmolality remains <400 mosmol/kg.

Thyroid function

Hormone assays

If abnormalities of thyroid function are suspected then plasma levels of TSH, T_4 and T_3 should be measured. Both thyroid hormones are measured because variations in thyroxine-binding globulin (TBG) levels can give inaccurate results. Further investigation is often not needed:

- Low levels of T_4 and T_3—hypothyroidism.
- High levels of T_4 and T_3—hyperthyroidism.

TSH is measured with T_3 and T_4 to locate the lesion. In hypothyroidism a low TSH suggests a pituitary/hypothalamic lesion while a high TSH suggests a thyroid gland problem. In hyperthyroidism TSH will almost always be low.

TSH is also measured to guide thyroxine treatment of thyroid disorders. The correct dose of thyroxine or carbimazole is being administered when TSH levels return to normal.

Thyrotrophin-releasing hormone stimulation test

This stimulation test is used if TSH deficiency is suspected. However TSH measurement is now so sensitive that it is rarely used. Hypothalamic TRH is administered intravenously and plasma TSH levels are measured before and after.

Thyroid autoantibody assays

ELISA can also be used to detect thyroid autoantibodies caused by the common autoimmune thyroid diseases:

- Thyroid-stimulating antibodies (TsAb) suggest Graves' disease.
- Anti-thyroid-peroxidase (anti-TPO) and anti-thyroglobulin (anti-TgAb) antibodies suggest Hashimoto's thyroiditis.

Management of thyroid nodules varies between hospitals. Findings of irregular firm nodules, lymph node involvement or tethering to surrounding structures on clinical examination are suggestive of malignancy. Ultrasound and thyroid biochemistry are usually used as the first-line investigations, Malignancy is more commonly associated with euthyroidism or hypothyroidism and hypo-echoic lesions on ultrasound. Isotope scans can reveal 'hot' (functioning – and less likely to be malignant) and 'cold' (non-functioning) nodules. If thyroid biochemistry is within the normal range and nodules are 'cold', fine needle aspiration biopsy (FNAC) can be performed as the most sensitive and specific test for confirming a diagnosis of malignancy.

Cortisol assays

24-hour urinary free cortisol

Urine is collected over a 24-hour period and the quantity of cortisol is measured; it is normally <280 nmol/24 h. This gives an accurate guide to plasma levels.

Basal plasma cortisol and adrenocorticotrophic hormone

These are measured at 09:00 and 22:00 because of circadian variation. This test is not as reliable as 24-hour urinary free cortisol.

Aldosterone assays

Plasma levels of aldosterone are measured, along with renin and potassium, to assess the appropriateness of aldosterone secretion. Aldosterone is normally secreted in response to high renin or high potassium. Conn's syndrome is suggested by high aldosterone in the presence of low renin and potassium.

Catecholamine assays

Catecholamine levels can be measured directly or, more commonly, by measuring their metabolites such as vanillylmandelic acid (VMA). Both tests are performed on 24-hour urine samples. Phaeochromocytoma causes VMA levels to rise above 48 mol/24 h.

Dexamethasone suppression test

This test is used if excess cortisol (Cushing's syndrome) is suspected. Dexamethasone is a synthetic corticosteroid that normally suppresses hypothalamic CRH and pituitary ACTH secretion causing cortisol secretion to drop. High or low doses of dexamethasone may be used, as described below.

Low-dose This is used to investigate excess cortisol (i.e. Cushing's syndrome). Plasma cortisol is measured in the morning then 0.5 mg/6 h dexamethasone is given orally for 48 hours. Plasma cortisol is measured again in the morning after the last dose. A 24-hour urinary cortisol is also collected on the 2nd day of stimulation. Cushing's syndrome is diagnosed if the test fails to suppress plasma cortisol.

High-dose This is used if the patient has clear signs of Cushing's syndrome or has had a positive low-dose test. 2 mg/6 h dexamethasone is given orally for 48 hours and the same measurements are collected as in the low-dose test.

- Slight cortisol depression—Cushing's disease; ACTH-secreting pituitary tumour.
- No cortisol depression—ectopic ACTH-secreting or adrenal tumour.

Synacthen® stimulation test

This test is used to investigate cortisol deficiency (e.g. Addison's disease). Synacthen® (also called tetracosactrin) is a synthetic analogue of ACTH that normally stimulates cortisol secretion. There are two versions of the test (see below).

Short Synacthen® test This test is used to exclude Addison's disease. 0.25 mg Synacthen® is given intramuscularly and plasma cortisol levels are measured before and 30 minutes later. Addison's is excluded if:

- First plasma cortisol level is >140 nmol/L.
- Second plasma cortisol is >500 nmol/L.
- Second plasma cortisol is >200 nmol/L higher than the first.

Prolonged Synacthen® test This test is used if the short test fails to exclude Addison's disease. 1.0 mg Synacthen® is given intramuscularly on three successive days and plasma cortisol levels are measured before and 6 hours after each injection. The diagnosis can be made from the plasma cortisol 6 hours after the third injection:

- <690 nmol/L—Addison's disease.
- >690 nmol/L—pituitary ACTH deficiency.

ACTH and cortisol tests are ordered in patients with symptoms or signs of cortisol excess (obesity, moon face and high blood pressure, low potassium, high bicarbonate, high glucose) or insufficiency (muscle weakness, skin pigmentation). This investigation helps to determine the level of the pathology that is contributing to the cortisol perturbation (adrenal, pituitary, ectopic sites or endogenous administration).

Pancreatic function

Random and fasting blood glucose assays

Endocrine investigation of the pancreas is aimed at diagnosing suspected diabetes mellitus. Insulin deficiency causes abnormally high plasma glucose levels (hyperglycaemia) and sometimes glycosuria. Insulin levels are never measured directly because blood glucose gives a more consistent measure of insulin action, especially if insulin resistance is present.

Diabetes mellitus is diagnosed using blood glucose measurements after an overnight fast on two occasions. Fasting blood glucose levels are normally 3.5–5.5 mmol/L. The results are interpreted as follows:

- >7.8 mmol/L—diabetes mellitus confirmed.
- 6–7.8 mmol/L—impaired glucose tolerance.
- <6 mmol/L—not diabetic.

Oral glucose tolerance test

If the fasting blood glucose measurements show impaired glucose tolerance then an oral glucose tolerance test (OGTT) is indicated. This is a stimulation test to check for insulin deficiency; however, glucose is measured not insulin. The patient fasts overnight and then drinks 75 g glucose in water. Plasma glucose is measured before and 2 hours after the drink. The results are shown in Figs 19.4 and 19.5. In patients with normal glucose tolerance the blood glucose should return to the fasting level within 2 hours.

Gonadal function and pregnancy testing

Hormone assays

Male

The male reproductive hormones are measured to exclude gonadal failure causing infertility following two abnormal sperm counts. Plasma levels of the following hormones are measured:

Fig. 19.4 Interpretation of blood glucose measurements during an oral glucose tolerance test

Blood glucose level (mmol/L)	Normal	Impaired fasting glycaemia (IFG)	Impaired glucose tolerance (IGT)	Diabetes mellitus
After overnight fast	<6.1	≥6.1 and <7	<7.0	≥7.0
2 hours after consumption of 75 g of anhydrous glucose	<7.8	–	≥ 7.8 (IGT)	≥ 11.1

IGT, impaired glucose tolerance

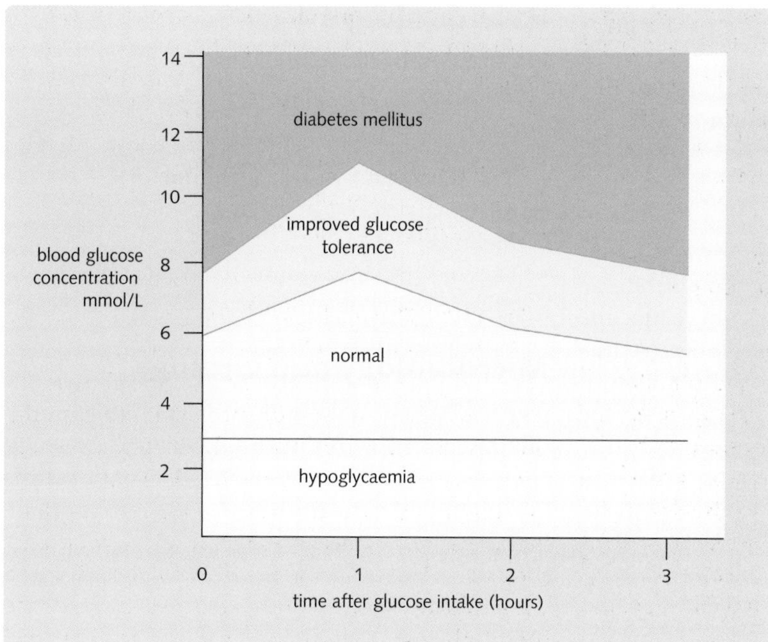

Fig. 19.5 Changes in blood glucose following an oral glucose tolerance test and interpretation of the results.

The diagnosis of diabetes mellitus can have significant lifestyle and legal implications for a patient. The diagnosis can be made in symptomatic patients (polyuria, polydipsia, unexplained weight loss, recurrent infection) on the basis of a single glucose measurement. A diagnosis is never made from a single measurement in an asymptomatic patient. An oral glucose tolerance test is used to establish a diagnosis in patients with borderline non-diagnostic glucose levels. Perturbations in random glucose levels under extreme stress (infection, haemorrhage) are not diagnostic in isolation.

- FSH and LH.
- Testosterone.
- Prolactin.

Testosterone requires three blood samples to be taken in the morning at 20-minute intervals because it is secreted in a pulsatile manner with a circadian rhythm.

Female

A similar set of hormones is investigated in a woman with amenorrhoea or infertility to exclude gonadal failure. Oestradiol-17β and progesterone are measured instead of testosterone. The stage of the menstrual cycle must be calculated because normal levels of FSH, LH, oestradiol-17β and progesterone vary throughout the cycle.

Primary gonadal failure

Low levels of gonadal steroids along with high levels of LH and FSH indicate primary gonadal failure.

Hypothalamic–pituitary dysfunction

Low levels of gonadal steroids with low or normal levels of LH and FSH indicate hypothalamic–pituitary dysfunction. Raised prolactin levels can cause this pattern.

Gonadotrophin-releasing hormone stimulation test

This test is used to investigate gonadal steroid deficiency (i.e. gonadal failure in both men and women). GnRH normally raises secretion of LH and FSH.

100 μg GnRH is injected intravenously and the plasma levels of the reproductive hormones are measured before and four times in the hour after the test. The levels of all the reproductive hormones should be increased following this test. Failure of LH and FSH levels to rise confirms pituitary dysfunction, while an excessive rise suggests hypothalamic dysfunction.

Pregnancy test

Pregnancy can be diagnosed by detecting human chorionic gonadotrophin (hCG) in the urine. The test will be positive approximately 10 days after conception.

OTHER INVESTIGATIONS

Information about endocrine and reproductive disorders can be gathered from tests not specifically designed to investigate hormone levels or organs.

Clinical chemistry

The clinical chemistry laboratory measures the concentrations of ionic and organic components in the blood and urine (e.g. UEs). Fig. 19.6 shows endocrine causes of disordered chemical levels. These results must be viewed alongside the history, examination and other tests, since endocrine diseases are rarely the most common cause.

Haematology

Investigations of the components that make up blood can suggest specific disorders:

- Low haemoglobin—chronic blood loss.
- Raised haematocrit—dehydration.
- Increased percentage of HBA_{1C}—diabetes mellitus.
- Raised erythrocyte sedimentation rate (ESR)—inflammation or infection.

Microbiology and virology

If an infection is suspected then an appropriate specimen can be tested for microorganisms. Specimens

Fig. 19.6 Normal concentration ranges for ionic organic components of the blood and endocrine causes of abnormally high or low concentrations

Component and its normal range	Endocrine causes of abnormally high concentration	Endocrine causes of abnormally low concentration
Plasma sodium: 135–145 mmol/L	Diabetes insipidus, Cushing's syndrome, Conn's syndrome	SIADH, Addison's disease, diabetes mellitus
Plasma potassium: 3.5–5.0 mmol/L	Addison's disease, diabetes insipidus, diabetes mellitus	Cushing's syndrome, hyperaldosteronism, SIADH, hyperthyroidism
Plasma urea: 2.5–7.5 mmol/L; plasma creatinine: <120 mmol/L	Diabetes insipidus, diabetes mellitus, Addison's disease	SIADH
Plasma osmolality: 270–300 mOsmol/kg	Diabetes insipidus, diabetes mellitus (NB abnormal aldosterone levels do not affect osmolality)	SIADH
pH: 7.35–7.45; bicarbonate: 24–30 mmol/L	Cushing's syndrome, Conn's syndrome	Addison's syndrome, diabetic ketoacidosis, hyperparathyroidism (mild)
Plasma calcium: 2.25–2.55 mmol/L	Hyperparathyroidism, vitamin D toxicity, hyperthyroidism, acromegaly, Addison's disease (NB abnormal calcitonin levels do not affect plasma calcium levels)	Hypoparathyroidism, vitamin D deficiency, Cushing's syndrome
Plasma phosphate: 0.8–1.5 mmol/L	Hypoparathyroidism, hyperthyroidism, acromegaly	Hyperparathyroidism, vitamin D deficiency, diabetes mellitus
Fasting blood glucose: 3.5–6.0 mmol/L	Diabetes mellitus, Cushing's syndrome, acromegaly, hyperthyroidism, phaeochromocytom	Exogenous insulin overdose, Addison's disease, pituitary insufficiency
Fasting plasma triglycerides: 0.55–1.90 mmol/L	Diabetes mellitus	
Plasma ketone bodies: not normally present in the blood	Diabetes mellitus	

SIADH, syndrome of inappropriate autidiuretic hormone secretion.

can be collected by swabbing, scraping or aspirating the infected region. Infections of endocrine organs are uncommon, but the reproductive system is prone to sexually transmitted diseases.

The following endocrine disorders can predispose to infection elsewhere in the body:

- Diabetes mellitus.
- Cushing's syndrome.
- Hypothyroidism.

Histopathology and cytology

Histopathological examination requires an intact sample of the tissue called a biopsy. Biopsies can be taken from many organs in the endocrine and reproductive systems if an abnormality or tumour is suspected. The specimens are examined for abnormal cells and tissue structure:

- Inflammatory cells—show the presence of inflammation or infection.
- Tissue structure changes (e.g. necrosis, hyperplasia).

Cytology only requires a cell sample (e.g. cervical smear). A full biopsy is not needed, but it can be used. The cells are examined for cancerous changes called dysplasia.

IMAGING OF THE ENDOCRINE AND REPRODUCTIVE SYSTEMS

Plain X-ray radiography

Plain X-rays demonstrate bony structures and calcified areas within organs because these tissues are radio-opaque (white), whilst soft tissues are radiolucent (grey to black). They are used to investigate endocrine and reproductive disorders that cause bone abnormalities:

- Acromegaly—thickened skull, enlarged jaw and hands (Fig. 19.7).
- Hyperparathyroidism and rickets—osteomalacia.
- Cushing's syndrome and thyrotoxicosis—osteoporosis.

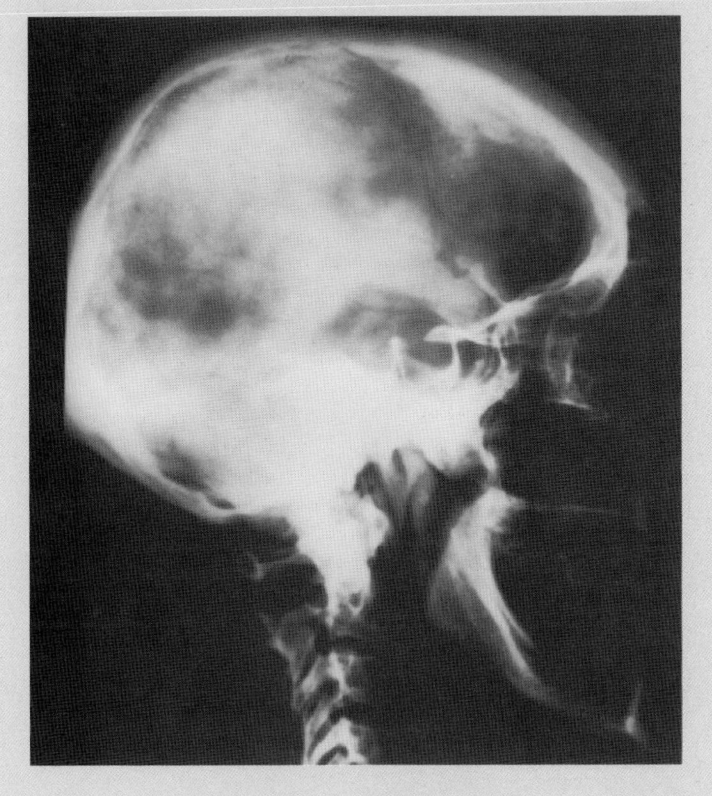

Fig. 19.7 Plain X-ray of the skull of a patient with acromegaly. It shows a large, protruding jaw, a large pituitary fossa and a thick skull (from Grainger & Allison, 4th edn).

- Prostate bony metastases—osteosclerotic lesions.
- Other bony metastases—osteolytic lesions.
- Size of the pituitary fossa—enlarged with large adenomas.
- Organ calcification—following disease in the adrenal glands.

Contrast media

Contrast media and dyes can be used to image soft tissues. Contrast media are used with X-rays, they must be radio-opaque and inert to prevent damage to the organ. The contrast medium or dye can be ingested or injected into a specific body compartment to allow visualization with X-rays.

Angiography

A contrast medium is injected into the arteries (intra-arterially) or veins (intravenously) allowing these blood vessels and the organs they supply to be visualized (Fig. 19.8).

Fluorescein angiography

This is a form of angiography used to visualize the retinal vessels. A fluorescein contrast medium is injected intravenously and the retina is photographed using ultraviolet light, which causes the fluorescein to fluoresce. This technique is especially useful in the investigation of diabetic retinopathy.

Hysterosalpingography

A contrast medium is injected into the uterus and uterine tubes via the cervix. Its progression along the uterine tubes is imaged using real time X-ray screening (Fig. 19.9).

Mammography

Mammography is one method of investigating and screening for breast lesions. Early detection of breast cancer by mammography may improve the prognosis. An example of a normal breast and one affected by cancer are shown in Fig. 19.10.

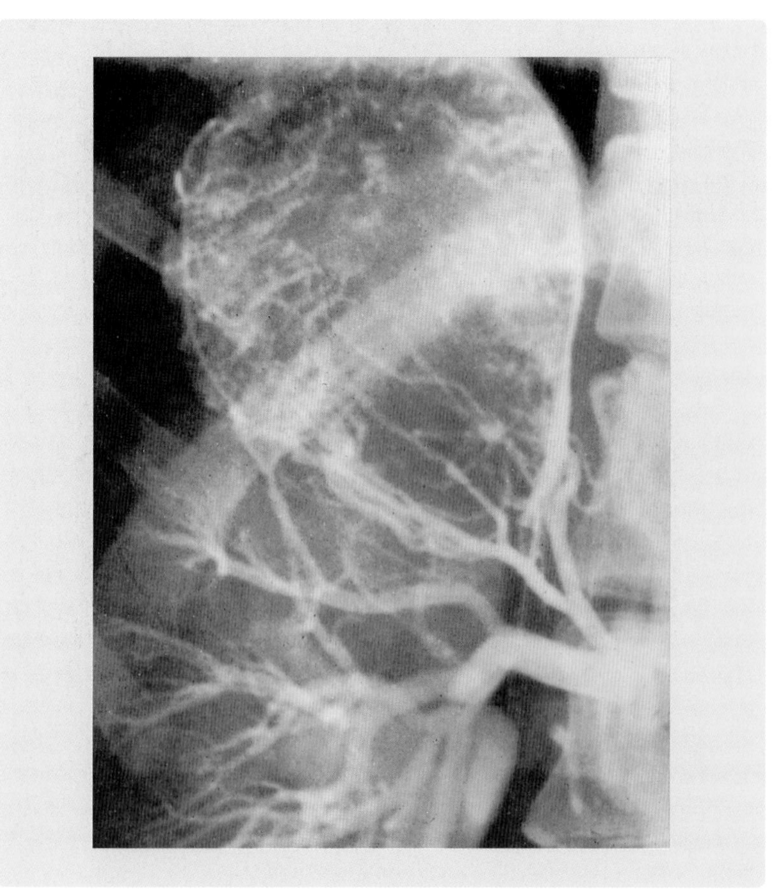

Fig. 19.8 Selective arteriogram of a phaeochromocytoma (from Sutton, 6th edn).

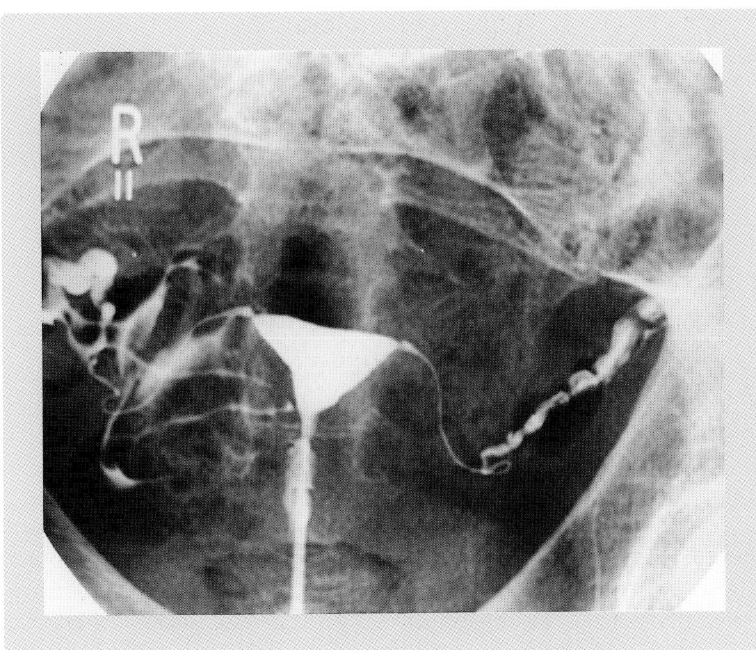

Fig. 19.9 Hysterosalpingogram of a normal uterus and fallopian tubes (from Grainger & Allison, 4th edn).

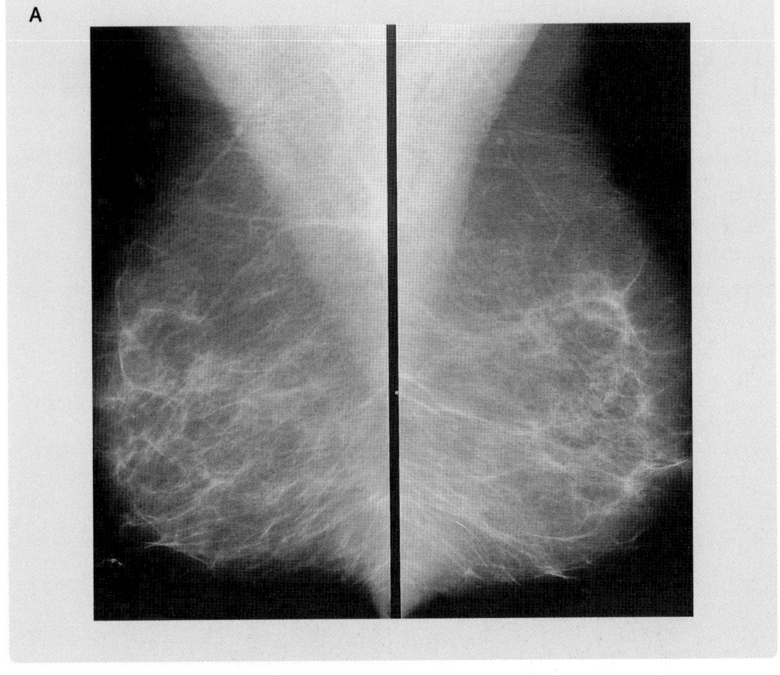

Fig. 19.10 (A) Mammogram of a normal breast.

(continued)

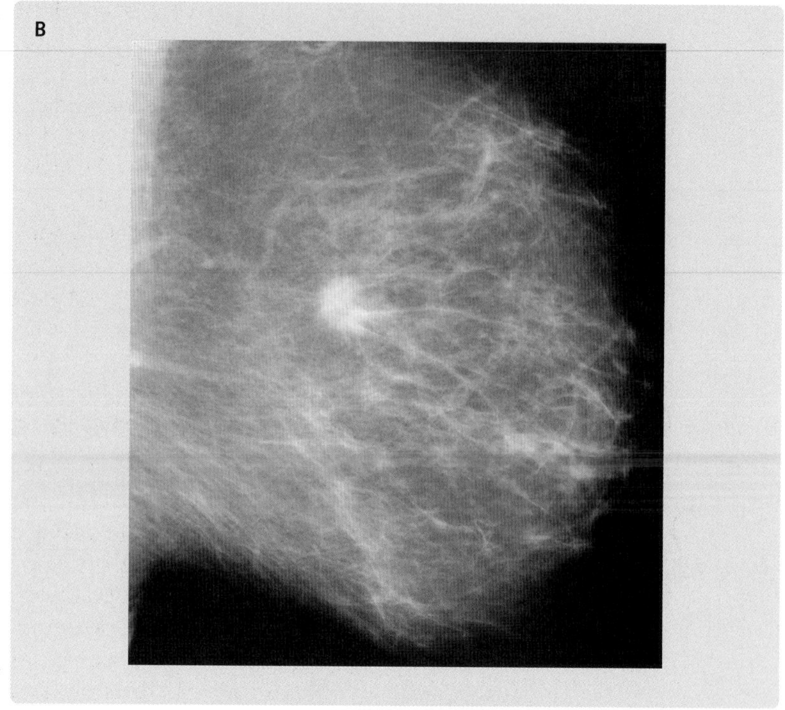

Fig. 19.10 Cont'd (B) Mammogram of a breast containing a carcinoma (from Sutton, 6th edn).

Ultrasonography

Ultrasonography uses the reflection of harmless, high-frequency sound waves to determine the composition of various tissues throughout the body. The reflected sound waves are processed to produce an image in which fluid appears black and denser structures appear white.

Ultrasonography may be used to evaluate the size and composition of masses, determining if they are cystic or solid. Masses are commonly examined by ultrasound in the breast, ovaries, testes, thyroid gland and adrenal glands. An example is shown in Fig. 19.11.

Ultrasound imaging is routinely used to examine the developing fetus and to investigate any abnormalities that may be suspected clinically. An example is shown in Fig. 19.12.

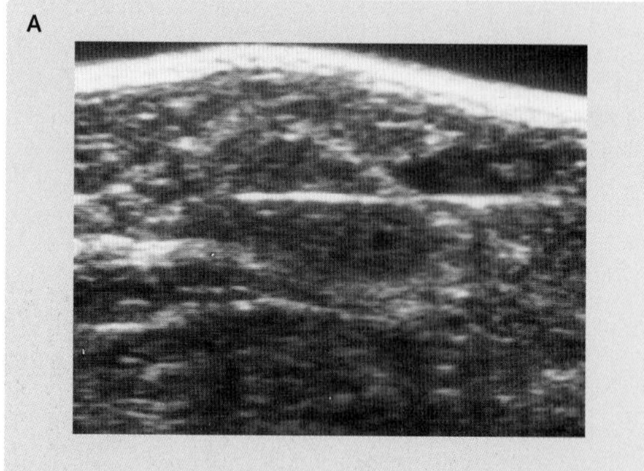

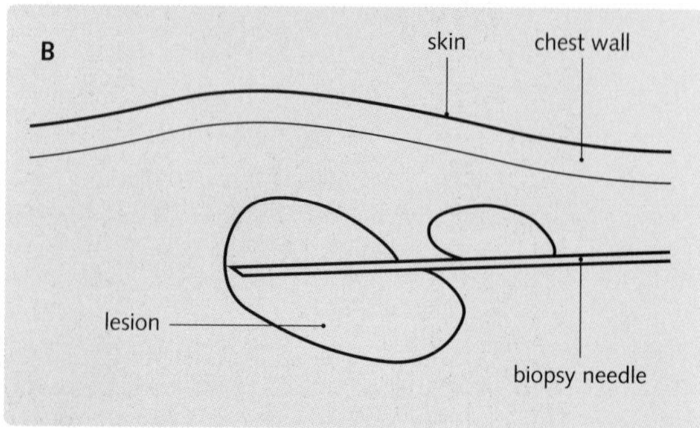

Fig. 19.11 (A) Ultrasound-guided needle biopsy of a breast mass. (B) Line drawing of A. Note that the needle is introduced parallel to the chest wall. (A, from Sutton, 6th edn.)

Computed tomography

Computed tomography (CT) produces cross-sectional images using X-rays, typically in the axial or horizontal plane. The X-ray emitter rotates about the patient and the computer reconstructs an image by combining views from the multiple X-ray detectors. The computer can differentiate over 2000 densities; this is significantly more than conventional

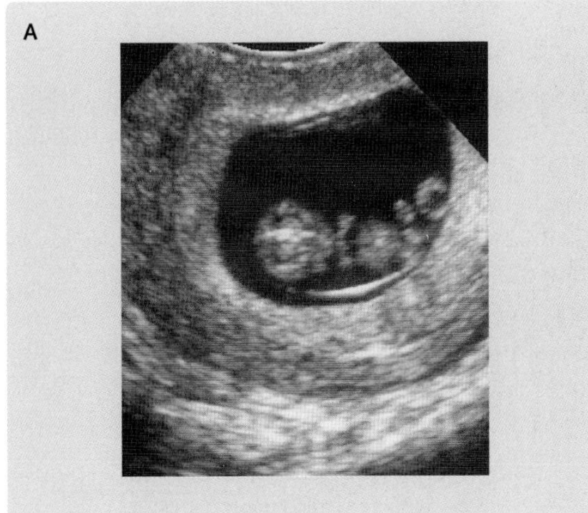

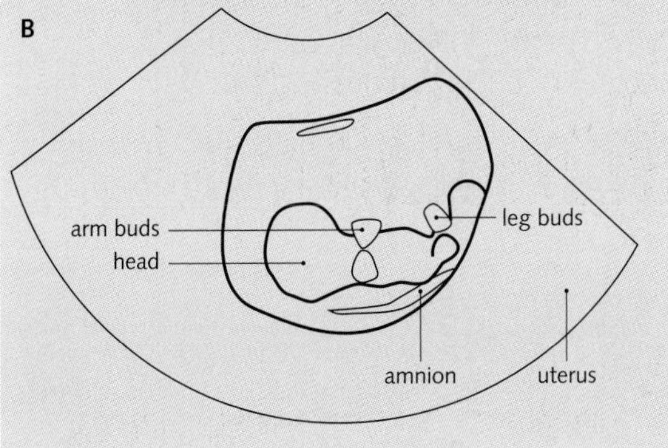

Fig. 19.12 (A) Transvaginal ultrasound scan of a normal 8- to 9-week fetus. (B) Line drawing of A. (A from Grainger & Allison, 4th edn.)

X-ray films. Bone appears white and other soft tissues are grey to black. An example is shown in Fig. 19.13.

CT scanning has applications in almost all disease processes, particularly oncology and neurology. It can also be used for planning accurate biopsy and interventions.

In a similar manner to conventional radiography, contrast media are routinely used in CT to enhance imaging of tissues and vasculature. The same contrast media can be used as for conventional radiography.

Magnetic resonance imaging

Magnetic resonance imaging (MRI) produces cross-sectional images without using ionizing radiation. MRI uses strong external magnetic fields formed by magnetic coils around the patient to manipulate the protons that form the nucleus of hydrogen atoms. The protons behave like miniature magnets, which line up to the strong magnetic field and gain energy in the process. Once the magnetic field is turned off, the protons release the energy they gained by inducing a current in the magnetic coils that produced the magnetic field. This current is detected and processed into a computerized image.

The hydrogen atoms detected are generally in water (H_2O). There are two main methods of processing the image:

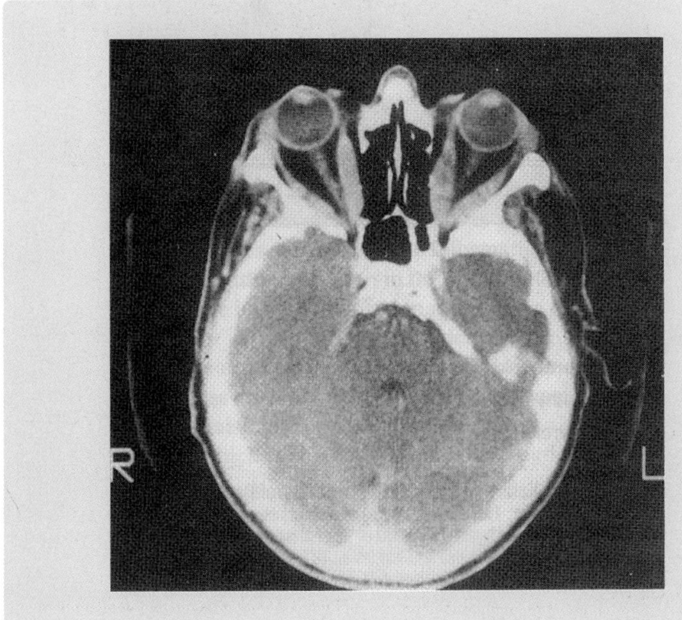

Fig. 19.13 CT scan showing exophthalmos in a patient with Graves' disease (from Edwards *et al.*, *Davidson's Principles and Practice of Medicine*, 17th edn).

- T1-weighted images: good anatomical detail; water is black.
- T2-weighted images: good detail for pathological changes; water is white.

An example is shown in Fig. 19.14.

Radioisotope scans

Certain chemicals are absorbed more rapidly by different tissues, for example iodine is actively absorbed by the thyroid gland. By tagging a chemical with a radioactive element (i.e. a radioisotope), uptake in the target tissue can be monitored using a gamma camera (this is called scintigraphy). This pattern of isotope uptake within the gland can expose abnormal areas.

This method is especially suitable for the thyroid gland because of the highly selective uptake of iodine. By administering an oral dose of ^{123}I (a radioactive isotope of iodine) the activity of different areas within the gland can be detected between 5 and 24 hours later. It allows measurement of:

- Hyperactivity.
- Abnormal anatomy.
- Tumours or nodules, including size and location.

Most tumours show up as inactive 'cold' spots; however, hypersecretory tumours show up as active 'hot' spots.

A better resolution can be achieved using intravenous technetium-99m pertechnetate. This substance is also less toxic and allows scanning just 20 minutes after injection. Examples are shown in Fig. 19.15.

Different substances can be used to scan the parathyroid and adrenal glands:

- Parathyroid glands—technetium-99m Sestamibi.
- Adrenal cortex—^{131}I-iodonorcholesterol (NP-59) or ^{75}Se-selenomethylnorcholesterol.
- Adrenal medulla—^{131}I-metaiodobenzylguanidine (mIBG).

Radioactive iodine is potentially harmful to the thyroid gland. Lugol's solution, which contains non-radioactive iodine, is given both the day before and on the test day to reduce the uptake of radioactive iodine by the thyroid gland.

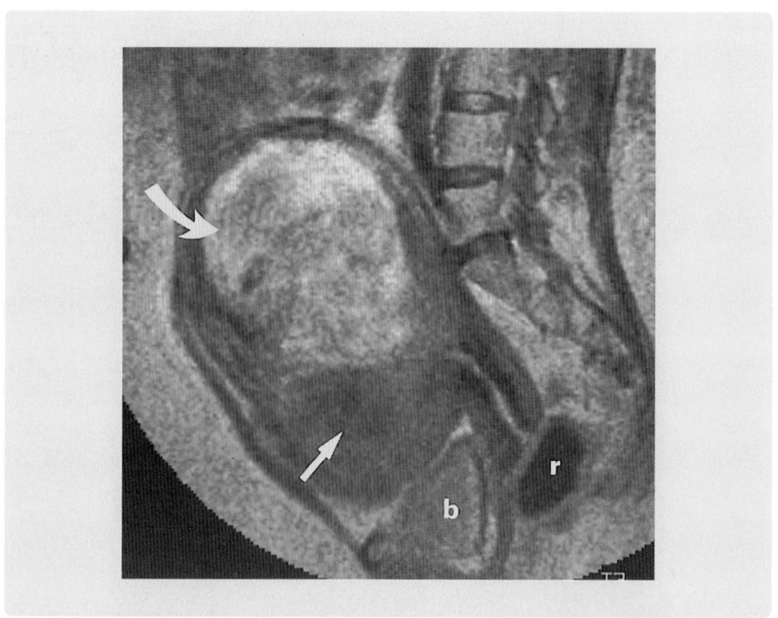

Fig. 19.14 MRI scan (T2-weighted spin echo image) of large uterine leiomyomas, showing areas of high signal (curved arrow) and low signal (straight arrow). b, bladder; r, rectum (from Sutton, 6th edn).

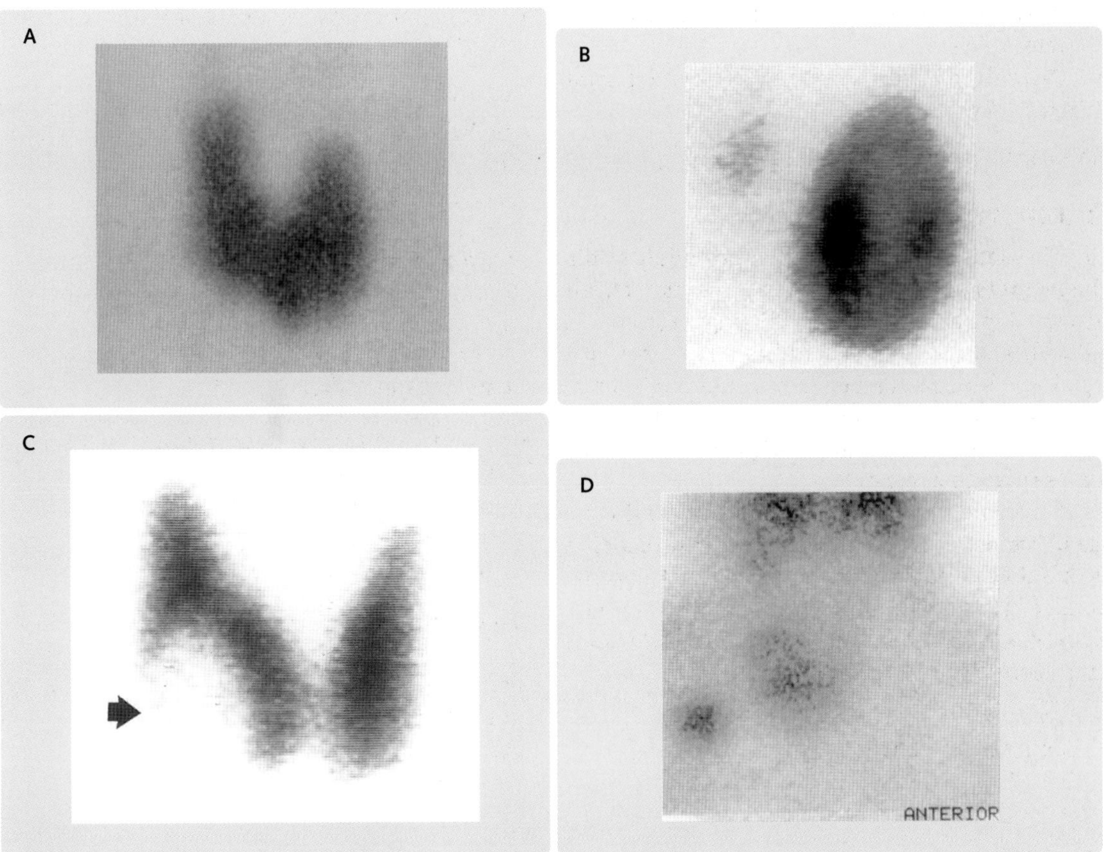

Fig. 19.15 Radioisotope thyroid images using technetium-99m pertechnetate. (A) Scan showing increased uptake throughout the gland in a patient with Graves' disease. (B) A patient with a single toxic nodule; the remainder of the gland is suppressed. (C) Increased uptake in a patient with Graves' disease but decreased uptake in a non-toxic (cold) lump (arrowed) consistent with a thyroid cancer or cyst. (D) ^{99m}Tc hexakis-2-methoxyisobutyl isonitrile (MIBI) scan of recurrent papillary thyroid carcinoma not seen on ^{131}I scanning (A, from Grainger & Allison, 4th edn; B–D, from Murray & Ell, 2nd edn).

SELF-ASSESSMENT

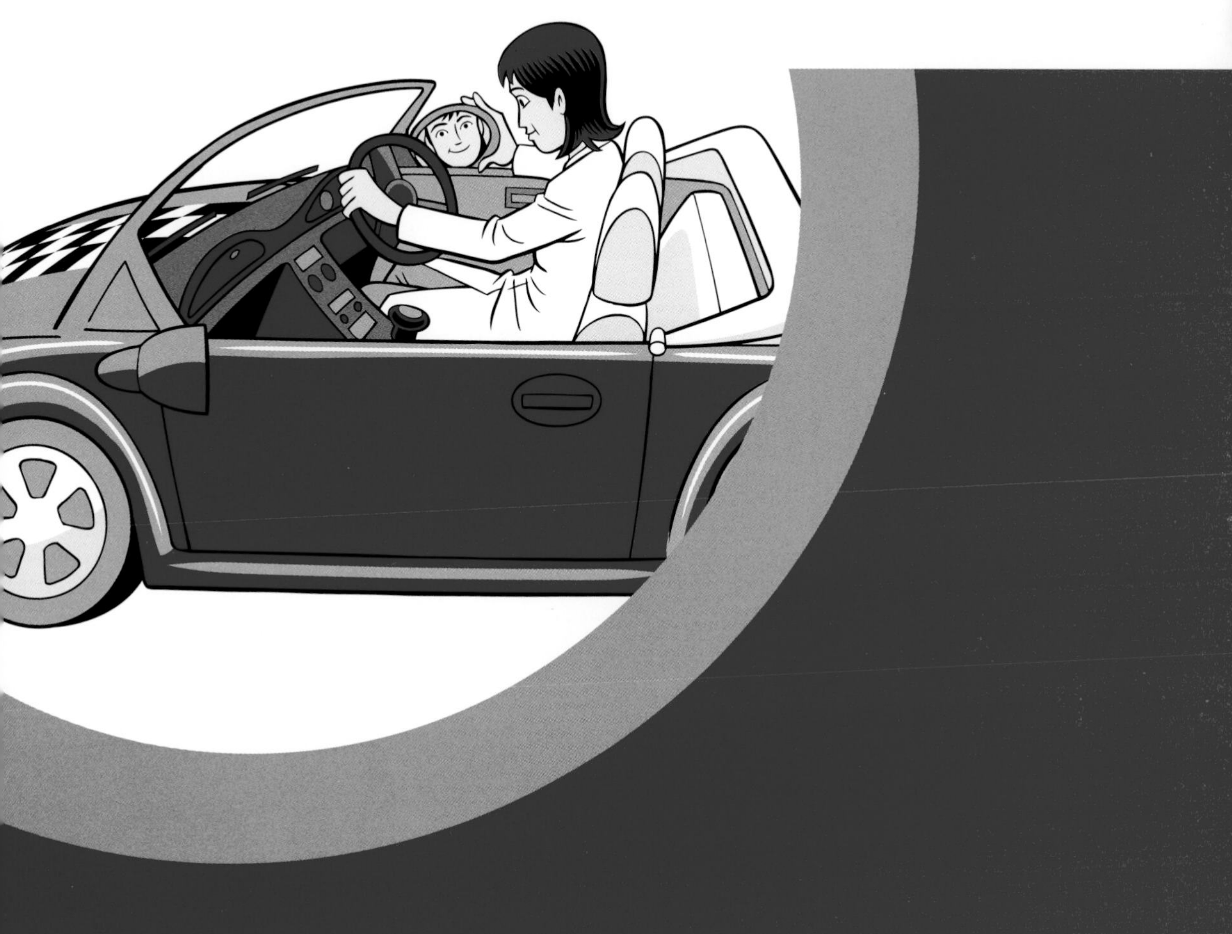

Multiple-choice questions (MCQs)

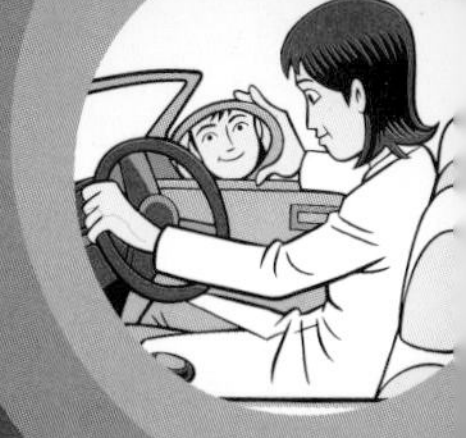

Indicate whether each answer is true or false.

Chapter 1 Overview of the endocrine system

1. **Concerning types of hormone:**
   a. Steroid hormones act through intracellular receptors.
   b. Polypeptide hormones readily cross plasma membranes.
   c. Many polypeptide hormones are synthesized by the cleavage of larger polypeptides.
   d. Several major hormones are synthesized by modification of the amino acid tyrosine.
   e. Steroid hormones are stored in secretory vesicles ready for release.

2. **Insulin receptors:**
   a. Insulin acts through tyrosine kinase receptors.
   b. Tyrosine kinase receptors are located in the surface of cells.
   c. This type of receptor is also used by adrenaline.
   d. The serine side chains of amino acid residues are phosphorylated.
   e. Their main effect is to stimulate protein synthesis directly.

3. **G-protein receptors:**
   a. Are located on the cell membrane.
   b. Often use cATP as a second messenger.
   c. G-proteins bind GDP in their resting state.
   d. When the receptor is active following stimulation the G-protein is attached to the receptor protein.
   e. The receptor protein is a type of glycoprotein.

4. **Concerning eicosanoids:**
   a. Prostaglandins are usually transported in the blood to act on distant cells.
   b. Prostaglandins are synthesized from a phospholipid found in the cell membrane.
   c. Leukotrienes are synthesized by the cyclooxygenase pathway.
   d. Prostaglandins are only synthesized by specialized cells.
   e. Eicosanoids are stored in secretory granules.

5. **Hormonal feedback:**
   a. Polypeptide hormones can readily cross the blood–brain barrier.
   b. Feedback to the hypothalamus is by intracellular receptors only.
   c. If a variable altered by a hormone (e.g. plasma osmolarity) affects the regulation of the same hormone this is considered to be feedback.
   d. The hypothalamus and pituitary gland are the only sites of hormonal feedback.
   e. In a healthy person thyroid hormones inhibit the synthesis of TSH at all times.

Chapter 2 The hypothalamus and the pituitary gland

6. **The hypothalamus:**
   a. Is located at the base of the brain either side of the 3rd ventricle.
   b. Secretes hormones that act directly on many endocrine organs.
   c. Synthesizes mainly steroid hormones.
   d. Stimulates ACTH secretion by direct neural stimulation of the pituitary gland.
   e. Contains nerve cells derived from the fetal ectoderm layer.

7. **The anterior pituitary gland:**
   a. Secretes the gonadotrophins LH and FSH.
   b. Is a direct extension of the hypothalamus.
   c. Is a relation of the optic chiasma.
   d. Secretes only polypeptide and glycoprotein hormones.
   e. Secretes a hormone that is the main regulator of aldosterone secretion.

8. **The posterior pituitary gland:**
   a. Secretes aldosterone, which regulates fluid balance.
   b. Is essential for breastfeeding.
   c. Synthesizes two small polypeptide hormones.
   d. Is covered superiorly by a layer of dura mater.
   e. Contains glial support cells called pituicytes.

9. **A 48-year-old woman presents with loss of her central vision:**
   a. This is a well-recognized symptom of pituitary adenomas.
   b. Pituitary adenomas are most commonly prolactinomas.
   c. Pituitary adenomas often present with disorders of several pituitary hormones.
   d. The diagnosis could be confirmed by ultrasound.
   e. Pituitary adenomas are often treated by surgical removal.

Chapter 3 The thyroid gland

10. Concerning thyroid hormones:

a. They regulate the rate of metabolism in cells.
b. They are transported in the blood bound to a plasma protein called thyroglobulin.
c. Most tissues in the body can add an iodine molecule to T_3 to form the more active molecule called T_4.
d. They act through intracellular receptors.
e. They are synthesized from the same amino acid as adrenaline.

11. The thyroid gland:

a. Responds to TSH secreted by the anterior pituitary gland.
b. Is drained by veins that are closely related to nerves to the larynx.
c. Is involved in the regulation of calcium.
d. Is bound to the trachea by the pre-tracheal fascia.
e. Usually has a pyramidal lobe, which joins the isthmus.

12. A 43-year-old woman presents with weight gain and lethargy. A blood test shows a raised level of TSH:

a. Hypothyroidism is a common disease, especially in women.
b. Hypothyroidism is responsible for 10% of obesity.
c. In children hypothyroidism causes dwarfism.
d. Hypothyroidism is often a long-term complication of the treatment of hyperthyroidism.
e. Hypothyroidism should be treated with thyrotrophin-releasing hormone (TRH) to return blood TSH levels to normal.

13. A 45-year-old woman presents with weight loss, irritability and sweating that is diagnosed as hyperthyroidism:

a. Graves' disease is an autoimmune disease that stimulates thyroid cells causing hyperthyroidism.
b. A history about what clothes she wears is of clinical interest.
c. The diagnosis of hyperthyroidism can be made by measuring TSH, T_3 and T_4 only.
d. The history of weight loss and excess thyroid hormone secretion makes carcinoma a likely diagnosis.
e. It could be treated with the drug bromocriptine.

14. A 79-year-old woman presents with a lump in her throat that has developed over the last few months. Thyroid function tests and fine-needle aspiration are performed:

a. A papillary carcinoma develops from the follicle cells.
b. If she also has features of Cushing's syndrome then it is more likely to be a medullary carcinoma.
c. If it is a carcinoma then her thyroid hormone levels are likely to be high.
d. Anaplastic carcinoma has a particularly poor prognosis.
e. Anaplastic carcinoma of the thyroid invades mainly by vascular spread.

15. A 53-year-old woman presents with a lump in the front of her throat:

a. If it rises when she protrudes her tongue, it is almost certainly part of the thyroid gland.
b. If the lump is a toxic adenoma her TSH levels will be raised.
c. Cardiac arrhythmia is a sign of hyperthyroidism.
d. A fine-needle aspiration should almost always be performed for cytology (having taken into account other factors).
e. Surgery could potentially result in chronic hypercalcaemia.

Chapter 4 The adrenal glands

16. The cortex of the adrenal gland:

a. Secretes hormones derived from cholesterol.
b. Develops from neural crest tissue.
c. Is arranged in follicles that contain stored hormone.
d. Responds directly to corticotrophin-releasing hormone (CRH).
e. The zona fasciculata secretes cortisol.

17. Adrenocorticotrophic hormone (ACTH):

a. Acts mainly on the medulla of the adrenal gland.
b. Secretion is stimulated by CRH and inhibited by cortisol.
c. Is secreted by corticotrophs in the hypothalamus.
d. The peak of secretion occurs early in the morning before waking.
e. Inhibits the release of adrenal androgens.

18. Stress:

a. Stimulates the release of growth hormone.
b. Stimulates the release of cortisol.
c. Causes a rise in blood glucose levels.
d. Can be tolerated better in the absence of cortisol.
e. Activates the parasympathetic nervous system.

19. Concerning the hormonal release of catecholamines:

a. These hormones prepare the body for fight or flight.
b. More adrenaline is secreted than noradrenaline.
c. They increase the heart rate and stroke volume.
d. They lower blood glucose.
e. They are secreted by cells that are equivalent to preganglionic sympathetic neurons.

20. A 59-year-old man has been taking corticosteroids for 7 years for an inflammatory condition, but he is starting to notice side effects:

a. He is suffering from Cushing's disease.
b. His blood glucose levels will probably be high.
c. He will probably have lost weight.
d. His skin will be thick and prone to bruising.
e. The steroids should be stopped immediately to prevent further complications.

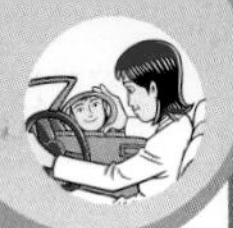

21. A 41-year-old man with vomiting, hypotension and confusion is diagnosed with Addison's disease.

a. This is an excess of aldosterone secretion.
b. If the cause was primary adrenal insufficiency the patient is likely to have increased skin pigmentation.
c. It can be diagnosed using the Synacthen® test.
d. A history of growing beetroot is of clinical interest.
e. The treatment must often be continued for life.

22. A 43-year-old man is investigated for hypertension; this reveals that he has Conn's syndrome.

a. Conn's syndrome is a type of primary hyperaldosteronism.
b. The plasma potassium levels will probably be low.
c. Conn's syndrome is an adenoma of the adrenal medulla.
d. About 27% of hypertension is caused by raised aldosterone levels.
e. Testing the blood levels of aldosterone alone can show hyperaldosteronism.

23. A 25-year-old man was admitted to hospital with a severe headache and found to have a very high blood pressure. This resolved spontaneously before treatment could be given:

a. You should measure the quantity of vanillylmandelic acid in his urine to exclude phaeochromocytoma.
b. Phaeochromocytoma is a tumour of the adrenal cortex.
c. Phaeochromocytoma can be treated with diuretics and ACE inhibitors and repeated scans to monitor growth.
d. The hypertensive episodes are caused by fluctuations in blood volume.
e. During the hypertensive attack his pupils were probably dilated.

Chapter 5 The pancreas and diabetes

24. Insulin:

a. Deficiency causes diabetes mellitus.
b. Is normally secreted after a meal.
c. Stimulates the uptake and use of glucose in muscle cells.
d. Is secreted by the α-cells of the islets of Langerhans in the pancreas.
e. Secretion ceases entirely during prolonged starvation.

25. The pancreas:

a. Has a retroperitoneal position.
b. Secretes hormones into the duodenum via the pancreatic duct.
c. Is a relation of the left kidney, stomach and spleen.
d. Develops from two buds that grow out of the endodermal digestive tract.
e. The hormone-secreting cells are richly innervated.

26. Concerning hypoglycaemia:

a. Is present if blood glucose levels are 3.7 mmol/L.
b. Stimulates the release of glucagon.
c. This glucagon is released by the exocrine pancreas.
d. Inhibits the release of adrenaline.
e. Can be detected directly by the islet cells of the pancreas.

27. Glucagon:

a. Consists of multiple glucose molecules.
b. Inhibits the secretion of insulin.
c. Inhibits the actions of insulin.
d. Secretion is inhibited by insulin.
e. Has a catabolic and antianabolic effect.

28. A 10-year-old boy presents with tiredness for the last 3 months, with malaise and vomiting in the last month:

a. This could be caused by diabetes mellitus (DM).
b. DM could be excluded if there is no glucose in his urine.
c. A history of weight gain and polyuria would increase the probability of this diagnosis.
d. His diabetes could be treated by carefully regulating his diet for several months until the type of diabetes is determined.
e. If diabetes mellitus is confirmed he will need an urgent referral to an ophthalmologist to treat retinopathy as this can cause irreversible blindness.

29. An elderly woman is referred from an ophthalmologist due to concerns about her vision:

a. This could be the presentation of a type of diabetes mellitus treatable with oral medications.
b. Retinopathy is a common microvascular complication of all types of diabetes mellitus.
c. Blindness caused by retinopathy can be prevented by frequent screening and treatment.
d. Microvascular complications of diabetes mellitus are associated with hyaline arteriolosclerosis.
e. Diabetes mellitus could be excluded by a urine dipstick test.

30. A 76-year-old man is found to have glycosuria:

a. His blood glucose levels must be above 10 mmol/L.
b. This is a common presentation of NIDDM.
c. If this is NIDDM he can be reassured that he will not need to inject insulin.
d. NIDDM is often associated with obesity and hypotension called syndrome X.
e. NIDDM is caused by autoantibodies against the β-cells of the islets of Langerhans.

Chapter 6 Up and coming hormones

31. Concerning leptin:

a. It is a hormone secreted by muscle cells.
b. It is essential for fertility and puberty.

c. It helps to regulate food intake.
d. Oral leptin will reduce food intake in the majority of patients.
e. Inherited leptin deficiency is a common cause of obesity.

32. Melatonin:

a. Is a polypeptide hormone.
b. Is secreted mainly by the pineal gland.
c. Increased secretion causes pigmentation of the skin.
d. Acts to reset the preoptic nucleus of the hypothalamus.
e. Is secreted in response to stimulation of the retina.

33. A 53-year-old man has suffered from recurrent peptic ulcers that are difficult to treat medically:

a. In Zollinger–Ellison syndrome there is a tumour in the stomach.
b. This condition affects about 1 in 1000 people.
c. The tumour secretes gastrin.
d. Gastrin stimulates the chief cells of the stomach to secrete acid.
e. This tumour is fairly often associated with MEN I.

Chapter 7 Endocrine control of fluid balance

34. Renin:

a. Is an enzyme secreted by the juxtaglomerular complexes in the kidney.
b. Is secreted in response to low sodium or low blood pressure.
c. Acts on angiotensinogen to form angiotensin I.
d. Release is inhibited by angiotensin-converting enzyme (ACE) inhibitors.
e. Indirectly stimulates aldosterone release.

35. Antidiuretic hormone (ADH):

a. Increases water excretion.
b. Is secreted from specialized neurons.
c. Acts on the proximal tubule of the kidney nephrons to raise permeability to water.
d. Secretion is stimulated by raised plasma osmolarity.
e. Causes vasodilation of arteries to control blood pressure.

36. The following factors cause a rise in blood pressure:

a. An increase in blood volume.
b. Reduced peripheral vascular resistance.
c. High renin levels.
d. High angiotensinogen levels.
e. High adrenaline levels.

37. A 27-year-old man has recently started to excrete large volumes of urine:

a. His fasting blood sugar should be measured in case he has diabetes mellitus.
b. It could be caused by hypocalcaemia.
c. He is likely to have reduced skin turgor.
d. It could be caused by a urinary tract infection.
e. The water stimulation test is used to confirm diabetes insipidus.

Chapter 8 Endocrine control of calcium homeostasis

38. The parathyroid glands:

a. In most people there are three pairs of parathyroid glands, which lie posterior to the thyroid gland.
b. Secrete parathyroid hormone and calcitonin to regulate calcium levels.
c. Are derived from the mesenchyme surrounding the thyroid gland.
d. Secrete parathyroid hormone in response to low blood calcium.
e. Are supplied by branches of the lingual artery.

39. Concerning calcium:

a. The majority of calcium within the body is stored in bone.
b. A rise in intracellular calcium levels stimulates muscle contraction.
c. A fall in intracellular calcium levels stimulates exocytosis (e.g. hormone secretion).
d. Osteoclasts release calcium by eroding bone.
e. Low calcium stimulates the activation of vitamin D by acting directly on the kidney.

40. Vitamin D:

a. Is derived from cholesterol.
b. Deficiency results in poor bone formation.
c. Acts mainly on the kidneys to increase the reabsorption of calcium.
d. Can be synthesized in the skin by the action of infra-red light.
e. Must be activated by conversion to 24,25-dihydroxy-vitamin D_3 in the kidney.

41. Parathyroid hormone:

a. Is usually secreted by four small glands located anteriorly to the thyroid gland in the neck.
b. Is secreted in response to low blood calcium levels.
c. Is a modified amino acid hormone.
d. Acts chiefly on the intestines to increase the absorption of calcium.
e. Stimulates the activation of 25-hydroxyvitamin D_3 by acting on 1α-hydroxylase in the kidney.

42. Calcitonin:

a. This hormone is secreted by parafollicular cells in the thyroid gland.
b. The main stimulus for calcitonin release is high blood calcium.
c. Is essential for normal calcium regulation.
d. Is a polypeptide hormone.
e. The secretory cells are types of APUD cells.

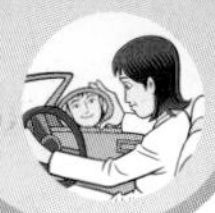

43. **A 52-year-old man presents with a fractured head of femur. A history is difficult to obtain as the patient seems confused but he does complain of abdominal pain:**
    a. Hypercalcaemia would be consistent with this history.
    b. Hypercalcaemia can be caused by secondary hyperparathyroidism.
    c. Hypercalcaemia can be caused by a parathyroid adenoma.
    d. Failure to treat parathyroid adenomas increases the risk of renal failure.
    e. If a parathyroid adenoma was found in a very young patient it could be a component of MEN I.

Chapter 9 Endocrine control of growth

44. **Growth hormone:**
    a. Is released from the posterior pituitary gland.
    b. Is a polypeptide hormone.
    c. Stimulates growth in many tissues by direct stimulation.
    d. Secretion usually increases at night.
    e. Secretion normally ceases after puberty.

45. **Insulin-like growth factors:**
    a. Are peptide hormones secreted mainly by the kidney.
    b. Blood levels are higher during sleep.
    c. Stimulate the uptake of glucose into cells.
    d. Stimulate the release of growth hormone.
    e. Act via tyrosine kinase receptors on the cell surface.

46. **A 32-year-old man is referred by his dentist with change in his jaw that the dentist cannot explain:**
    a. This could be because the jaw has enlarged due to an excess of growth hormone.
    b. If there is an excess of growth hormone he is likely to be taller than he was 5 years ago.
    c. This excess of growth hormones is called gigantism.
    d. He has an increased risk of insulinomas.
    e. The most common cause is a somatotroph adenoma of the anterior pituitary gland.

Chapter 10 Endocrine disorders of neoplastic origin

47. **A 79-year-old man has been diagnosed with lung cancer. This is may be associated with secretion of:**
    a. Parathyroid hormone, causing hypercalcaemia.
    b. Cortisol, causing hypoglycaemia.
    c. Prolactin, causing gynaecomastia.
    d. Testosterone, causing aggression.
    e. ADH, causing diabetes insipidus.

48. **The man in question 23 is investigated further:**
    a. The adrenal tumour will probably be palpable on abdominal examination.
    b. He also has a lump in his neck: this suggests MEN II.
    c. You should order a CT scan to exclude pancreatic tumours found in MEN II.
    d. The thyroid lump probably has a papillary pattern.
    e. Other members of his family may have similar tumours.

Chapter 11 Development of the reproductive system

49. **Regarding development of the male reproductive system:**
    a. The vas deferens develops from the mesonephric (Wolffian) ducts.
    b. Early differentiation from the indifferent stage is caused by expression of the sex-determining region (SRY) on the X chromosome.
    c. The scrotum develops from the same structures that form the labia majora in the female.
    d. The testes have a blood supply directly from the aorta.
    e. The primordial germ cells originate on the dorsal body wall of fetal abdomen.

50. **Regarding development of the female reproductive system:**
    a. The ovaries are derived from the same structure that forms the testes in the male.
    b. Müllerian inhibiting substance (MIS) is secreted to cause the male reproductive system to regress.
    c. The primordial oocytes begin a meiotic division before birth that is not completed until after puberty.
    d. Female and male development is the same until the sixth week.
    e. Ovarian stroma develops as an outgrowth of the paramesonephric ducts.

51. **Concerning male puberty:**
    a. Puberty occurs at an earlier age in boys than girls.
    b. Testosterone stimulates growth of the long bones.
    c. Hypothalamic GnRH secretion is inhibited prior to puberty.
    d. Puberty is said to have started when the testes reach 12 mL.
    e. When the gonads begin to secrete sex steroids at puberty it is called adrenarche.

52. **Concerning female puberty:**
    a. Body weight is a better predictor of when menarche will occur than age.
    b. Menarche is the first sign of female puberty.
    c. Pubic and axillary hair grow as a result of adrenal androgens.
    d. The first ovulation usually occurs at menarche.
    e. The ovarian follicles mature into secondary follicles during puberty.

Chapter 12 The female reproductive system

53. Concerning the ovaries:

a. They are located on the posterior of the broad ligament of the uterus.
b. New follicles can be formed until puberty.
c. Each month several follicles develop in response to FSH.
d. At ovulation, the oocyte leaves the ovary and enters the peritoneal cavity.
e. All blood vessels, lymphatics and nerves reach the ovary via the hilum.

54. Concerning the uterine tubes:

a. They form the superior border of the broad ligament.
b. Fertilization usually occurs in their uterine section.
c. Their blood supply is derived from the ovarian and uterine arteries.
d. They open into the peritoneal cavity forming a connection to the outside world via the vagina.
e. They develop from the paramesonephric (Müllerian) ducts.

55. Concerning the cervix:

a. The cervix is considered to be a section of the vagina.
b. The opening of the cervix into the vagina is called the internal os.
c. The endocervix is usually lined by columnar epithelium.
d. During childbirth the cervix dilates to 5 cm diameter.
e. The action of progesterone allows the cervix to dilate at childbirth.

56. Concerning the vagina:

a. The acidic environment is maintained by commensal *Candida* yeast.
b. The epithelial lining of the vagina is shed during menstruation.
c. It is lined by simple columnar epithelium throughout.
d. It is a posterior relation of the bladder.
e. It develops as an outgrowth from the urethra.

57. Concerning the breast:

a. The glandular tissue of the breast is derived from specialized hair follicles.
b. Until puberty the male and female breasts are structurally indistinguishable.
c. A single lactiferous duct opens at each nipple.
d. The breast tissue can move freely over the underlying muscle.
e. Progesterone stimulates the development of the secretory tissue during puberty.

58. Concerning oestrogen:

a. Blood levels are usually higher in females than males.
b. It acts via cell-surface receptors.
c. It is essential for the normal development of female external genitalia.
d. It is not secreted in the luteal phase of the menstrual cycle.
e. It acts on the anterior pituitary gland where it has a variable effect of LH and FSH secretion.

59. Concerning progesterone:

a. Blood levels are low between menstruation and ovulation.
b. Progesterone causes smooth muscles to relax during pregnancy.
c. In the non-pregnant female, the main source of progesterone is the endometrium.
d. Progesterone is a complex steroid hormone that is synthesized in many steps from cholesterol.
e. Progesterone's main role is to promote growth of the reproductive organs.

60. Hormones during the menstrual cycle:

a. LH levels are highest during menstruation.
b. Oestrogen and progesterone stimulate the release of gonadotrophins around the middle of the cycle.
c. Human chorionic gonadotrophin (hCG) rises in the follicular phase of the menstrual cycle.
d. LH is a glycoprotein hormone released by the anterior pituitary gland.
e. Oestrogen stimulates the synthesis of progesterone.

61. Concerning ovarian follicles:

a. Each follicle contains a single oocyte.
b. They develop into primary follicles from primordial follicles during puberty.
c. The thecal cells are the major site of oestrogen secretion.
d. Just before ovulation the follicles contain a fluid filled cavity called the antrum.
e. Several follicles begin to develop at the start of each menstrual cycle.

62. The corpus luteum:

a. Is the main source of hCG for the first 6 weeks after fertilization.
b. Is formed by the remaining granulosa and thecal cells of the mature follicle after ovulation.
c. Regresses in the absence of fertilization due to falling LH levels.
d. Has a characteristic blue colour due to the rapid metabolism required for hormone synthesis.
e. Is usually found in both ovaries during early pregnancy.

63. Concerning cyclical changes in the endometrium:

a. The endometrium begins to proliferate after ovulation.
b. The uterine glands secrete a fluid that is rich in glycogen in response to oestrogens.

c. Approximately 30 mL blood is lost during menstruation.
d. The entire endometrium is shed during menstruation.
e. Menstruation is caused by contraction of the uterine arteries causing ischaemia of the uterus.

Chapter 13 Disorders of the female reproductive system

64. A woman presents with infertility and amenorrhoea. On investigation this is diagnosed as polycystic ovarian syndrome:

a. She is likely to have the features of Cushing's syndrome.
b. Ultrasound is very useful for diagnosis.
c. This diagnosis would have been suspected if she had galactorrhoea.
d. This diagnosis would have been suspected if she had hirsutism.
e. Her blood levels of LH and FSH are likely to be raised.

65. A 32-year-old woman presents with menorrhagia and pre-menstrual abdominal pain that is diagnosed as endometriosis:

a. Endometriosis can be caused by bacterial infections following trauma.
b. She has a higher risk of infertility.
c. Endometriosis is usually diagnosed through ultrasound.
d. Endometriosis is often associated with hirsutism.
e. Adhesions can develop causing constant pain.

66. A 46-year-old woman presents with abdominal pain and tenderness a month after having an IUD inserted:

a. She probably has chronic pelvic inflammatory disease.
b. The most common cause of pelvic inflammatory disease is from STDs.
c. In this woman's disease, the infectious organism is probably *Chlamydia*.
d. Pelvic inflammatory disease sometimes causes damage to the uterine tubes.
e. The woman will probably need a laparoscopy.

67. A 37-year-old woman presents with menorrhagia and deep dyspareunia. On bimanual vaginal examination, a lump is felt outside the uterus on the left:

a. The lump is likely to be palpable on careful abdominal examination.
b. A fluid-filled cyst will have a dark centre on an ultrasound scan.
c. If the lump is found to contain tissues that resemble teeth and skin it is probably malignant.
d. A yellow-coloured cyst would suggest the woman has endometriosis.
e. Most ovarian neoplasia originates from the epithelial component of the ovary.

68. A 27-year-old woman presents with an intensely itchy vulva and vaginal discharge:

a. This is a common presentation of herpes simplex infection.
b. A vaginal swab showing the presence of lactobacilli would prompt antibiotic treatment with metronidazole.
c. A thick, white discharge is commonly caused by the fungal infection often called thrush.
d. Thrush is normally a sexually transmitted infection.
e. If *Chlamydia* infection is not treated it can cause pelvic inflammatory disease.

69. A 51-year-old woman presents with menorrhagia that is diagnosed as leiomyoma:

a. This is a common, benign tumour often called a fibroid.
b. Fibroids form in the myometrium.
c. Fibroids grow mainly in the presence of progesterone.
d. They can progress into endometrial carcinoma.
e. After the menopause it will probably get better.

70. A 49-year-old woman presents with a lump in her left breast:

a. This is likely to be a cyst caused by fibrocystic change.
b. It is likely to be a fibroadenoma.
c. The presence of skin dimpling on the breast when the woman leans forwards suggests breast cancer.
d. The presence of a red eczema-like rash around the nipple suggests an infection.
e. The possibility of breast cancer can often be excluded by careful examination.

71. A 50-year-old woman presents with nipple discharge in her right breast:

a. If a lump is palpable near the nipple this is likely to be mammary duct ectasia.
b. If the lump is malignant the breast may have the appearance of an orange skin.
c. The appearance in (b) is caused by local invasion of the sweat glands.
d. A strong family history of ovarian cancer would prompt investigation for a *BRAC* mutation.
e. Early menarche is a risk factor for breast cancer.

72. A 51-year-old woman is suffering from oligomenorrhoea and hot flushes that are diagnosed as the early stages of the menopause. She has previously had two children and no gynaecological surgery:

a. This is quite early to start the menopause.
b. If she desires HRT, oestrogen should be given alone.
c. If she took HRT it would lower her risk of fracturing the neck of her femur.
d. HRT is associated with an increased risk of cardiovascular disease.
e. Her gonadotrophin levels are probably reduced.

Chapter 14 The male reproductive system

73. Concerning the testes:

a. After puberty they continuously produce sperm.
b. The seminiferous tubules are lined by testosterone-secreting Leydig cells.
c. They are surrounded by the tunica vaginalis, which is derived from the peritoneum.
d. They are divided into lobes, each of which contains 20 seminiferous tubules.
e. Blood from the right testis usually drains into the right renal vein.

74. The epididymis:

a. Is 'Z' shaped.
b. Is a major site of spermatogenesis.
c. Is formed from a single tube.
d. Is found within the testis.
e. Transmits sperm to the seminal vesicles where they are stored in preparation for ejaculation.

75. Concerning the penis:

a. It is composed of two corpora cavernosa and one corpus spongiosum.
b. The body of the penis is derived from the genital tubercle.
c. Erection is maintained by the parasympathetic innervation.
d. The structures that transmit sperm and urine are on opposing sides of the penis.
e. The penis enters the cervix during sexual intercourse.

76. Concerning spermatogenesis:

a. Spermatocytes are stem cells that develop into spermatozoa.
b. As they develop spermatids migrate between the Sertoli cells.
c. FSH stimulates the Sertoli cells to synthesize testosterone receptors.
d. Spermatogenesis can only take place at temperatures of 37°C or above.
e. Spermatozoa only complete their second meiotic division when they reach the epididymis.

77. Concerning spermatozoa:

a. The front of the nucleus is surrounded by a giant lysosome.
b. Mitochondria are found mainly in the head of the sperm.
c. The tail contains microtubules derived from a centriole.
d. The spermatozoon is only motile after maturation in the epididymis.
e. The end piece forms the majority of the spermatozoon's length.

78. An elderly man presents with recurrent urinary tract infections and on questioning he admits he has difficulty urinating:

a. He probably has carcinoma of the prostate gland.
b. Prostatic cancer usually develops in the larger peripheral zone glands.
c. hCG is a useful tumour marker for prostatic cancer.
d. Prostatic cancer can be treated by transurethral resection of the prostate.
e. Prostate cancer is known to metastasize to bones, where it forms characteristic osteosclerotic lesions.

79. A 20-year-old man presents with a lump on the surface of his right testicle:

a. If the lump is malignant it is probably a seminoma.
b. If the lump is a teratoma it is probably benign.
c. Teratomas commonly spread to the lungs.
d. Seminomas are very sensitive to radiotherapy.
e. 50% of testicular tumours are derived from the germ cells of the testes.

80. A 16-year-old boy presents with a swollen, tender, and painful right testicle:

a. This is consistent with epididymo-orchitis.
b. A history of recent ballet lessons is relevant.
c. This condition can be diagnosed from the history and treated with antibiotics.
d. This history is consistent with a varicocoele.
e. Varicocoeles can reduce fertility.

81. On a well baby check a transluminable lump is found in the scrotum:

a. This condition is much more common on the left of the scrotum.
b. If the testis is not distinguishable from the lump, it is probably a hydrocoele.
c. Congenital hydrocoeles are caused by absorption of amniotic fluid.
d. The majority of congenital hydrocoeles will resolve without treatment.
e. If a hydrocoele develops in an adult, the entire testicle should be removed.

82. A 7-year-old boy presents with a non-retractile foreskin:

a. This is called paraphimosis.
b. The boy will need a circumcision.
c. The foreskin usually becomes retractile by 5 years of age.
d. Before performing a circumcision it is important to check for hypospadias.
e. Infection of the glans with *Candida albicans* is called balanitis xerotica obliterans (BXO).

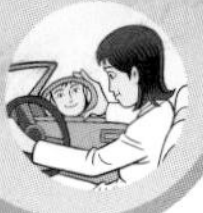

Chapter 15 The process of reproduction

83. Concerning fertilization:

a. It usually occurs in the uterus.
b. The sperm are capable of fertilization as soon as they enter the uterus.
c. The oocyte only completes the first meiotic division when the sperm penetrates the plasma membrane.
d. The sperm penetrates the zona pellucida by the secretion of acrosin from the acrosome.
e. Polyspermy (repeated fertilizations) is prevented by depolarization of the oocyte membrane and changes in the zona pellucida.

84. Hormonal contraception:

a. Oestrogen is used as a hormonal contraceptive agent on its own.
b. Progesterone can prevent implantation of the blastocyst.
c. The main contraceptive action of oestrogen is to inhibit follicle development.
d. Both oestrogen and progesterone inhibit LH to prevent ovulation.
e. Progesterone directly inactivates sperm.

85. Concerning the contraceptive pill:

a. The combined contraceptive pill must be taken without breaks to be effective.
b. The combined pill contains oestrogens and progesterone, both of which suppress ovulation.
c. The combined pill causes fewer adverse side effects than the progesterone-only pill.
d. Using the combined pill reduces the risk of ovarian cancer.
e. Small amounts of irregular bleeding in the first month requires urgent referral to a specialist.

86. Early fetal development:

a. At ovulation, the oocyte has completed its meiotic divisions.
b. For the first 4 days after conception the zona pellucida prevents an increase in embryo size.
c. After the first mitotic division the cells are called blastomeres.
d. Compaction is the process by which an inner and outer layer of cells is formed.
e. The zona pellucida is shed from the morula when it enters the uterus.

87. Implantation:

a. At the point of implantation the embryo is called a blastocyst.
b. The blastocyst is formed from two layers and a fluid-filled cavity.
c. The embryoblast splits into two layers, one of which has many nuclei but no dividing cell membranes.
d. The cytotrophoblast initially invades the functional endometrium.
e. The blastocyst normally implants with the embryoblast closest to the uterine cavity.

88. Development of the placenta:

a. When the first finger-like projections of the blastocyst develop spaces filled with maternal blood they are called primary chorionic villi.
b. The secondary chorionic villi invade the myometrium.
c. The lacunar spaces are eventually supplied by the spiral arteries.
d. The tertiary villi contain fetal blood vessels.
e. Before birth, the maternal and fetal blood supplies are separated by just three layers of cells.

89. Concerning the placenta:

a. It is derived mainly from maternal tissue.
b. The chorionic villi secrete hCG.
c. It is expelled from the uterus during the second stage of labour.
d. It contains a large space in which maternal and fetal blood can mix.
e. It is divided into cotyledons by fibrous septa from the fetal side.

Chapter 16 Pregnancy and birth

90. Regarding maternal adaptations to pregnancy:

a. The uterine myometrial cells hypertrophy.
b. Initial adaptations by the circulatory system are mostly due to an increase in blood volume.
c. Blood pressure rises throughout pregnancy.
d. The maternal metabolism uses more glucose, to conserve fat for storage.
e. The immune system becomes more active to prevent the risk of infection.

91. Labour and birth:

a. Progesterone inhibits contractions of the uterus.
b. When the baby's head is first seen, it usually faces the mother's thigh.
c. The pain of early labour is caused by stretching of the cervix.
d. Stimulation of the cervix causes oxytocin release.
e. Oxytocin stimulates the release of locally acting thromboxanes that cause contractions.

92. Regarding lactation:

a. Suckling during breastfeeding stimulates the secretion of oxytocin but inhibits prolactin secretion.
b. Colostrum has a lower fat content than normal maternal milk.
c. Oxytocin initiates the production of milk.
d. During pregnancy, oestrogen inhibits the production of milk.
e. Prolactin inhibits LH and FSH release, lowering fertility.

93. A young woman had her last period 7 weeks ago; she now has abdominal pain; an ectopic pregnancy is suspected:

a. Raised hPL would suggest that this could be an ectopic pregnancy.
b. In ectopic pregnancy the embryo almost always implants in a uterine tube.
c. Vaginal bleeding would alter this diagnosis.
d. Pelvic inflammatory disease predisposes to ectopic pregnancy because the zygote travels more slowly in the damaged uterine tube.
e. Rupture almost always causes a life-threatening intra-pelvic haemorrhage.

94. A pregnant woman of 34 weeks gestation presents with a headache and a blood pressure of 156/104:

a. She probably has eclampsia.
b. Her urine probably has more than 300 mg/L protein.
c. Antihypertensive treatment could cure this condition.
d. She should be treated as an emergency.
e. Magnesium sulphate would be an appropriate treatment.

95. A 6-week pregnant woman presents with vaginal bleeding, a blood pressure of 142/98 and severe vomiting most mornings:

a. A likely diagnosis is a hydatidiform mole.
b. This diagnosis could be largely excluded if she has high levels of hCG.
c. This diagnosis would be corroborated by an abnormally large uterus.
d. An ultrasound scan could confirm this diagnosis.
e. The woman has an increased risk of developing choriocarcinoma.

96. A young couple present in clinic with a failure to conceive after a year of unprotected sexual intercourse:

a. The cause of infertility will almost certainly be an abnormality in the woman.
b. Female infertility is usually caused by amenorrhoea or abnormalities of the uterine tubes.
c. The blood levels of several hormones are routinely investigated for infertility.
d. In-vitro fertilization (IVF) has an 80% success rate per cycle.
e. IVF is the main fertility treatment for women with obstructed uterine tubes.

97. Concerning male and female sterilization:

a. In a vasectomy the epididymis is separated from the testis.
b. Reliable contraception occurs more rapidly with a vasectomy than tubal ligation.
c. Vasectomies are more effective at preventing pregnancy than tubal ligation.
d. Tubal ligation is normally performed by laparotomy.
e. Both procedures are irreversible.

98. A 28-year-old woman is 8 weeks pregnant when she experiences a small amount of bleeding from her vagina. She presents in floods of tears saying she has had a miscarriage:

a. She is probably right.
b. An amniocentesis should be performed to assess the state of the baby.
c. If her cervix is dilated then urgent medical treatment is needed to prevent spontaneous abortion.
d. The spontaneous abortion probably occurred because of a fetal abnormality.
e. Therapeutic abortion can legally be performed up to 24 weeks gestation.

Chapter 17 Common presentations of endocrine and reproductive disease

99. The following conditions can cause weight loss:

a. Cushing's syndrome.
b. Diabetes mellitus.
c. Addison's disease.
d. Amenorrhoea.
e. Hypothyroidism.

Chapter 19 Investigations and imaging

100. Concerning the investigation of endocrine pathology:

a. Thyroid hormone levels can be measured directly using ELISA.
b. A stimulation test is used to investigate a deficiency of hormone levels.
c. The triple stimulation test is used to investigate the function of the adrenal cortex.
d. The water deprivation test is used to investigate diabetes mellitus.
e. An MRI scan involves the use of X-rays.

Short-answer questions (SAQs)

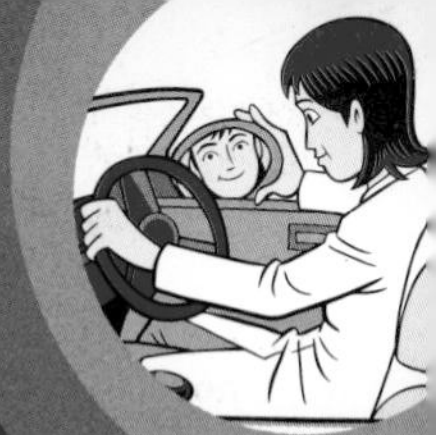

1. Describe the mechanism of action of a G-protein linked receptor.

2. Describe the possible presentations of a pituitary tumour.

3. Briefly describe what negative feedback is and how it can be employed in hormonal regulation? Draw a flow diagram to show the negative feedback inhibition involved in cortisol release.

4. Describe the synthesis of thyroid hormones.

5. Explain the actions of parathyroid hormone, vitamin D and calcitonin.

6. Briefly describe the divisions of the adrenal glands and the hormones they secrete.

7. What is the role of progesterone in pregnancy?

8. Draw a diagram which illustrates the molecular progression of prostate cancer.

9. Discuss the neuroendocrine control of lactation.

10. Describe the endometrial changes that occur over a 28-day menstrual cycle if fertilization does not occur.

11. A 15-year-old boy is concerned about his short height. Describe how growth hormone regulates growth and determines final height.

12. A 49-year-old woman has gone through the menopause and wants to know about hormone replacement therapy (HRT). List reasons for prescribing HRT to women during and after the menopause and the type of HRT used.

13. A 19-year-old woman has recently had unprotected sex with a man she met on holiday. She has developed lower abdominal pain and tenderness. How is pelvic inflammatory disease (PID) caused, diagnosed and treated?

14. A 74-year-old man with a fractured neck of femur is investigated for secondary hyperparathyroidism. What is this condition and how is it caused?

15. A 30-year-old man presents with a scrotal lump. List five conditions that this could be and discuss how they can be differentiated on examination.

16. A 25-year-old woman wants to go on the 'Pill' but doesn't know which type to use. How does the progestogen-only pill provide contraceptive protection? List its advantages and disadvantages compared with the combined oral contraceptive pill.

17. An abnormality of the adrenal gland is seen on a CT scan of a 65-year-old man. In preparation for the radiologist's report, what are: Addison's disease, Cushing's syndrome, Cushing's disease and Conn's syndrome?

18. A thyroid function test of a 54-year-old woman gives the following results:

Thiroid function test results

Hormone	Result	Normal levels
TSH	7.8 mU/L	0.5–5.7 mU/L
T_4	55 nmol/L	70–140 nmol/L
T_3	0.8 nmol/L	1.2–3 nmol/L

What type of thyroid disease is this and what symptoms would you expect?

19. A 78-year-old woman presents with tiredness, polyuria and weight loss. State what disease this is likely to be. How is it diagnosed, and what are the treatment options?

20. It is time to witness your first delivery, but the midwife expects you to know what is going on. Describe the three stages of labour.

Extended-matching questions (EMQs)

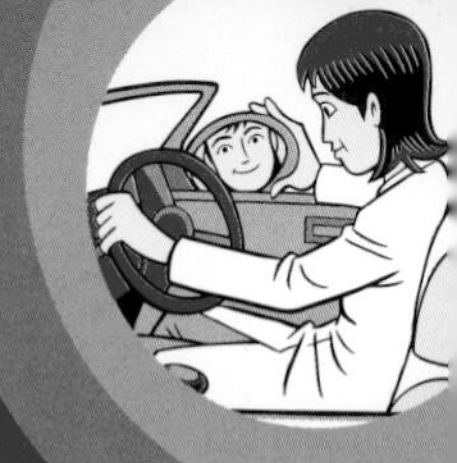

For each scenario described below, choose the *single* most likely diagnosis from the list of options. Each answer may be used once, more than once or not at all.

1. **The pancreas and diabetes.**

   A. Type 2 diabetes
   B. Gestational diabetes mellitus
   C. Hyperosmotic non-ketotic diabetic coma (HONK)
   D. Diabetic ketoacidosis
   E. The metabolic syndrome
   F. Maturity onset diabetes of the young (MODY)
   G. Hypoglycaemia

   Instruction: Match the diagnosis to the following clinical scenarios:

   1. A 60-year-old women whose recent-onset diabetes is entirely controlled by diet, metformin and sulphonylureas.
   2. A 15-year-girl with diabetes who is known to suffer from a mutation in the glucokinase gene.
   3. A 50-year-old man suffering from mild fasting hyperglycaemia, hypertriglyceridaemia and central adiposity who has deranged function tests.
   4. A 10-year-old boy who is found in his room drowsy, vomiting, severely dehydrated, suffering from acidotic breathing (Kussmal breathing).
   5. A 42-year-old pregnant women with hyperglycaemia who has family history of history of NIDDM and has previously given birth to a large baby.

2. **The hypothalamus and the pituitary gland.**

   A. Supraoptic nucleus
   B. Antidiuretic hormone
   C. Sheehan's syndrome
   D. The syndrome of inappropriate ADH secretion
   E. Oxytocin
   F. Gonadotrophs
   G. Prolactinoma
   H. Pars distalis
   I. Lactotrophs
   J. Pituicytes

   Instruction: Match the appropriate letter to the following numbered statements:

   1. The cells which produce prolactin.
   2. The hormone which does not function appropriately in diabetes insipidus.
   3. A common cause of galactorrhoea.
   4. A cause of hyponatraemia in a woman suffering from post-partum haemorrhage.
   5. The cells which secrete follicule-stimulating hormone

3. **The adrenal glands.**

   A. Phaeochromocytoma
   B. Conn's syndrome
   C. Renal artery stenosis
   D. Cushing's syndrome
   E. Congenital adrenal hyperplasia
   F. Addison's disease
   G. Bartter's syndrome

   Instruction: Match the diagnosis to the following clinical scenarios:

   1. A 45-year-old woman with buccal hyperpigmentation, weakness, abdominal pain, hyperkalaemia and hypernatraemia.
   2. A 36-year-old man with a hypocholoremic metabolic alkalosis, low serum renin and a mass in the adrenal glands on MRI.
   3. A 30-year-old female who presents with episodic pallor, chest pain and hypertension. A cause of hyponatraemia in a woman suffering from post partum hemorrhage.
   4. A rheumatology patient on long-term steroids who presents with weight increase, moon face, menstrual irregularity and purple striae.
   5. A young girl presenting with virilism and hirsutism.

4. **Endocrine disease.**

   A. Cushing's disease
   B. Acromegaly
   C. Graves' disease
   D. Dwarfism
   E. Diabetes mellitus
   F. Adipsic diabetes insipidus

   Instruction: Decide which endocrine disease may be implicated in each of these scenarios:

1. A 55-year-old man who presents with a large jaw and bitemporal hemianopia.
2. A 25-year-old woman who presents with excessive micturition who does not become thirsty on hyperosmolar stress testing.
3. A 50-year-old woman with an irregular irregular pulse (i.e. atrial fibrillation), tremor and exophthalmos.
4. A 76-year-old woman with rheumatoid arthritis who presents depression and a fractured neck of femur.
5. A 63-year-old patient with renal failure, angina and deteriorating sight.

5. Thyroid disease.

A. Thyrotoxicosis
B. Papillary thyroid cancer
C. Myxoedema
D. Hyperthyroidism
E. Ophthalmoplegia
F. Follicular thyroid cancer
G. Adipsic diabetes insipidus

Instruction: Decide which of A–G best matches each of the statement below:

1. A disease of the thyroid which is often associated with the production of a fusion protein.
2. A sign of Graves' disease.
3. A disease of the thyroid which is often associated with activation of the *RET* proto-oncogene.
4. A symptomatic patient with high serum thyroid hormone which is being produced by a struma ovarii.
5. Puffiness on the anterior surface of the lower leg.

6. Symptoms of pregnancy.

A. Rising oestrogen levels
B. Progesterone-induced smooth muscle relaxation
C. Raised serum TSH
D. Oestrogen-induced ligament softening
E. Raised melanocyte-stimulating hormone level
F. Impaired glucose tolerance due to the actions of cortisol

Instruction: Match each of these conditions with the appropriate physiological change from the list above:

1. Gestational diabetes.
2. Morning sickness.
3. Goitre.
4. Back ache.
5. Constipation.

7. Disorders of pregnancy.

A. Placental abruption
B. Placenta praevia
C. Pre-eclampsia
D. Ectopic pregnancy
E. Hydatidiform mole
F. Sheehan's syndrome

Instruction: Match each of these characteristics with the appropriate condition from the list above:

1. A women in the third trimester of her pregnancy presents with high blood pressure, oedema and proteinuria.
2. A pregnant women presents with pelvic inflammatory disease presents with severe abdominal pain and sudden collapse.
3. A pregnant women with polyhydramnios presents with vaginal bleeding and abdominal pain. Ultrasound reveals serious intrauterine blood clots.
4. A pregnancy in which the placenta is located over the lower uterine segment.
5. A condition in which chorionic villi form grape-like vesicles.

8. Signs of endocrine disease.

A. Acromegaly
B. Cushing's disease
C. Goitre
D. Pituitary tumour
E. Congenital adrenal hyperplasia
F. Infection with *Candida albicans*
G. Hypopituitarism
H. Rickets

Instruction: Match each of these signs or symptoms with the appropriate endocrine disease:

1. Bilateral decrease in breast size.
2. Clitoromegaly.
3. Thick, white, cottage-cheese-like inflammation of the skin a mucous membranes.
4. 'Pigeon' chest.
5. Papilloedema.

9. Signs of endocrine disease.

A. Blood glucose of 7.3 mmol/L 2 hours after glucose intake
B. No cortisol suppression on high dose dexamethasone suppression test after a positive low-dose test
C. Thyroid-stimulating antibodies in the blood
D. Slight depression of cortisol on high-dose dexamethasone suppression test after a positive low-dose test

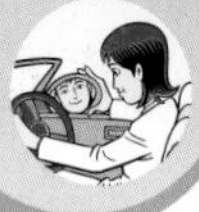

E. Fasting blood glucose of 6.5 mmol/L
F. Anti-thyroid peroxidase and anti-thyroglobulin antibodies

Instruction: Match each of these diseases to the appropriate findings on investigation:

1. Hashimoto's thyroiditis.
2. ACTH-secreting tumour.
3. Normal glucose tolerance.
4. Graves' disease.
5. Impaired glucose tolerance.
6. Ectopic ACTH-secreting tumour or adrenal tumour.

10. Imaging and endocrine disease

A. Osteosclerotic lesions
B. Osteolytic lesions
C. Osteoporosis
D. Osteomalacia
E. Enlarged sella turcica
F. Organ calcification

Instruction: Match each of these pathologies with the appropriate bone conditions suggested by X-ray findings from the list above:

1. Prostate bony metastases.
2. Thyrotoxicosis.
3. Pituitary adenoma.
4. Adrenal disease.
5. Hyperparathyroidism.

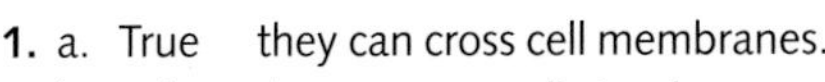

1. a. True they can cross cell membranes.
b. False they are generally too large.
c. True the larger proteins are called prohormones.
d. True for example, thyroid hormones and adrenaline.
e. False steroid hormones are secreted immediately, but polypeptide hormones are stored in vesicles.

2. a. True as do insulin-like growth factors.
b. True insulin is a polypeptide, so it cannot cross the cell membrane.
c. False adrenaline acts via G-protein receptors.
d. False as the name suggests, it is the tyrosine side chains that are phosphorylated.
e. False that is the action of an intracellular receptor, instead it activates preformed proteins.

3. a. True they bind many polypeptides that cannot cross this membrane.
b. False it is cAMP that is the common second messenger.
c. True hence the name; GDP is released when the receptor is active.
d. False the G-protein leaves the receptor protein to split and activate effectors.
e. True it is a cell-surface receptor with glycoprotein binding sites.

4. a. False prostaglandins act locally, usually by diffusion through extracellular fluid.
b. True arachidonic acid is a phospholipid.
c. False they are synthesized by the lipoxygenase pathway.
d. False most cells in the body secrete prostaglandins.
e. False they are released immediately after synthesis.

5. a. False they often need special transporter proteins.
b. False individual hormones use similar receptors all over the body.
c. True negative feedback does not have to be directly hormonal.
d. False feedback is used in many different cells throughout the body.
e. True it is only the feedback to oestrogens and progesterones that changes.

6. a. True it forms a 'V' shape beneath the thalamus.
b. False the hormones secreted by the hypothalamus act on the anterior pituitary gland.
c. False they are polypeptides and modified amino acids.
d. False ACTH is an anterior pituitary hormone, so the stimulation is hormonal via the portal veins.
e. True nerve cells are derived from the neuroectoderm.

7. a. True in response to GnRH.
b. False that is the posterior pituitary; the anterior pituitary comes from the endodermal Rathke's pouch.
c. True it is directly below the optic chiasma.
d. True it does.
e. False ACTH regulates aldosterone, but angiotensin II is the main regulator.

8. a. False aldosterone is from the adrenal cortex; the posterior pituitary secretes ADH, which regulates fluid balance.
b. True it secretes oxytocin to stimulate milk ejection.
c. False ADH and oxytocin are both made of 9 amino acid residues; they are synthesized in the hypothalamus and stored in the posterior pituitary.
d. True this layer is called the diaphragma sellae.
e. True it is made of neural tissue with these glial cells.

9. a. False it is the peripheral vision that is lost: a bitemporal hemianopia.
b. True functioning prolactinomas are the most common pituitary adenomas.
c. True they grow to a large size causing hypopituitarism.
d. False a CT scan of the pituitary fossa is needed.
e. True the pituitary gland can be accessed through the nose leaving no visible scar.

10. a. True this is their primary function.
b. False thyroglobulin is the stored form found in the follicles; thyroid-binding globulin is the relevant plasma protein.
c. False most tissues can remove an iodine from T_4 to make T_3.
d. True thyroid hormones readily cross the cell membrane.
f. True these hormones are made from tyrosine.

11. a. True as its name suggests, TSH stimulates the thyroid gland.
b. False it is the arteries that are closely related to these nerves.
c. True calcitonin is released from the parafollicular cells.
d. True this is why it moves with the larynx on swallowing.
e. False it is only found in about 10% of people.

12. a. True it is about three times more common in women than men.
b. False most obesity has no known cause.
c. False it causes cretinism.
d. True ablation of the thyroid gland by surgery or radioactive iodine often results in hypothyroidism with time.
e. False it should be treated with thyroxine (T_4) to return TSH levels to normal.

13. a. True the autoantibodies stimulate the TSH receptors.
b. True she may suffer from heat intolerance causing her to wear few clothes despite cold weather.
c. True TSH will be low despite raised T_3 and T_4.
d. False thyroid carcinoma rarely causes hyperthyroidism.
e. False carbimazole is used to treat hyperthyroidism.

14. a. True these cells would be seen on fine-needle aspiration.
b. True these can secrete ectopic ACTH.
c. False thyroid carcinoma usually causes hypothyroidism.
d. True the 5-year survival is very low.
e. False it invades locally and rarely causes distant metastases.

15. a. False this is the description of a thyroglossal cyst.
b. False they will be lowered due to the excess thyroid hormones.
c. True especially atrial fibrillation.
d. True thyroid carcinoma cannot be excluded by history, examination or blood tests.
e. False loss of the parathyroid glands can cause chronic hypocalcaemia.

16. a. True all steroid hormones are derived from cholesterol.
b. False that is the adrenal medulla, the cortex is from surrounding mesenchyme.
c. False that is the thyroid gland; the adrenal cortex is arranged in cords.
d. False CRH stimulates the anterior pituitary to release ACTH, which stimulates the adrenal cortex.
e. True remember GFR—the middle layer secretes cortisol.

17. a False it acts mainly on the adrenal cortex as suggested by its name.
b. True CRH is a hypothalamic stimulant, and cortisol has a negative feedback effect.
c. False it is secreted by the corticotrophs, which are found in the anterior pituitary gland.
d. True ACTH has a very marked circadian rhythm that peaks in the early morning.
e. False it stimulates adrenal androgen release (e.g. in congenital adrenal hyperplasia).

18. a. False it inhibits growth hormone release.
b. True to cope with the stress.
c. True adrenaline and cortisol inhibit the actions of insulin to raise blood glucose
d. False cortisol allows the body to cope with stresses.
e. False it is the sympathetic nervous system that is activated.

19. a. True they have similar actions to the sympathetic nervous system.
b. True the sympathetic neurons secrete mainly noradrenaline while the adrenal gland secretes mainly adrenaline.
c. True so that cardiac output increases.
d. False they raise blood glucose; only insulin can lower blood glucose.
e. False they are secreted by cells that are equivalent to postganglionic sympathetic neurons.

20. a. False Cushing's disease is caused by a pituitary tumour. Exogenous corticosteroids may cause a presentation similar to Cushing's syndrome.
b. True corticosteroids raise blood glucose.
c. False he will probably have gained weight.
d. False his skin will probably be thin and prone to bruising.
e. False long-term steroid therapy must never be stopped suddenly as ACTH would be suppressed.

21. a. False it is a deficiency of cortisol and aldosterone.
b. True due to the excess ACTH secretion.
c. True this is a stimulation test using synthetic ACTH.
d. False it is completely irrelevant.
e. True he will probably need life-long cortisol replacement.

22. a. True it is a disease of the adrenal gland, so it is a primary disease.
b. True aldosterone increases potassium excretion but retains sodium.
c. False it is an adenoma of the adrenal cortex.

d. False it is a rare cause of hypertension.
e. False renin and potassium levels should also be measured.

23. a. True severe hypertensive episodes like this need investigating.
b. False it is found in the adrenal medulla and secretes catecholamines.
c. False the phaeochromocytoma should be removed as soon as possible, though this is a dangerous operation.
d. False adrenaline causes vasoconstriction which raises blood pressure.
e. True adrenaline causes pupil dilation.

24. a. True especially IDDM.
b. True in response to the high blood glucose.
c. True this acts to lower blood glucose.
d. False these secrete glucagon; the β-cells secrete insulin.
e. False in most people, insulin secretion is always maintained at basal levels.

25. a. True it is located on the back wall of the abdomen with the duodenum behind the peritoneum.
b. False it secretes digestive enzymes via the pancreatic ducts, but pancreatic hormones enter the blood directly.
c. True it passes over the left kidney, under the stomach, to touch the spleen with its tail.
d. True the ventral and dorsal buds.
e. False the hormone-secreting cells are sparsely innervated since their activity is mainly regulated by blood glucose levels.

26. a. False this is the lower end of the normal glucose range.
b. True to raise blood glucose.
c. False it is released by the endocrine pancreas.
d. False it stimulates adrenaline release, which also raises blood glucose.
e. True glucose is the main regulator of insulin and glucagon release.

27. a. False it is a polypeptide; it is glycogen that is made from glucose molecules.
b. False it stimulates the secretion of insulin.
c. True it prevents glucose uptake and use.
d. True this allows insulin to act unopposed after a meal.
e. True it causes large molecules (e.g. glycogen) to be broken down, whilst preventing them from being synthesized.

28. a. True this is a common presentation.
b. False glycosuria is a poor diagnostic measure; his fasting blood glucose should be measured on two occasions.
c. False weight loss and polyuria would be expected.
d. False his young age suggests that he has IDDM and will almost certainly need insulin injections.
e. False in IDDM diabetic complications take several years to develop so the appointment does not need to be urgent.

29. a. True this is a presentation of NIDDM.
b. True though it can only be a presenting feature in NIDDM.
c. True good glucose control also helps prevent retinopathy.
d. True this is the hyalinization of arterioles.
e. False glycosuria is not a good diagnostic measure for diabetes.

30. a. False the threshold for glycosuria is very variable.
b. True though NIDDM can be present without glycosuria.
c. False he may well need insulin for good glucose control.
d. False syndrome X is hypertension, obesity and insulin resistance.
e. False these are found in IDDM, but NIDDM is usually due to insulin resistance.

31. a. False it is a hormone secreted by fat cells.
b. True it permits the synthesis of GnRH in the hypothalamus.
c. True it causes satiety (fullness).
d. False leptin must be injected as it is a protein.
e. False it is incredibly rare.

32. a. False it is a modified amino acid made from tryptophan.
b. True found at the back of the 3rd ventricle.
c. False melatonin is not the same as melanin.
d. False it acts to reset the suprachiasmatic nucleus of the hypothalamus.
e. False melatonin is secreted in response to the dark when the retina is not stimulated.

33. a. False the tumour is in an islet of Langerhans within the pancreas.
b. False it is a very rare condition.
c. True it is called a gastrinoma.
d. False it stimulates the parietal cells to secrete acid.
e. True about 30% of gastrinomas are caused by MEN I.

34. a. True it is also considered to be a hormone.
b. True it acts to raise blood volume.

c. True it forms angiotensin I from angiotensinogen.
d. False renin secretion increases due to the loss of negative feedback.
e. True via angiotensin II.

35. a. False increases water reabsorption; its name gives the answer
b. True the neurons in the hypothalamus and posterior pituitary.
c. False it has this action, but on the collecting duct.
d. True it lowers blood osmolarity by retaining water.
e. False it can cause vasoconstriction following severe hypotension.

36. a. True conversely, severe haemorrhage causes hypotension.
b. False increased peripheral resistance can raise blood pressure.
c. True causes vasoconstriction via angiotensin II.
d. False has no effect without the presence of renin.
e. True causes vasoconstriction.

37. a. True this is a good diagnostic indicator of diabetes mellitus.
b. False but hypercalcaemia is associated with polyuria.
c. True this is a sign of the resulting dehydration.
d. False this causes urinary frequency, but the volume of urine remains relatively constant.
e. False it is the water deprivation test that is used.

38. a. False there are two pairs of parathyroid glands.
b. False they only secrete parathyroid hormone.
c. False they are derived from APUD cells.
d. True it raises calcium levels.
e. False their blood supply is mainly from the arteries supplying the thyroid.

39. a. True over 99%, in fact.
b. True this is true in all types of muscle throughout the body.
c. False it is a rise in calcium that stimulates this process.
d. True so excess osteoclast activity can weaken bones.
e. False it acts via parathyroid hormone.

40. a. True it has the same characteristics as a steroid hormone.
b. True e.g. the disease rickets.
c. False its main site of action is the gastrointestinal tract, where it stimulates calcium absorption.
d. False it is ultraviolet light.
e. False it is activated from 25-hydroxyvitamin D_3.

41. a. False the four small parathyroid glands are located posterior to the thyroid gland.
b. True it raises blood calcium in response.
c. False it is a polypeptide.
d. False that is the action of vitamin D, instead it acts on the kidneys and bones.
e. True PTH stimulates the activation of vitamin D.

42. a. True as their name suggests, these are found next to the follicles.
b. True it has the opposite role to that of parathyroid hormone.
c. False excess or absence have no clinical effects on calcium regulation.
d. True it is.
e. True they secrete the characteristic polypeptides.

43. a. True remember 'bones, stones, abdominal groans and psychic moans'.
b. False secondary hyperparathyroidism is a result of hypocalcaemia.
c. True this is a relatively common cause.
d. True chronic hypercalcaemia is associated with renal failure.
e. True though parathyroid hyperplasia is more common.

44. a. False it is from the anterior pituitary gland.
b. True all anterior pituitary hormones are polypeptides or glycoproteins.
c. False it acts mostly via insulin-like growth factors.
d. True it follows a circadian rhythm and is stimulated by sleep.
e. False growth hormone secretion continues throughout life to maintain tissues.

45. a. False the liver is the main site of synthesis, though other tissues are important too.
b. True growth hormone is stimulated during sleep.
c. False they have the opposite action on glucose metabolism to that of insulin.
d. False they inhibit growth hormone release by negative feedback.
e. True they act on similar receptors to insulin.

46. a. True the jaw is not a long bone, so it can continue to grow with excess growth hormone.
b. False the growth plates of his long bones will have fused.
c. False it is called acromegaly in adulthood.
d. False he has an increased risk of insulin resistance.
e. True this can cause visual disturbances.

47. a. True this is a polypeptide and it is also secreted from APUD cells, making it more common as an ectopic hormone.
b. False ectopic hormones are usually polypeptides as these only require the activation of a single gene. Cortisol would cause hyperglycaemia anyway.
c. True this is a polypeptide.
d. False this is a steroid.
e. False it is the deficiency of ADH that causes diabetes insipidus.

48. a. False the adrenal glands are posterior in the abdomen and endocrine tumours do not need to grow large to cause symptoms.
b. True these are both features of MEN II and he has multiple tumours at a young age.
c. False these are a feature of MEN I.
d. False it will almost certainly have a medullary pattern.
e. True MEN syndromes often have an autosomal dominant inheritance.

49. a. True as do most of the internal genitalia.
b. False this gene is found on the Y chromosome.
c. True the labioscrotal folds.
d. True the testes retain their abdominal blood supply when they pass through the inguinal canal.
e. False they originate outside the embryo in the yolk sac and migrate into the fetal gonads.

50. a. True the indifferent gonads.
b. False MIS causes regression of female ducts.
c. True this division is completed just before ovulation; the second division is only completed on fertilization.
d. True this is called the indifferent stage of development.
e. False it develops from the mesenchyme.

51. a. False girls typically go through puberty earlier than boys.
b. True it also stimulates fusion of the growth plates.
c. True puberty is the reactivation of GnRH secretion.
d. False it has started at 4 mL.
e. False this is called gonadarche; adrenarche is when the adrenal glands start secreting androgens.

52. a. True 47 kg is the average weight at menarche, and this is relatively constant.
b. False it is a relatively late sign; breast budding or the growth spurt are noticed first.
c. True in females, adrenal androgens are an important androgen source.
d. False it occurs 10 months later, on average.
e. False they mature from primordial follicles into primary follicles.

53. a. True they are held by the mesovarium and ligaments.
b. False no new follicles are formed after birth.
c. True but only one reaches full maturity.
d. True the oocyte bursts out of the ovary into the peritoneal cavity. It remains close to the ovarian surface.
e. True this is the site of the mesovarium.

54. a. True they are surrounded by the fold of peritoneum that makes up the broad ligament.
b. False fertilization normally occurs in the ampulla of the uterine tubes.
c. True there are anastomoses between these vessels.
d. True though the cervix prevents easy access.
e. True these are mesenchymal structures.

55. a. False it is a section of the uterus.
b. False it is the external os.
c. True though squamous metaplasia can occur.
d. False it dilates to 10 cm.
e. False it is the action of oestrogens and relaxin that do this.

56. a. False it is the commensal lactobacilli bacteria that maintain the acidic environment.
b. False it is the uterine lining (the functional endometrium) that is shed during menstruation.
c. False the lining is a stratified squamous epithelium.
d. True it is located between the bladder and rectum.
e. True it is an endodermal structure.

57. a. False the glandular tissue is derived from apocrine sweat glands.
b. True it is only at puberty that the female breast changes.
c. False there about 15–20 lactiferous ducts opening onto each nipple.
d. True if it becomes tethered it is a sign of neoplasia.
e. False oestrogen stimulates the growth of the lobules and acini.

58. a. True it is a female sex steroid.
b. False it crosses cell membranes to act on intracellular receptors.
c. True it is secreted during development and puberty.
d. False it is secreted along with progesterone.

e. True feedback is normally negative, but it becomes positive before ovulation.

59. a. True progesterone is mainly secreted in the second half of the menstrual cycle.
b. True it inhibits contractions in the uterus, but it also causes oesophageal reflux and urinary incontinence.
c. False it is the corpus luteum.
d. False it only requires two steps from cholesterol, via pregnenolone.
e. False that is oestrogen's main role; progesterone maintains the endometrium and promotes secretion.

60. a. False LH peaks just before ovulation.
b. True this positive feedback causes the LH and FSH surge.
c. False this hormone is only found during pregnancy.
d. True it is secreted in response to GnRH.
e. False it is LH that stimulates progesterone release.

61. a. True though several follicles and oocytes begin to develop each month.
b. True the primordial follicles are present at birth.
c. False thecal cells secrete androgens that granulosa cells convert to oestrogens.
d. True the fluid is under pressure to allow the oocyte to be ejected.
e. True but only one reaches full maturity.

62. a. False during early pregnancy hCG is secreted by the chorionic villi, as its name suggests.
b. True they secrete progesterone.
c. True after fertilization hCG replaces the falling LH.
d. False lutein means yellow in Greek and this is its characteristic colour.
e. False only one follicle ovulates, so only one corpus luteum is formed.

63. a. False it begins to proliferate after menstruation under the influence of oestrogen.
b. False they secrete this fluid in response to progesterone.
c. True up to 80 mL is considered normal.
d. False only the functional layer is shed.
e. False it only causes ischaemia in the functional endometrium.

64. a. False cortisol levels are unaffected by POS.
b. True it shows the multiple cysts.
c. False that would suggest a prolactinoma.
d. True this is a recognized symptom of the high androgen levels.
e. False LH will be raised, but FSH should be low.

65. a. False that is endometritis.
b. True this is an association of endometriosis.
c. False laparoscopy is the best means of diagnosis.
d. False polycystic ovarian syndrome is associated with hirsutism.
e. True caused by rupture of the ectopic endometrial lining.

66. a. False but this *could* be acute pelvic inflammatory disease.
b. True especially *Chlamydia* and *Gonococcus*.
c. False it is more likely to be *Staphylococcus* or *Streptococcus*.
d. True in about 10% of infections.
e. False the IUD's location should be checked by feeling the threads and the PID should be treated with antibiotics.

67. a. False only very large pelvic masses are palpable on abdominal examination.
b. True fluid appears dark on ultrasound scans.
c. False this is the presentation of a benign cystic teratoma.
d. False it is a brown (chocolate) cyst that suggests endometriosis leading to endometrioid tumours.
e. True including cystadenomas and endometrioid tumours.

68. a. False herpes forms itchy, red blisters; it does not cause a vaginal discharge.
b. False lactobacilli are normal residents of the vagina and they prevent infection.
c. True this is the classic presentation of *Candida albicans* infection.
d. False *Candida albicans* is commonly found in the vagina; it has purely overgrown.
e. True it is the most common organism causing PID.

69. a. True they are the most common neoplasia of the female reproductive tract.
b. True they are tumours of the smooth muscle cells.
c. False it is oestrogen that mainly stimulates their growth.
d. False these two conditions occur in different layers of the uterus.
e. True in the absence of oestrogen they begin to regress and menorrhagia will no longer be a problem.

70. a. True this is the most probable diagnosis, but it cannot be assumed.
b. False these mainly affect younger women.
c. True this is caused by interference with the connective tissue.

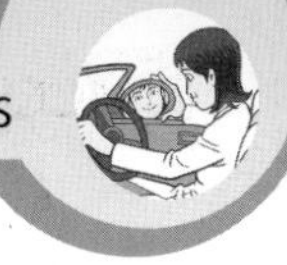

d. False it suggests Paget's disease; it is another sign of malignancy.

e. False breast cancer can only be excluded by ultrasound scan with fine-needle aspiration.

71. a. True these are most common just before the menopause.

b. True peau d'orange is a classic sign of breast cancer.

c. False it is caused by interference with lymphatic drainage.

d. True *BRAC* mutations increase the risk of both breast and ovarian cancer.

e. True it increases the lifetime oestrogen exposure.

72. a. False 51 years is the average age of menopause.

b. False she must use oestrogen and progestogen to protect her endometrium from carcinoma.

c. True oestrogen reduces the risk of osteoporosis.

d. True HRT increases the risk of cardiovascular disease.

e. False they will be increased in the early stages of menopause due to reduced feedback of oestrogen.

73. a. True this is continuous until death.

b. False they are lined by Sertoli cells; the Leydig cells lie between the seminiferous tubules.

c. True this is the tissue cavity in which hydrocoeles develop.

d. False each lobe contains 1–4 seminiferous tubules.

e. False it usually drains into the inferior vena cava. It is the left testis that drains to the left renal vein.

74. a. False they have a comma shape.

b. False spermatogenesis only occurs in the testes.

c. True this tube is about 5 m long.

d. False it is within the scrotum next to the testes.

e. False sperm are stored in the epididymis.

75. a. True these are the erectile components.

b. False it is derived from the urogenital folds.

c. True remember 'point and shoot'.

d. False both fluids are transmitted by the urethra.

e. False hopefully not; it should only enter the vagina.

76. a. False the spermatogonia are the stem cells.

b. True they reach the lumen surface as they develop.

c. True this allows them to respond to testosterone that stimulates spermatogenesis.

d. False spermatogenesis requires temperatures below 37°C, this is why the testes are outside of the abdominal cavity.

e. False they complete meiosis as they become spermatids.

77. a. True this is called the acrosome.

b. False they are arranged in spirals in the middle piece.

c. True they are arranged in the characteristic 9+2 pattern.

d. True the membrane phospholipids are rearranged allowing motility.

e. False it is the principal piece that is the longest.

78. a. False benign prostatic hyperplasia is much more common.

b. True while benign prostatic hyperplasia affects the periurethral glands.

c. False it is prostate-specific antigen (PSA) that is a useful marker.

d. True though the staging determines treatment.

e. True most bony metastases are osteolytic; osteosclerotic lesions suggest prostatic carcinoma.

79. a. False due to his young age it is likely to be a teratoma.

b. False male teratomas are almost always malignant.

c. True by vascular spread.

d. True while teratomas respond well to chemotherapy.

e. False 97% are derived from the germ cells, including seminomas and teratomas.

80. a. True this is an infection of the testis and epididymis.

b. True any intensive exercise can predispose to testicular torsion.

c. False testicular torsion must be excluded surgically.

d. False varicocoeles are non-tender and they are felt in the spermatic cord.

e. True they raise the temperature of the testes.

81. a. False it is varicocoeles that are more common on the left.

b. True this is the most common testicular lump at all ages.

c. False they are caused by patency of the processus vaginalis.

d. True though they can need surgery if they do not.

e. False though it suggests there is an infection or malignancy.

82. a. False it is phimosis; paraphimosis is when the foreskin becomes stuck behind the glans.

b. False this is only needed if BXO is present.

c. True but it is a common disorder after 5 years of age.

d. True the foreskin is essential for the repair of hypospadias.
e. False it is called balanitis; the cause of BXO is not known.

83. a. False the ampulla of the uterine tubes is the most common site.
b. False they must undergo capacitation.
c. False it completes the second meiotic division at this point.
d. True this is stimulated by binding to ZP3 receptors.
e. True the fast and slow block.

84. a. False oestrogen is only used with progesterone, but progesterone can be used alone. Oestrogen alone would cause endometrial hyperplasia.
b. True this is one of its main contraceptive effects.
c. True oestrogen inhibits FSH, which is required for follicle development.
d. True this is a contraceptive action that both hormones can cause.
e. False this is the action of a copper IUD.

85. a. False it is only taken for 21 days with a 7 day break; progesterone-only pills are taken continuously.
b. True both hormones inhibit LH secretion.
c. False it is more effective, but it causes more side effects.
d. True it also reduces the risk of endometrial carcinoma.
e. False this is a common side effect.

86. a. False the second meiotic division is only completed if the oocyte is fertilized.
b. True only after the zona pellucida is shed can the blastocyst begin to grow.
c. True the zygote splits into two blastomeres.
d. False is the process when tight junctions develop at the 8 cell stage.
e. False the zona pellucida is shed from the blastocyst in the uterus.

87. a. True it has a blastocyst cavity, which distinguishes it from the morula.
b. True the trophoblast, embryoblast and blastocyst cavity.
c. False the trophoblast splits into the syncytiotrophoblast and cytotrophoblast.
d. False it is the syncytiotrophoblast that invades the functional endometrium.
e. False the embryoblast usually faces the endometrium.

88. a. False this is the lacunar phase; the primary villi are formed when the cytotrophoblast invades the syncytiotrophoblast.
b. False further invasion by the placenta is prevented by the decidua basalis.
c. True failure of this invasion predisposes to pre-eclampsia.
d. True the chorionic villi enter their tertiary phase when the fetal mesenchyme forms blood vessels.
e. False there are only two layers because the cytotrophoblast regresses.

89. a. False the chorionic villi and umbilical cord are fetal tissues.
b. True this is essential for maintaining the corpus luteum and progesterone in early pregnancy.
c. False expulsion of the placenta and membranes is the third stage of labour.
d. False the fetal and maternal blood are separated by the syncytiotrophoblast and fetal blood vessel walls.
e. False these septa come from the maternal tissue and are incomplete on the fetal side.

90. a. True this allows the uterus to enlarge and prepare for birth.
b. False blood volume rises mostly in the second half of pregnancy; stroke volume increases initially.
c. False blood pressure initially decreases, then rises back to normal levels.
d. False the metabolism relies on fat more than normal to spare glucose for the fetus.
e. False the immune system is less active.

91. a. True it prevents early expulsion.
b. False the head usually faces backwards, but then it turns to the thigh.
c. False the pain of early labour is caused by hypoxia of the uterus during contractions; stretching of the cervix usually causes pain in the second stage.
d. True this is called the Ferguson reflex.
e. False it is prostaglandins, especially PGE_2, that are stimulated by oxytocin.

92. a. False both prolactin and oxytocin are stimulated.
b. True this is why it doesn't appear white.
c. False it is prolactin that does this; oxytocin stimulates the ejection of milk.
d. True though many women express small amounts towards the end of pregnancy.
e. True breastfeeding has a contraceptive effect.

93. a. False it is a raised hCG that is used to diagnose pregnancy.
b. True 99% of ectopic pregnancies are in the fallopian tubes.
c. False this would suggest that a tubular abortion of an ectopic pregnancy has occurred.

d. True any disease process that slows the transport along the uterine tube predisposes to ectopic pregnancies.
e. False this is a rare complication.

94. a. False eclampsia is seizures following pregnancy induced hypertension or pre-eclampsia; it is pre-eclampsia that she probably has.
b. True she has severe hypertension, so she will probably have proteinuria.
c. False it may help prevent eclampsia, but the only cure is birth.
d. True this is a very serious condition.
e. True this should help bring her blood pressure down and reduce the risk of a seizure.

95. a. True she has early pre-eclampsia and severe morning sickness, so this is a likely diagnosis.
b. False hCG levels are massively raised in the presence of hydatidiform moles.
c. True another symptom of 'excessive pregnancy'.
d. True it will show a snow-storm-like uterine cavity.
e. True recurrent moles often become malignant.

96. a. False both men and women can be responsible for infertility.
b. True these are the two most common causes.
c. True including prolactin, oestrogen, progesterone, testosterone, LH and FSH.
d. False it has a 20–30% success rate.
e. True it is the only means of implanting an embryo in the uterus.

97. a. False it is the vas deferens that is cut.
b. False other contraceptive measures should be used for a couple of months after a vasectomy.
c. True the failure rate for vasectomies is 10 times lower.
d. False it is usually a laparoscopic procedure.
e. False there is a 50% chance of being able to restore fertility.

98. a. False usually the bleeding is from other causes, but miscarriage is high on the list of differential diagnoses.
b. False an ultrasound scan will be less harmful and more useful.
c. False miscarriage is inevitable at this point; the fetus and afterbirth should be expelled and checked.
d. True 60% of miscarriages are due to fetal abnormalities, especially chromosome defects.
e. True although the majority are performed before 14 weeks.

99. a. False associated with weight gain.
b. True due to the inhibition of anabolism and unopposed catabolism.
c. True due to the deficiency of cortisol.
d. False this can be caused by weight loss.
e. False it is hyperthyroidism that causes weight loss.

100. a. True ELISA is the main technique for measuring many hormone levels.
b. True while suppression tests are used for excess secretion.
c. False it is used to investigate hypopituitarism.
d. False it is used to investigate diabetes insipidus.
e. False CT scans use X-rays; MRI uses magnets and radio waves.

1. G-protein coupled receptors consist of two main elements: a glycoprotein receptor and an associated protein bound to GDP. The receptor spans the membrane with a hormone binding site on the extracellular surface and a G-protein binding site on the intracellular surface. Binding of the hormones stimulates a change in shape that affects the attached G-protein. The G-protein has two components: the α-subunit that binds GDP in the resting state and the βγ-complex that is bound to the α-subunit in the resting state. The change in shape of the receptor causes the α-subunit to exchange GDP for GTP. The G-protein then leaves the receptor and splits into the two subunits described above, both of which bind to effector proteins also found on the inside of the cell membrane. The effector proteins stimulate other molecules (e.g. ATP is converted to cAMP) that act as second messengers (see Fig. 1.9).

2. Pituitary tumours can present with symptoms due to 'the mass effect' of the tumour and/or with endocrine symptoms, which can involve distant organs. Endocrine manifestations can be the result of overproduction or underproduction of hormones by the tumour. These commonly include excess growth hormone, prolactin or ACTH or a deficiency in growth hormone or gonadotrophins. A broader deficiency in pituitary hormones, panhypopituitarism, presents with symptoms of multiple deficiencies and requires replacement of the full complement of hormones. As these hormones act differently at different stages in the life cycle the clinical manifestation of perturbations can vary greatly. For instance growth hormone deficiency in an adult causes acromegaly in an adult and dwarfism in a child.

3. A hormone is said to be regulated by negative feedback when it inhibits its own production / release. Negative feedback is a good way of maintaining a system in a steady state, homeostasis. Negative feedback and other forms of feedback are becoming increasing fundamental to the study of intracellular signalling, so-called systems biology. For an example, see Fig. 4.1.

4. T_3 and T_4 are derived from the amino acid tyrosine and iodine. Tyrosine is converted into the glycoprotein thyroglobulin, which is secreted into the follicle lumen. Iodine ions are actively transported into the follicular cells where they are oxidized into reactive iodine atoms that are also secreted into the follicle lumen. The iodine binds to thyroglobulin by the action of thyroperoxidase resulting in monoiodothyrosine and diiodotyrosine. These molecules are coupled together to form tri-iodothyronine and thyroxine. These are secreted by reabsorbing the thyroglobulin and breaking down this large molecule in lysosomes. The thyroid hormones are released. See Fig. 3.6.

5.

Actions of parathyroid hormone, vitamin D, and calcitonin

Hormone	Parathyroid hormone (PTH)	Vitamine D	Calcitonin
Secreted/activated in response to:	Low blood calcium	PTH	High blood calcium
Kidneys	Calcium reabsorbed vitamine D activited	Calcium reabsorbed	Calcium excreted
Bones	Calcium released	Calcium trapped	Calcium trapped
Intestines	Negligible	Calcium absorbed	Negligible

6. The adrenal gland is divided into two regions: the adrenal cortex and the adrenal medulla. The adrenal cortex is further divided into three layers:

- Zona glomerulosa—secretes mineralocorticoids (e.g. aldosterone).
- Zona fasciculata—secretes glucocorticoids (e.g. cortisol).
- Zona reticularis—secretes glucocorticoids and androgens (e.g. testosterone).

The adrenal medulla secretes catecholamines (e.g. noradrenaline and adrenaline).

7. Progesterone induces the uterine glands to secrete nutrient-rich 'milk' for the developing embryo. It also prepares and maintains the endometrium for implantation. Progesterone secretion increases continually as pregnancy proceeds and is essential for its maintenance. After implantation its effects include:

- The prevention of premature labour by inhibiting prostaglandin secretion, which stimulates contractions in the myometrium.
- Promotes the storage of body fat.
- Maintenance of the functional endometrium.
- Physiological adaptation to pregnancy, e.g. changes in cardiovascular, renal and respiratory systems.
- Relaxation of smooth muscle throughout the body.

8. See Fig. 14.12 on page 168.

9. The nipples are stimulated during suckling and this stimulus is conveyed to the hypothalamus via neural pathways. It causes the secretion of oxytocin from the posterior pituitary gland and prolactin from the anterior pituitary gland. Prolactin initiates the synthesis of milk in the acini once the plasma oestrogen levels decline after pregnancy; it also maintains the secretory ability of the breast. Oxytoxin stimulates milk ejection by the contraction of the myoepithelial cells. Lactation is maintained by frequent suckling via a positive feedback loop. See Fig. 16.7.

---

10. There are three phases to the menstrual cycle in the endometrium:
    1. Menstrual phase (days 1–4)—the absence of progesterone causes spiral arteries to constrict and coil causing the functional endometrium to become ischemic and necrotic. It is shed through the vagina, along with blood from the damaged blood vessels, in a process called menstruation.
    2. Proliferative phase (days 4–13)—cells in the basal epithelium proliferate in response to oestrogen to form a new functional endometrium with new spiral arteries. Endometrial glands are formed within this layer, but they do not secrete.
    3. Secretory phase (days 14–28)—progesterone causes the endometrial glands to enlarge and develop a corkscrew shape. They begin to secrete a glycogen-rich fluid in preparation for implantation. The endometrium continues to thicken and becomes oedematous. Towards the end of this phase, low progesterone levels cause the spiral arteries to contract causing ischaemia.

---

11. Growth hormone stimulates the production of insulin-like growth factors (IGFs) in many tissues, but especially the liver. These polypeptide hormones stimulate the growth of soft tissues and bones. They stimulate the uptake and anabolism of amino acids, causing cell growth that also stimulates cell division. In the bones, IGFs stimulate growth of the chondrocytes at the epiphyseal growth plates causing the bone to lengthen. The growth factors also stimulate fusion of this growth plate preventing further growth. Final height is determined by the rate of growth and the time at which these growth plates fuse.

---

12. Hormone replacement therapy (HRT) preparations are prescribed during and after the menopause to:
    - Treat menopausal symptoms such as hot flushes and sweating.
    - Protect against osteoporosis caused by chronic oestrogen deficiency.
    - Protect against collagen loss, which can cause uterovaginal prolapse, immobility, muscle weakness, and skin wrinkling.

    There may be slightly increased risks of breast and ovarian cancer and heart attack or stroke.

    In most women, oestrogen can only be given with progesterone to prevent the risk of endometrial carcinoma. This causes withdrawal bleeding similar to that when using the pill. If the woman has had a hysterectomy then oestrogen can be given alone.

---

13. Pelvic inflammatory disease (PID) is an infection of the endometrium, fallopian tubes or ovaries. It is most commonly caused by sexually transmitted disease including *Chlamydia trachomatis* (60% of PID) or *Neisseria gonorrhoeae* (30% of PID). The remaining 10% comes from other routes:
    - Direct infection following trauma due to childbirth, surgical abortion or insertion of a coil.
    - Blood-borne infection (e.g. tuberculosis).
    - Transperitoneal infection (e.g. from appendicitis).

    It is diagnosed from the history and examination followed by screening the urine for signs of the infectious agent and taking vaginal and cervical swabs. It is treated with doxycycline and metronidazole.

---

14. Secondary hyperparathyroidism is a disorder where parathyroid hormone (PTH) secretion is elevated in response to persistent hypocalcaemia. Persistent hypocalcaemia and secondary hyperparathyroidism can be caused by:
    - Calcium malabsorption (e.g. vitamin D deficiency or coeliac disease).
    - Renal failure causing uncontrolled calcium excretion and a failure to activate vitamin D (called renal osteodystrophy).

---

15. Indirect hernia, testicular tumour (seminoma or teratoma), hydrocoele, varicocoele, epididymal cyst:
    - Indirect hernia arises in the abdomen so you cannot feel above the mass in the scrotum; it may be reducible or tender.
    - A mass that is solid and feels to be part of the testis is likely to be a testicular tumour.
    - A hydrocoele is cystic (i.e. translucent when a light is shone through it) and surrounds the testis (i.e. the testis is indistinguishable).
    - A mass caused by a varicocoele lies above the testis, feels like a 'bag of worms' and often reduces when the patient lies flat.
    - A mass caused by an epididymal cyst is small, firm, cystic and lies within the epididymis (i.e. it feels separate from the testis).

---

16. The progestogen-only pill does not reliably suppress ovulation; it provides contraceptive protection by:
    - Inhibiting the changes in the cervical mucus that normally occur around ovulation so that the passage of sperm is reduced.
    - Increasing the rate of ovum transport so it reaches the endometrium before implantation can take place.

- Inhibiting endometrial proliferation so that implantation does not occur.

The progestogen-only pill does not cause an increased risk of cardiovascular disease, breast cancer or other side effects associated with oestrogen. It must be taken at the same time every day ±3 hours and it is still less effective than the combined pill, especially in younger women. It often causes irregular bleeding and may cause symptoms of premenstrual syndrome (PMS).

The combined pill carries the risks and side effects associated with oestrogen, but it is more effective, does not need to be taken at the same time each day, and reduces the risk of ovarian and endometrial cancer.

---

17. These four conditions are disorders of the adrenal cortex hormones:.

- Addison's disease—a deficiency of glucocorticoids (cortisol) and mineralocorticoids (aldosterone) caused by destruction of the adrenal gland, often by an autoimmune process.
- Cushing's syndrome—an excess of glucocorticoids (cortisol) caused by any disease causing a characteristic set of symptoms.
- Cushing's disease—an ACTH-secreting pituitary adenoma that causes Cushing's syndrome along with hyperpigmentation.
- Conn's disease—an adenoma of the zona glomerulosa causing primary hyperaldosteronism.

---

18. Raised TSH and low thyroid hormones indicates primary disease of the thyroid gland causing hypothyroidism. The symptoms are shown in Fig. 3.10.

---

19. It is probably non-insulin dependent diabetes mellitus (NIDDM). It is diagnosed by blood glucose levels above 7.8 mmol/L after an overnight fast on two occasions. There are three treatment options:

- Diet alone.
- Diet and oral hypoglycaemic agents.
- Diet and injected insulin.

---

20. **First stage**—from the onset of labour until full cervical dilatation (10 cm). The uterine contractions become stronger and more frequent and they push the fetal head into the pelvis towards the cervix. The woman feels pain due to hypoxia of the uterus caused by occlusion of the blood vessels following the muscular contractions. The amniotic membrane often ruptures during this stage.

Second stage—from full cervical dilatation until the birth of the baby. The fetal head descends sideways through the pelvis and it rotates 90° so that it faces the sacrum. Contractions continue and are assisted by voluntary pushing by the mother. Once the head is born it rotates back 90° to face the mother's leg and the rest of the baby is born shortly afterwards. The pain is most severe during this stage; it is caused by stretching of the cervix, vagina and perineum.

Third stage—from birth of the baby until the delivery of the placenta and membranes. The entire placenta and decidua basalis detach and are expelled, causing haemorrhage from the ruptured blood vessels. The haemorrhage is stopped by the muscle fibre arrangements within the uterus. The contractions slowly subside once the afterbirth has been expelled.

1. The pancreas and diabetes.

1. A
2. F
3. E
4. D
5. B

2. The hypothalamus and the pituitary gland.

1. I
2. B
3. G
4. C
5. F

3. The adrenal glands.

1. F
2. B
3. A
4. D
5. E

4. Endocrine disease.

1. B
2. F
3. C
4. A
5. E

5. Thyroid disease.

1. F
2. E
3. B
4. A
5. C

6. Symptoms of pregnancy.

1. F
2. A
3. C
4. D
5. B

7. Disorders of pregnancy.

1. C
2. D
3. A
4. B
5. E

8. Signs of endocrine disease.

1. G
2. E
3. F
4. H
5. D

9. Signs of endocrine disease.

1. F
2. D
3. A
4. C
5. B

10. Imaging and endocrine disease.

1. A
2. C
3. E
4. F
5. D

Index